Dyslexia, Speech and Language

A Practitioner's Handbook

Second Edition

Edited by

MARGARET J. SNOWLING

Department of Psychology, University of York

JOY STACKHOUSE

Department of Human Communication Sciences,
University of Sheffield

W
WHURR PUBLISHERS
LONDON AND PHILADELPHIA

Other Wiley Editorial Offices

John Wiley & Sons Inc., 111 River Street, Hoboken, NJ 07030, USA

Jossey-Bass, 989 Market Street, San Francisco, CA 94103-1741, USA

Wiley-VCH Verlag GmbH, Boschstr. 12, D-69469 Weinheim, Germany

John Wiley & Sons Australia Ltd, 42 McDougall Street, Milton, Queensland 4064, Australia

John Wiley & Sons (Asia) Pte Ltd, 2 Clementi Loop #02-01, Jin Xing Distripark, Singapore 129809

John Wiley & Sons Canada Ltd, 22 Worcester Road, Etobicoke, Ontario, Canada M9W 1L1

Wiley also publishes its books in a variety of electronic formats. Some content that appears in print may not be available in electronic books.

A catalogue record for this book is available from the British Library

ISBN -13   978-1-86156-485-6 (PB)
ISBN -10   1-86156-485-6 (PB)

Printed and bound in Great Britain by TJ International Ltd, Padstow, Cornwall

This book is printed on acid-free paper responsibly manufactured from sustainable forestry in which at least two trees are planted for each one used for paper production.

Contents

Preface to the Second Edition

We were pleased to be asked by Colin Whurr to do a second edition of our book. We wondered first how much had changed and then how we would go about reflecting this. And so we embarked on this new edition focusing on the relationship between spoken and written language difficulties. This second edition continues the theme of linking theory and practice. It is particularly aimed at practitioners in the fields of education, speech and language therapy and psychology. All the original chapters have been updated, and new authors have joined us to reflect current developments.

The first part of the book focuses on the nature of spoken and written language difficulties and includes chapters on current research into dyslexia, the dyslexic brain, speech, phonological awareness and spelling problems, and the predictors of literacy difficulties. We then turn to the assessment of speech and language difficulties, reading and spelling skills, and reading comprehension, before moving on to consider techniques for training memory, contemporary approaches to reading intervention, and the teaching of spelling and handwriting skills. Finally, we consider how to manage the needs of people with dyslexia in the mainstream setting, including their psychosocial needs, and the interdisciplinary training of early-years workers.

We hope that this book will reach a wide range of practitioners and provide valuable advice to all those engaged in work with children who have problems of reading and language. We are indebted to many colleagues for their input, both those who have made formal contributions to this book and others who, through valuable discussion and joint assessments, have taught us much. We again thank our children, James, Laura and Christopher (now much grown), and our husbands, Charles and Bill, for their continuing support and tolerance!

Maggie Snowling and Joy Stackhouse
February 2005

Preface to the First Edition

This book focuses on the relationship between spoken and written language difficulties and represents the culmination of our thinking over some 15 years. The book is aimed at the practitioner in the field of children's language and learning difficulties and aims to forge links between theoretical advances and clinical issues in this field. Our collaborators on this project include former students and professional colleagues who share the same theoretical framework as ourselves and also the desire to improve the educational opportunities of children who have language difficulties.

We are indebted to the many children who have participated in our research, and who have provided us with invaluable insights into the nature and the developmental course of their difficulties. We have enjoyed many valued discussions with too many people to mention by name, but we would particularly like to thank colleagues associated with the Department of Human Communication Science at University College London (formerly the National Hospital's College of Speech Sciences). Most of all, we thank Charles Hulme and Bill Wells for their inspiration, support and encouragement, and our children James, Laura and Christopher for giving us another perspective on speech, language and literacy development!

Maggie Snowling and Joy Stackhouse

Contributors

Hilary Gardner Department of Human Communication Sciences, University of Sheffield.

Nata K. Goulandris Department of Human Communication Science, University College London.

Janet Hatcher Dyslexia Institute and University of York.

Peter J. Hatcher Department of Psychology, University of York.

Claire Jamieson Department of Human Communication Science, University College, London.

W.A. Lishman Emeritus Professor of Neuropsychiatry, Institute of Psychiatry, London.

Jane E. Mitchell Communication and Learning Skills Centre, Sutton, Surrey.

Valerie Muter Consultant Clinical Psychologist, Great Ormond Street Hospital for Children, London and Department of Psychology, University of York.

Poppy Nash Department of Psychology, University of York.

Kate Nation Department of Experimental Psychology, and Fellow of St John's College, University of Oxford.

Sarah Simpson Department of Human Communication Science, University College London.

Margaret J. Snowling Department of Psychology, University of York.

Joy Stackhouse Department of Human Communication Sciences, University of Sheffield.

Jane Taylor Handwriting Consultant, Weymouth, Dorset.

Maggie Vance Department of Human Communication Science, University College London.

Janet Wood Department of Human Communication Science, University College London.

Jannet A. Wright Department of Human Communication Science, University College London.

Conventions used in this book

TIE	Words in small capitals are target words (or non-words) that a child is being asked to say, read or write.
/tai/	Slanting brackets contain phonetic script.
"tie"	Double speech quotation marks show when an item is spoken by the child or adult.
<tie>	< > Indicates a written target or response.
➤	An arrow indicates 'is realized as'; for example TIE ➤ "die" means that the target word TIE was spoken by the child as "die"; <tie> ➤ "die" means that the written word TIE was read out loud as "die"; and TIE ➤ <di> means that the target word TIE was written as <di> by the child.

CHAPTER 1

Language skills and learning to read: the dyslexia spectrum

MARGARET J. SNOWLING

Children vary in the age at which they first start to talk. For many families, late talking might go unnoticed, particularly if the child in question is the first born of the family and no comparisons can be made. Later in the pre-school years, children may be difficult to understand; they might have a large repertoire of their 'own words' that others find unintelligible. Such utterances are often endearing, the source of family amusement, and no one worries much because an older sibling can translate. But speech or language delay can be the first sign of reading difficulties, difficulties that will come to the fore only when the child starts school; a key issue therefore is when is 'late talking' a concern, and when is it just part of typical variation?

Language is a complex system that requires the coordinated action of four interacting subsystems. *Phonology* is the system that maps speech sounds on to meanings, and meanings are part of the *semantic system*. *Grammar* is concerned with syntax and morphology (the way in which words and word parts are combined to convey different meanings), and *pragmatics* is concerned with language use. An assumption of our educational system is that by the time children start school, the majority are competent users of their native language. This is a reasonable assumption, but those who are not 'very good with words' start out at a disadvantage, not only in speaking and listening skills, but also, as this book will demonstrate, in learning to read.

Thus, oral language abilities are the foundation for later developing literacy skills. It is, however, important to distinguish *speech skills* from *language abilities* when considering literacy development. Learning to read in an alphabetic system, such as English, requires the development of mappings between speech sounds and letters – the so-called *alphabetic principle* – and this depends on speech skills. Wider language skills are required to understand the meanings of words and sentences, to integrate these into texts and to make inferences that go beyond the printed words. Before examining evidence concerning how language difficulties compromise literacy in dyslexia and related disorders, we begin with a short historical review of the concept of dyslexia.

The concept of dyslexia

Arguably, the scientific study of dyslexia first came to prominence in the late 1960s when one of the main issues of debate was whether 'dyslexia' was different from plain poor reading. Studies of whole-child populations, notably the epidemiological studies of Rutter and his colleagues, provided data about what differentiated children with *specific* reading problems (dyslexia) from those who were slow in reading but for whom reading was in line with general cognitive ability (Rutter and Yule, 1975). The results of these studies were not good for proponents of the 'special' condition of dyslexia. In fact, there were relatively few differences in aetiology between children with specific reading difficulty and the group they described as generally 'backward readers'. The group differences that were found included a higher preponderance of males among children with specific reading difficulties and more specific delays and difficulties with speech and language development. On the other side of the coin, the generally backward group showed more hard signs of brain damage, for example cerebral palsy and epilepsy. Important at the time, the two groups differed in the progress they had made at a 2 year follow-up. Contrary to what might have been expected on the basis of their IQ, the children with specific reading difficulties (who had a higher IQ) made less progress in reading than the generally backward readers. This finding suggested that their problems were intransigent, perhaps because of some rather specific cognitive deficit. Note, however, that this differential progress rate has not been replicated in more recent studies (Shaywitz et al., 1992), perhaps because advances in knowledge have led to better interventions (see Snowling, 2000, for a review).

Following on from these large-scale studies, the use of the term 'dyslexia' became something of a taboo in educational circles. Instead, children were described as having specific reading difficulties or specific learning disability if there was a *discrepancy* between their expected attainment in reading, as predicted by age and IQ, and their actual reading attainment. The use of IQ as part of the definition of 'dyslexia' has, however, fallen from favour. First, IQ is not strongly related to reading. Indeed, many children with a low IQ can read perfectly well even though they may encounter reading comprehension difficulties. Second, and perhaps more importantly, measures of verbal IQ may underestimate cognitive ability among poor readers who have mild language impairments. As a result, adherence to the 'discrepancy definition' of dyslexia can disadvantage those children with the most severe problems whose apparently low verbal IQ may obscure the 'specificity' of the reading problem.

Another problem with the discrepancy definition of dyslexia is that it cannot be used to identify younger children who are too young yet to show a discrepancy. In fact, many children who fail to fulfil diagnostic criteria at one age may do so later in the school years (Snowling, Bishop and Stothard, 2000). Moreover, the definition is silent with regard to the 'risk' signs for dyslexia, and how to diagnose dyslexia in young people who may have overcome basic literacy difficulties. What is needed to get around these difficulties is a set of positive diagnostic criteria for dyslexia. It is just such criteria that have been sought by psychologists working in the field of reading disabilities.

Cognitive deficits in dyslexia

At about the same time as the first epidemiological studies were being conducted, cognitive psychologists began comparing groups of normal readers and readers with dyslexia using a range of experimental paradigms. In a landmark review, Vellutino (1979) synthesized the extant evidence to propose the *verbal deficit hypothesis*. According to this hypothesis, children with dyslexia are subject to problems centring on the verbal coding of information that create specific problems for learning to read in an alphabetic script. Arguably, since that time, the most widely accepted view of dyslexia has been that it can be considered to be part of the continuum of language disorders. There has, however, been a gradual shift from the verbal deficit hypothesis to a more specific theory: that dyslexia is characterized by phonological processing difficulties (see Vellutino et al., 2004, for an updated review).

Children with dyslexia typically have difficulties that primarily affect the phonological domain; the most consistently reported phonological difficulties are limitations of verbal short-term memory and, more directly related to their reading problems, problems with phonological awareness. There is also evidence that children with dyslexia have trouble with long-term verbal learning. This problem may account for many classroom difficulties, including problems memorizing the days of the week or the months of the year, mastering multiplication tables and learning a foreign language. In a similar vein, this problem may be responsible for the word-finding difficulties and poor vocabulary development often observed in children with dyslexia.

Before proceeding, it is important to note that a number of authors have argued that difficulties with phonological awareness are not a universal phenomenon in dyslexia. Instead, children learning to read in more regular or transparent orthographies than English, in which the relationships between spellings and their sounds are consistent (e.g. German, Italian, Spanish or Greek), learn to decode quickly, while at the same time rapidly acquiring an awareness of the phonemic structure of spoken words (Ziegler and Goswami, 2005). It follows that, in these languages, deficits in phonological awareness are less good markers of dyslexia. Instead, impairments of phonological processing, such as rapid naming or poor verbal memory, are more sensitive diagnostic signs in these writing systems. Notwithstanding this proviso, the strength of the evidence pointing to the phonological deficits associated with dyslexia has led Stanovich and his colleagues to propose that dyslexia should be defined as a core phonological deficit. Importantly, within the *phonological core-variable difference* model of dyslexia (Stanovich and Siegel, 1994), poor phonology is related to poor reading performance irrespective of IQ and also, it seems, irrespective of language background (Caravolas, 2005; Goulandris, 2003).

Phonological representations, learning to read and dyslexia

Although the role of visual deficits in dyslexia continues to be debated (Stein and Talcott, 1999), the best candidate for the cause of dyslexia is an underlying phonological deficit. A useful way in which to think about this is that children with dyslexia come to the task of learning to read with poorly specified phonological representations – the way in which their brain codes phonology is less efficient than that of normally developing readers. As we have seen, this problem at the level of phonological representation causes a range of typical symptoms, such as those described above. It is, however, important to understand why a deficit in *spoken* language should affect the acquisition of *written* language.

Studies of normal reading development offer a framework for considering the role of phonological representations in learning to read and for understanding the problems of dyslexia. At the basic level, learning to read requires the child to establish a set of mappings between the letters (graphemes) of printed words and the speech sounds (phonemes) of spoken words. These mappings between orthography and phonology allow novel words to be decoded and provide a foundation for the acquisition of later and more automatic reading skills. In English, they also provide a scaffold for learning multi-letter (e.g. 'ough', 'igh'), morphemic ('-tion', '-cian') and inconsistent ('-ea') spelling–sound correspondences. Indeed, the early developing ability of the child to 'invent' spellings that are primitive phonetic transcriptions of spoken words (e.g. <LEVNT> for ELEPHANT) is one of the best predictors of later reading and spelling success (Caravolas, Hulme and Snowling, 2001). More broadly, there are strong relationships between phonological skills and reading ability throughout development and into adulthood, when the phonological deficits of people with dyslexia persist (Bruck, 1992).

More formally, the relationship between oral and written language skills has been simulated in computational models of the reading process. In the triangle model of Plaut and colleagues (shown in Figure 1.1), reading is conceptualized as the interaction of a *phonological pathway* mapping between letters and sounds and a *semantic pathway* mapping between letters and sounds via meanings (Plaut et al., 1996). In the early stages of learning to read, children's attention is devoted to establishing the phonological pathway (*'phonics'*). Later, children begin to rely increasingly on word meanings to gain fluency in their reading. We can think of this as an increase in the role of the semantic pathway, something which is particularly important for reading exception words in English, such as YACHT and PINT, words that cannot be processed efficiently by the phonological pathway. Arguably, however, this model is limited for considering the risk of reading difficulties among children with spoken language impairments; the model is of single-word reading, but most reading takes place in context. Language skills that encompass grammar and pragmatics are needed for making use of context. Children with dyslexia do not typically have problems with these processes, but children with wider language difficulties almost certainly do.

Within this model of reading development, deficits at the level of phonological representation constrain the reading development of children with dyslexia (Snowling, 2000). A consequence is that although such children

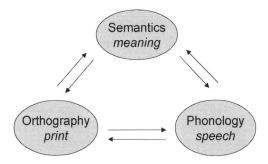

Figure 1.1 Triangle model of reading (after Seidenberg and McClelland, 1989). In this model, the mappings between orthography to phonology comprise the phonological pathway; mappings between orthography and phonology via semantics comprise the semantic pathway.

may learn to read words by rote (possibly relying heavily on context), they have difficulty generalizing this knowledge. For English readers with dyslexia, a notable consequence is poor non-word reading (Rack, Snowling and Olson, 1992). In contrast, the semantic skills of readers with dyslexia are, by definition, within the normal range, and these can be used to facilitate the development of word reading (Nation and Snowling, 1998a).

In short, learning to read is an interactive process to which the child brings all of his or her linguistic resources. It is, however, phonological processing that is most strongly related to the development of reading and the source of most dyslexic problems in reading and spelling. The phonological representations hypothesis therefore provides a parsimonious explanation of the disparate symptoms of dyslexia that persist through school to adulthood. It also makes contact with theories of normal reading development and with scientific studies of intervention. Here, the consensus view is that interventions that promote phonological awareness in the context of a highly structured approach to the teaching of reading have a positive effect in both preventing reading failure and ameliorating dyslexic reading difficulties (see Chapter 9 in this volume; Troia, 1999). There is also biological evidence in support of the theory.

Biological evidence in support of the phonological deficit hypothesis

It has been known for many years that poor reading tends to run in families, and there is now conclusive evidence that dyslexia is heritable. Gene markers have been identified on chromosomes 6, 15 and 18, but we are still a long way from understanding the precise genetic mechanisms involved. What we do know is there is as much as a 50 per cent probability of a boy becoming dyslexic if his father is dyslexic (about 40 per cent if his mother is affected) and a somewhat lower probability of a girl developing dyslexia. What is inherited is not of course reading disability *per se* but the risk of reading problems, mediated via speech and language delays and difficulties. The results of large-scale twin studies suggest that there is heritability of the phonological ('phonic') aspects of reading and that phonological awareness shares heritable variance with this (Olson, Forsberg and Wise, 1994).

Studies of readers with dyslexia using brain imaging techniques also supply a piece in the jigsaw (see Chapter 3 in this volume). In one such study, we investigated differences in brain function between dyslexic and normal readers while they performed two phonological processing tasks (Paulesu et al., 1996). This study involved five young adults with a well-documented history of dyslexia; all of these people had overcome their reading difficulties, but they had residual problems with phonological awareness. Under positron emission tomography scanning, they completed two sets of parallel tasks. The phonological tasks were a rhyme judgement and a verbal short-term memory task; the visual tasks were visual similarity judgement and visual short-term memory. Although these adults with dyslexia performed as well as controls on the experimental tasks, they showed different patterns of left hemisphere brain activation from controls during performance on the phonological processing tasks. The brain regions associated with reduced activity were those involved in the transmission of language and, plausibly, allowed the translation between the perception and the production of speech. It is therefore possible to speculate that this area may be the 'seat' of the problems viewed at the cognitive level, as a difficulty in setting up phonological representations.

Individual differences in dyslexia

A significant issue for the phonological representation view is that of individual differences. The phonological deficit theory has no difficulty explaining the problems of a child with poor word attack skills, who cannot read non-words and whose spelling is dysphonetic (Snowling, Stackhouse and Rack, 1986). There are also, however, children with dyslexia who appear to have mastered alphabetic skills. Such children have been referred to as developmental 'surface' dyslexics. The classic characteristic of these children is that, in single-word reading, they rely heavily upon a phonological strategy. They thus tend to pronounce irregular words as though they were regular (e.g. <glove> ➤ "gloave", <island> ➤ "island"), they have particular difficulty distinguishing between written homophones such as <pear> _ <pair> and <leek> _ <leak>, and their spelling is usually phonetic (e.g. BISCUIT ➤ <biskt>, PHARMACIST ➤ <farmasist>).

Although evidence in favour of distinct subtypes is lacking, most systematic studies of individual differences among children with dyslexia have revealed variations in their reading skills (Castles and Coltheart, 1993). One way of characterizing children's reading strategies is to assess how well they can decode words they have not seen before (e.g. using a non-word reading test) and to compare this with how well they recognize words that they cannot 'sound out', such as irregular or exception words that do not conform to English spelling rules. A number of studies have now shown that poor readers who have relatively more difficulty in reading non-words than exception words (phonological dyslexia) perform significantly less well than younger, reading age-matched controls on tests of phonological awareness. In contrast, children who have more difficulty with exception words than non-words (surface dyslexia) perform at a similar level to that of controls on these tests.

Arguably, findings of individual variation have directed the field in different ways. Some theorists have hypothesized that deficits other than the phonological deficit must be implicated in the aetiology of dyslexia, whereas others have proposed dimensions of variation. Two prominent alternate theories are the magnocellular deficit (Stein and Talcott, 1999) and the cerebellar deficit (Fawcett and Nicolson, 1999) theories. However, in contrast to the phonological deficit hypothesis, evidence in support of these theories is equivocal (Ramus et al., 2003). Moreover, it is important to note that neither theory refutes the evidence for the phonological processing problems of dyslexia. Instead, they seek a more basic cause for these deficits. It falls to these theorists to demonstrate that their theories explain both a necessary and a sufficient cause of dyslexia.

More generally, however, it does not seem useful to classify children with dyslexia into subtypes because all taxonomies leave a substantial number of children unclassified. Instead, individual differences in phonological processing, as measured by performance on tests of phonological awareness and phonological memory, predict individual differences in non-word reading, even when reading age has already been taken into account (Griffiths and Snowling, 2002). In essence, the more severe a child's phonological deficit, the greater his or her impairment in non-word reading. In contrast, variations in exception word reading appear to be tied to reading experience, reflecting the fact that print exposure is required to learn about the inconsistencies of the English orthographic system. As we saw earlier, exception-word reading builds on a foundation of grapheme–phoneme mappings, but it is also supported by semantics. To this extent, exception-word reading may develop independently of decoding skill in some children with dyslexia, forging a pattern of 'phonological dyslexia' at the behavioural level.

The issue of co-morbidity

Some of the apparent difference between children with dyslexia may depend on what is known as *co-morbidity*. Co-morbidity refers to the fact that there is a high probability that any developmental disorder will co-occur with at least one other disorder. Commonly co-occurring with dyslexia are difficulties with coordination (dyspraxia) or with attention control (attention-deficit hyperactivity disorder, or ADHD). The cause of this co-morbidity may be the sharing of brain mechanisms involved in the two disorders or the sharing of similar risk factors (e.g. family adversity).

In cases of children with co-morbid disorders, it is easy to mistake a behavioural symptom of one disorder for that of the other. Many children with dyslexia are clumsy, but not all are, by any means. It is therefore important not to build a theory of dyslexia on the assumption that motor impairments play a causal role. Similarly, one of the key cognitive features of ADHD is a difficulty in controlling and allocating attention, both aspects of executive function. A behavioural marker of poor executive skill is a problem of organization. Many children with dyslexia are poorly organized; it is not yet known whether this difficulty is central to their dyslexia, a consequence of it or a problem associated with a mild form of co-morbid ADHD.

Finally, and of considerable theoretical importance, the behavioural profile of children with dyslexia may change with age. Studies of the early language development of the children who go on to become dyslexic point to language impairments outside the phonological system, encompassing slow vocabulary development and grammatical delays (Scarborough, 1990). In the same way, children who have specific difficulties in reading comprehension may develop decoding problems at a later stage in their development because their language skills are not sufficiently strong to bootstrap word recognition (Snowling, Bishop and Stothard, 2000).

Language skills and learning to read: risk and protective factors

Given that we can now take as established the fact that children with dyslexia have phonological deficits, the research agenda turns to a consideration of how this risk is shared by other groups of vulnerable children. Furthermore, we need to understand how the risk of reading problems can be modified in children who compensate well. In order to understand the interplay between risk and protective factors in children's literacy development, it is important to begin by considering the reading impairment that affects children who have been called 'poor comprehenders'. Such children (who are considered in detail in Chapter 7 in this volume) have normal decoding skills but impaired reading comprehension. Important for the present argument is the fact that poor comprehenders perform at the normal level for their age on phonological tasks but have semantic processing deficits. Indeed, as we have argued elsewhere, poor comprehenders can be considered to be the 'mirror image' of those with dyslexia (Nation and Snowling, 1998a). Where children with dyslexia have phonological deficits, poor comprehenders have semantic deficits; where children with dyslexia have decoding deficits, poor comprehenders decode well but have problems of comprehension not shared with dyslexia; where children with dyslexia reap a huge benefit from reading in context, poor comprehenders do not.

Thus, findings from children with dyslexia and children with selective deficits of reading comprehension (in its extreme form referred to as *hyperlexia*) suggest that there is a degree of modularity in the developing reading system. Furthermore, they confirm the fact that poor phonology should be considered to be a risk factor for problems of word recognition, whereas semantic impairments (principally poor vocabulary) carry the risk of poor reading comprehension. But pure disorders are rare in development, and children's reading difficulties more commonly reflect the balance of their language strengths and weaknesses, modified by any interventions they have received.

The interaction of different language skills in determining the literacy outcomes of children at risk of reading failure can be seen clearly in studies of children at family risk of dyslexia. For example, Snowling, Gallagher and Frith (2003) followed the progress of preschool children, recruited just before their fourth birthday, who were considered to be 'at risk' of dyslexia. The risk in this case was carried by virtue of the fact that they had a parent with a history of reading difficulties, and it is interesting to note that some 38 per cent of these children were late talkers. The children in the 'at-risk' study were assessed at 4, 6 and 8 years of age on a large battery of tests of language and reading-related tasks. At each point in time, they were compared with children in a control group who came from families with no history of reading impairment but of similar socioeconomic status. As predicted, at 8 years of age, there was an increased risk of poor reading and spelling among the children at family risk of dyslexia. The definition of poor literacy was having literacy skills one standard deviation below the average of the control group of similar socioeconomic status. In relation to this norm, 66 per cent of the family sample was affected.

It was then possible to compare the developmental profiles of the at-risk affected children (who became poor readers), those 'at-risk' children who became normal readers and the control group. Figure 1.2a shows the performance of the three groups of children on the language and phonological tasks at 4 and at 6 years of age. At 4 years, the oral language development of the poor readers was slow compared with that of the two normal reader groups. At 6 years, the poor readers were already showing difficulty with phonological awareness tasks, particularly phoneme awareness, after only a short time of reading instruction. On phonological awareness tasks, the 'at-risk' normal readers were not statistically different from the control group, but it is interesting to note that there was a trend for them to be slightly worse than controls, which was not seen for oral language development.

Figure 1.2b shows the performance of the groups on tests of early literacy skill. Here, the picture is somewhat different. As expected, the poor readers were impaired in letter knowledge and on a test of phonic skill (derived from the number of non-words they could read and the phonetic accuracy of their spellings). However, the performance of the 'at-risk' children who went on to be normal readers was also less good than that of controls: it was midway between that of the controls and the poor readers on the test of letter knowledge, and as poor as the affected group on the phonetic spelling test.

In summary, the 'at-risk' children who went on to be poor readers had impairments on a wide range of measures, including phonological awareness and letter knowledge, as well as in measures of oral language skills including vocabulary and expressive grammar. The 'at-risk' children who

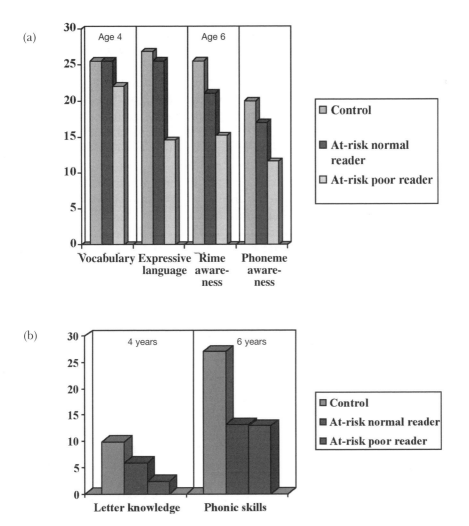

Figure 1.2 Performance of control, at-risk normal and at-risk poor readers on tests of reading and language (after Snowling, Gallagher and Frith, 2003). (a) The 'at-risk' children who went on to be poor readers were delayed in their early language development (at 4 years) and in the development of phonological awareness (at 6 years). (b) The 'at-risk' children who went on to be normal readers at 8 years of age showed early literacy problems; their letter knowledge was moderately impaired at 4 years, and they were impaired in translating between graphemes and phonemes at 6 years.

went on to be normal readers were as poor as the poor readers in phono-logical reading and spelling skills (phonics), and they were moderately impaired in letter knowledge, but their (non-phonological) oral language development was normal. Because these children did not succumb to reading deficits at 8 years of age, we must assume that they were able to compensate for the phonic decoding deficit they experienced, possibly by relying on their good language skills.

We can conclude that the risk of reading impairment is not all or none. Among children whose parents are dyslexic, there are a number of differ-ent outcomes. These include: a pervasive reading impairment affecting both word recognition and reading comprehension associated with poor language; classic dyslexia; a 'hidden' (compensated) reading impairment; and a pattern of normal reading. It seems that the developmental out-come for children at risk of poor reading depends not only on how severe their phonological difficulties are, but also on the other language skills they bring to the task of learning. Those who have good vocabulary and wider language skills are likely to be able to compensate better, modifying the genetic risk they carry of becoming dyslexic.

The findings of high-risk studies, such as the one described above (see also Pennington and Lefly, 2001) have implications for the way in which we conceptualize dyslexia. Throughout its history, dyslexia has defied def-inition, and perhaps rightly so. There are no strict criteria that can be used to make a cut-off between dyslexia and other forms of reading diffi-culty that affect decoding skills. In almost all such cases, the disorders are associated with phonological deficits, albeit to varying degrees. Although it is true that a relatively small proportion of children (the prevalence depending upon the exact criteria used) fulfil the formal criteria for read-ing disorder (e.g. American Psychiatric Association, 1994), others may fulfil the criteria at one time and not another, and others may be just below the threshold for 'diagnosis'. One way out of this dilemma is to talk of degrees of dyslexia, for example *mild*, *moderate* and *severe*, but again the criteria would not be readily agreed. Instead, it seems appropriate to begin to aban-don categorical diagnoses for cognitive disorders that are, by definition, both developmental and interactive (Bishop and Snowling, 2004).

In short, children come to the task of learning to read with differing patterns of language strength and difficulty. The language skills they bring to reading will determine how easily they can learn, the pitfalls they will face and the compensatory strategies they will use. But learning to read does not take place in a vacuum. The nature of children's difficulty in learning to read will be conditioned by the language in which they learn – some languages are 'transparent' and easier to learn than others – and the family, school and culture in which they learn will also have a profound influence. Importantly for children who have phonological weaknesses and are therefore at risk of reading problems, wider language skills can mitigate that risk. It goes without saying that another critical protective factor is early intervention, as clearly demonstrated by the evidence reviewed in Chapter 9 in this volume.

Conclusions

This chapter began by distinguishing the role of speech and of language skills in the development of reading: whereas phonological skills are the foundation of word-recognition processes in reading, wider language skills are critical to text comprehension (Muter et al., 2004). We currently know something about the role of vocabulary and semantic skills in learning to read, but grammar and pragmatics are likely to be important too, particularly in explaining how children use context during their reading. The findings from developmental disorders suggest that speech and language skills work in interaction to determine literacy outcomes. At the core of reading difficulties are phonological problems, but children with good language skills can use these to bootstrap their ineffective phonic skills, probably by using context in reading. This is why interventions that train phoneme awareness and at the same time encourage children to make full use of phonological, semantic and syntactic cues in text are effective for children with reading difficulties (Hatcher, Hulme and Snowling, 2004).

Given the evidence that we have reviewed, the concept of dyslexia might be usefully reinterpreted as a spectrum of disorder, as depicted in Figure 1.3. In line with the large body of evidence suggesting that phonological skills are the foundation of decoding skills and are deficient in classic

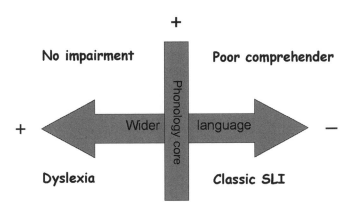

Figure 1.3 The dyslexia spectrum. SLI, specific language impairment.

forms of 'discrepancy-defined' dyslexia, phonological skills are the core dimension in this spectrum. Children with poor phonology (irrespective of IQ or other wider forms of language impairment) are at high risk of reading problems; this risk may be mitigated when wider language skills are proficient and exacerbated when oral language skills are also impaired, as for example in specific language impairment (Bishop and Snowling, 2004).

Finally, let us return to our initial question: When does 'late talking' become a cause for concern? Findings from recent research on children who have speech difficulties suggest that, for them too, having good language mitigates the risk of reading failure (Raitano et al., 2004; Stothard et al., 1998). However, as Stackhouse argues in this volume (see Chapter 2), if a speech difficulty is severe and persists into the school years, poor literacy is a likely concomitant regardless of whether wider language skills are also impaired (Carroll and Snowling, 2004; Nathan et al., 2004a).

Speech and spelling difficulties: what to look for

JOY STACKHOUSE

> Over one million children and young people in the UK have a speech, language or communication impairment. That's an average of 2 children in every classroom. (AFASIC promotion leaflet)

Although it is difficult to be precise about the incidence of speech and language difficulties, it is clear that there are sufficient numbers to warrant further investigation of the scale of the problem and what can be done to support children with such problems. A systematic review of the literature by Law et al. (2000a) reports prevalence rates of speech and language difficulties in children to be as high as 24.6 per cent. Speech difficulties are one of the most common communication problems in children. It is estimated that 5 per cent of primary school children have speech difficulties (Weiss, Gordon and Lillywhite, 1987) and that 3.8 per cent of children in the USA in the age range 3–11 years old have 'phonological problems' (Shriberg, Tomblin and McSweeny, 1999). Based on a study of children referred to a mainstream paediatric speech and language therapy service in the north of England, Broomfield and Dodd (2004) estimate that 48 000 children per year in the UK present with 'primary' speech difficulties. The rise of inclusive education policies has resulted in teachers being confronted more than ever before by children with speech and language difficulties in their classrooms (Lindsay et al., 2002), and teachers are reported to be concerned about their level of training in this area (Marshall, Stojanovik and Ralph, 2002).

School-age children rarely have isolated difficulties with their speech or language skills. More typically, their spoken language difficulties are associated with difficulties in other domains. Their difficulties may impede access to the curriculum, in particular by causing difficulties in reading, spelling and often maths. Some children have associated psychosocial difficulties (see Chapter 13 in this volume), and in the longer term there can

15

be problems with relationships and employment (Clegg et al., 2005). The link between spoken and written language difficulties is well established and forms the main theme of this volume. Young children with speech and language difficulties may well go on to have difficulties with reading and spelling. Older children with dyslexic difficulties may have had earlier speech and language difficulties that may persist in sometimes subtle ways. It is, however, not the case that all children with a history of speech and language difficulties go on to have associated problems in the classroom and with their learning. This chapter explores the relationship between speech and literacy difficulties and how children at risk of persisting speech and literacy problems might be identified.

How do you know if a child has a speech difficulty?

Recognizing a child's speech difficulty is not always as easy as one might imagine. Although everyone recognizes when 'sounds' are omitted or not produced 'correctly', there are more subtle signs to look out for, particularly as the child gets older. By the time children start school, they should be using a full range of sounds and be intelligible most of the time. By around 5 years of age, any children who stand out as being different in their speech production skills should be assessed, and the development of their spoken and written language skills should be monitored. However, children's speech at this age will not necessarily be adult-like, so what are the warning signs?

Sounds and blends

Children of school age should not be omitting sounds in simple words, for example the beginning or final sound of a word (e.g. CAT pronounced as "at" or "a", and TAP as "ta"), or substituting sounds (e.g. "tar" for CAR or "tea" for SEA). They should certainly not be reducing simple words like FISH to, for example, "bi" or "pi". They should also be able to manage two element blends (also called 'clusters') most of the time, such as at the beginning of STAR and SKY. Three-element blends such as SCRAP and SPLASH may not be perfect, but they should be clearly differentiated from RAP and LASH. Being able to produce words in isolation does not, however, guarantee intelligible speech. There may still be times when a flow of connected speech is unclear, but the young school-age child should be generally understood.

In English, particularly difficult sound contrasts to hear and to make are 'th' versus 'f', 'the' versus 'v' and 'r' versus 'w'. It is very common for young children to produce 'th' as "f", 'the' as "v" and 'r' as "w". A child's accent also needs to be taken into account when deciding whether or not a failure to make this contrast is a problem because some accents of English have these 'substitutions' as acceptable productions: in the south of England and in particular London, for example, "fin" for THIN and "vat" for THAT is typical of adult speech. Similarly, there are many acceptable variations in production of 'r' across accents in the UK (compare Scotland, Dorset and London) and between the UK and the USA. Such productions should not be labelled as speech errors; a child's language environment, locality and place of origin need to be taken into account when deciding whether a child has speech difficulties – particular if the teacher or therapist has a different accent!

The child's accent can, however, mask an underlying problem. If there is concern that a child's production of e.g "f" for TH or "v" for THE may be part of a persisting speech difficulty rather than part of an accent, the first question to ask concerns how the child's performance compares with that of peers who have the same accent. A check should be made on whether the child can:

- identify the different mouth postures for each sound made by the teacher or therapist (e.g. compare the production of 'f' and 'th');
- make the postures him- or herself and produce a contrast between two similar sounds (e.g. copy the sounds 'f' and 'th');
- hear the difference between similar sounds.

The child's spellings should then be examined for a differentiation between similar sounds (e.g. 'f'/'th', 'v'/'the' 'r'/'w') and compared with the spellings in the peer group. For example, Robert, aged 9 years, had unclear speech as well as reading and spelling problems. He had never been referred for speech and language therapy, and in single words his only persisting speech sound errors were "f" for 'th' and "v" for 'the'. These were described as errors as this pattern was not typical of his local accent or of his family's speech. In spelling, this substitution was reversed – the digraph was used to represent the sound "f": for example, TRAFFIC was spelt as <trathic>, FINGER as <thinger> and NERVE as <nerth>. This confusion should alert us to the need for further investigation. Indeed, when spelling multisyllabic words with blends, more serious problems became evident when Robert's imprecise speech did not allow an effective rehearsal of target words prior to spelling them: DISCOVERY was spelt as <dicoary>, and UMBRELLA as <upbla>.

Any words that contain the sounds 'w', 'r', 'l' or 'y' (e.g. LIBRARY, GORILLA, YELLOW WELLINGTONS) may be understandably tricky for young, normally developing children but persist as a specific difficulty for older children with subtle speech problems. These sound combinations are particularly difficult to segment for spelling because they are difficult to produce clearly in speech (e.g. LIBRARY spelt as <libily>, or SLIPPERY spelt as <sliply>). Similarly, words containing blends may be difficult to spell because the child has difficulty segmenting the components of the blend. It helps if a child can pronounce the elements of a word clearly in order to segment it into its bits and then apply the appropriate letters and conventions for spelling. If a child is still producing, for example, CLEAN as "te-lean", STREAM as "tweam" or WASP as "waps", he or she is disadvantaged when needing to spell the word.

Sequencing

Speech problems not only manifest at the sound level, but may also be evident in children who cannot sequence sounds in the right order even though they can produce all the sounds perfectly well. Christopher, for example, was 16 and a half years old when he was referred to speech and language therapy for the first time. He had been diagnosed as having dyslexia and was receiving support at school. Christopher was communicative but had generally unclear speech. An assessment showed that he had no difficulties with single sounds and simple words but that he could not produce sequences of sounds in more complex words, for example MELANIE pronounced as "Menelie" and SYSTEMATIC pronounced "synstemacit". As Christopher was approaching important examinations and interviews, his teachers and family were becoming concerned that his unclear speech would disadvantage him. Fortunately, because of his supportive home and school environment, as well as the opportunity to attend a course of speech and language therapy, he progressed well.

Connected speech

It is interesting to note the labels that are assigned to the speech production of children or adolescents such as Christopher. Many times, teachers or parents have not considered the existence of a speech difficulty because the child in question can pronounce all sounds perfectly well. They are therefore mystified as to why a child can at times be difficult to understand. A child's speech is often described as 'unclear', 'mumbly', 'muffled', 'jerky', 'hesitant' or 'non-fluent'. This description of a child's speech warrants further investigation if the child is also experiencing difficulties with other aspects of spoken language such as vocabulary development; new word learning in projects or school subjects, for example science (Wellington and Wellington, 2002); literacy and in particular spelling. If a speech assessment only includes tests of sounds and single words, important information about a child's speech difficulties will be missed. In particular, connected speech needs to be examined to establish what is happening at the junction between words and between sentences (Howard, 2004; Wells, 1994), and intervention for intelligibility may need to focus on the phrase and sentence level (Pascoe, Stackhouse and Wells, 2005).

Word-finding difficulties

Another warning sign of a speech-processing difficulty is jerkiness or non-fluency when a child appears to be struggling to get a word out or trying to improve its pronunciation through repeated attempts to self-correct. Katy, aged 7;7 with dyslexic difficulties, did just this. She pronounced SCREWDRIVER as "screw griver, str griver", and MICROSCOPE as "micostope, mi mictospoke". Assessment revealed that she had difficulties discriminating between sounds in words and between similar-sounding words. When trying to name pictures, she clearly had difficulties getting the word for an object that she knew. For example:

> BINOCULARS: "Kind of glasses. You put them on your eyes.
> You can put them round your hand and you can see really close."

> SADDLE: "Kind of seat when you go on a horsie.
> And you put your feet through there."

These word-finding difficulties are typical of children with speech, language and literacy difficulties and need careful investigation and support (see Constable, 2001, for a further discussion).

Stammering

A non-fluency is sometimes frequent or obvious enough to be labelled as a 'stammer'. It is not the case that all children who stammer have associated literacy difficulties, but there is evidence to suggest that some children who stammer have underlying speech-processing difficulties that interfere with their phonological awareness development and thus their literacy progress (Bernstein Ratner, 1997; Nippold, 2001).

Stephen was such a boy. He was referred for speech and language therapy at 7 years of age because of his stammer. An initial assessment revealed that he had a moderately severe stammer in need of attention. Phonological awareness activities were included as part of the routine assessment. When playing 'I Spy' with him, it was clear that he had underlying difficulties. When asked "I Spy with my little eye something in this room beginning with 'd'" (the target being DOOR), he looked around intently and replied "de-floor?", "de-window?", "de-telephone?" Contact with the school revealed that his teacher was indeed very concerned about his literacy development but had not connected this with his speech difficulties.

Prosody

Finally, another sign of speech difficulty may be manifested in a child's intonation, or prosody. This may be noticed because of unusual pitch changes and stress patterns. Tom came to our attention because of his unusual-sounding speech. He had a history of speech and language delay, specific expressive difficulties and severe verbal dyspraxia. At an age of 7;8, Tom had a performance IQ of 118 and a verbal IQ of 98 on the *Weschler Intelligence Scale for Children* (Wechsler, 1992). By 8;6, he had made considerable progress with his reading and language skills. He had an age equivalent of 8;8 on the *British Picture Vocabulary Scales* (Dunn et al., 1997) and performed at the 9;1 year level overall on the *Clinical Evaluation of Language Fundamentals* (*CELF-III*; Semel, Wiig and Secord, 2000). His reading was no longer a problem for him, but his spelling was still behind the level of his other skills. Although Tom's speech was now intelligible in that a listener could understand what he was saying, his speech still sounded 'different' because of its jerky rhythm and wide pitch changes. In particular, one pattern of errors seemed to be reflected in his spelling. He produced the 'sh', 'ch' and 's' sounds as "th", and the 'z' sound as "the", so SHADOW was pronounced "thadow" and MAGAZINE as "magathine". However, when the target sound in a word was 'th' or 'the', Tom pronounced it as "f" or "v" respectively: THUMB was pronounced "fum" and WITH as "wiv". As he demonstrated that he could produce all of the sounds, albeit not necessarily in the right place, his errors could not be explained by articulatory (i.e. production) difficulties alone.

When spelling these sounds, 'sh' was transcribed as <ch> as follows:

Target	Pronounced	Spelling
SHADOW	"thadow"	<chadow>
MEMBERSHIP	"memberthip"	<memberchip>

Furthermore, 'sh' and 's' were also written as <s> in the following:

Target	Spelling
REFRESHMENT	<refresment>
MACHINERY	<misnery>
POLITICIAN	<polltisn>
ADVENTURE	<edvenser>

These examples revealed that Tom had good syllable segmentation skills and was showing signs of developing sound segmentation skills.

The specific difficulty with the fricatives ('f', 's', 'sh', 'th') and affricates ('ch', 'j') needed further investigation. A series of spoken words beginning or ending with 'sh', 'ch' and 'j' were presented, and Tom was asked to decide which words began or ended with these sounds. He confused 'ch' and 'sh' on this task. For example, he thought that CHEAP and CHAIR began with 'sh' and MASH ended with 'ch'. He was then presented with a series of pictures beginning with 'j', 'sh', and 'ch' to sort into piles of the same onsets. There was slightly more confusion on this task when Tom had to generate words for himself from his own representations, compared with the first task where the words were spoken for him by the tester. He classified CHAIN, CHICKEN and JUMPER as beginning with 'sh', and SHORTS and SHE as beginning with 'ch'. On an auditory discrimination task, he also had difficulty differentiating between vowel sounds, sequences of sounds within clusters (as in LOTS versus LOST) and within unfamiliar words (as in the nonwords IBIKUS versus IKIBUS). These input problems may well have been more widespread in the past and affected the precision of Tom's stored phonological representations of words.

Therapy aimed at sharpening up the representations not only improved his speech, but also spontaneously carried over to the spelling of these sounds in words. By 9 years of age, Tom had no difficulties in pronouncing or spelling the target sounds; a reminder of the importance of combining speech input and production work with associated and targeted phonological awareness activities (Bernhardt and Major, 2005; Stackhouse et al., 2002).

In summary, identifying children with speech difficulties, particularly as they get older, involves more than listening for individual speech sound errors. Table 2.1 summarises the signs to look for when investigating

Table 2.1 Signs of speech difficulties in school-age children

'Sound' omissions and substitutions
    CAT – "at"; TAP – "ta"
    CAR – "tar"; FISH – "pish"

Blends
    CLEAN – "telean"
    STREAM – "tweam"
    SPLASH – "ba"

Sequencing
    SYSTEMATIC – "synsemacit"
    CAR PARK – "par cark"

Connected speech
    Often omits end of syllables/unstressed syllables and speech sounds
    Mumbley, jerky, hesitant, or non-fluent

Word-finding
    MOUSTACHE – "beeyer", "stash", "boustashe", "beeyer", "beeyerd", "stash", "stas", "boustase"*

Stammering

Prosody

*Data from Constable, 2001.

speech difficulties in school-age children in particular (see Chapter 5 in, this volume for discussion of useful speech and language assessments).

A psycholinguistic perspective on speech and spelling

The examples above of children with speech and literacy difficulties reveal that speech production problems can arise from different sources. Some children have difficulties with speech input (e.g. differentiating between similar sounding words); others have an imprecise storage of words that makes it difficult to access them or programme a clear production because of missing elements; still others have difficulty pronouncing speech at an articulatory level even though they know the words involved perfectly well. Children with persisting difficulties, however, may well have pervasive problems that involve all of these aspects of speech-processing: input, representations and output. Figure 2.1 is a simple psycholinguistic speech-processing model that attempts to illustrate how speech difficulties arise.

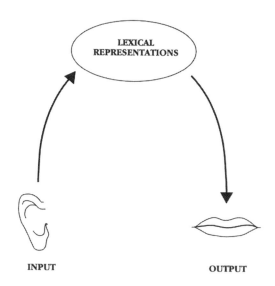

Figure 2.1 The basic structure of the speech-processing system (from Stackhouse and Wells, 1997).

The essence of the psycholinguistic approach to understanding speech difficulties is an assumption that a child receives information of different kinds (e.g. auditory and visual) about a spoken utterance or written form, remembers it and stores it in a variety of *lexical representations* (a means of keeping information about words) within the *lexicon* (a store of words), and then selects and produces spoken and written words. On the left of Figure 2.1, there is a channel for the input of information via the ear; on the right, there is a channel for the output of information through the mouth. At the top of the model, there are the lexical representations that store previously processed information, whereas at the bottom there is no such store.

This speech-processing system is not only the basis for speech development, but also the foundation for literacy development; 'written language' being an extension of 'spoken language'. An important link between the two is the development of phonological awareness, i.e. 'an ability to reflect on and manipulate the structure of an utterance as distinct from its meaning (Stackhouse and Wells, 1997, p. 53). If you consider tasks typically used to investigate or develop phonological awareness skills, for example judging whether or not two spoken words begin with the same sound, or producing a string of words that rhyme with CAT, then it becomes clear that all tasks draw on input and output speech-processing skills as well as stored representations in some form or degree. Any difficulty that children have in their basic speech-processing system will thus result not only in spoken difficulties, but also in problematic phonological awareness development, which will in turn impact on their literacy performance. The precise nature of the speech and literacy problems will, however, depend on the location of the deficit(s) in the speech-processing system (Snowling, Stackhouse and Rack, 1986; and see Chapter 1 in this volume).

When children start school at around 5 years of age, they should ideally have an intact speech-processing system in order to deal with spoken language. The child should be able to listen, attend and discriminate between similarly sounding words. They should also be able to produce intelligible speech, even if it is not identical to the adult form. They should have semantic, phonological and grammatical representations stored for common words, together with the motor programmes for producing them. A main aim for the teacher is to utilize this functioning and intact speech-processing system in order to develop the associated written forms (stored as orthographic representations) for what the child already knows, i.e. to teach children about the printed word, ensuring that the right orthographic representation is linked with the other representations of the target word. Put like this, it does not sound too onerous a task. In reality of course, it is one of the most challenging jobs a teacher has to face, not least because many of the children they are working with do not have a well-developed and stable foundation of spoken language on which to build written language.

The aim of a psycholinguistic assessment is to find out exactly where on the speech-processing model (presented in Figure 2.1) a child's speech-processing skills are breaking down, how this might affect his or her speech and literacy development, and how speech-processing strengths might be utilized in an intervention programme (Stackhouse and Wells, 2001). A psycholinguistic assessment thus investigates a child's underlying processing skills and involves both input and output tasks that also tap how a child is storing and accessing information (see Stackhouse and Wells, 1997).

Speech and spelling development

If a child has the necessary spoken language skills, written language develops broadly in three phases (Frith, 1985; and see Chapter 6 in this volume). A *logographic* or whole-word recognition strategy of reading initially relies predominantly on visual skills. However, emerging phonological awareness allows the child to crack the alphabetic code and move into an *alphabetic* phase utilizing phoneme–grapheme correspondences, and then finally to an *orthographic* phase dependent on the segmentation of larger units such as morphemes.

In the first phase, children can only recognize words that they know and are not able to decode unfamiliar words. When spelling, they have some learnt programmes for familiar words (e.g. their own name), but in general spelling does not show phoneme–grapheme correspondences, for example ORANGE spelt as <oearasrie>. Breakthrough to the alphabetic stage occurs when a child can apply phoneme-grapheme rules to decoding new words. Spelling becomes more logical: it demonstrates that the child is segmenting the word successfully and applying letter knowledge but has not yet learned (or been taught) the conventions of English spelling, for example ORANGE spelt as <orinj>. Finally, in the orthographic stage, the child is able to recognize larger chunks of words such as prefixes and suffixes (e.g. ADDITION), and to read more efficiently by analogy with known words.

Moving beyond the logographic phase of literacy development is thus dependent on understanding that spoken utterances can be segmented into smaller elements and that these elements can be represented via sound–letter correspondences. This is the key to cracking the alphabetic code. Figure 2.2 illustrates what this might look like. It is the spontaneous writing of a 6-year-old girl describing 'A Special Place'. Although not conventionally correct in terms of English spelling rules, it shows that she has cracked the code at a speech sound level. She is able to reflect on the sound structure of a word and assign letters of the alphabet to her perception of the word. Her writing is therefore logical. She shows a use of letter names for sounds (e.g. the letter <r> to denote a long 'ah' sound in GARDEN and PLANT). She shows typical cluster reduction in PLACE, LOTS and PANSY. She marks syllable structure correctly even though not necessarily with the appropriate vowels.

Laura's writing shows that normal spelling development is mapped in some way on to a speech foundation. She has intact speech skills, which are

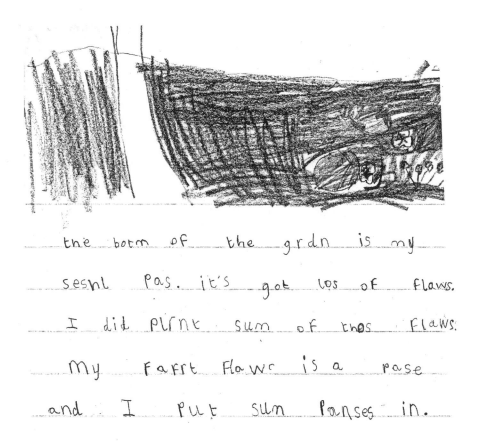

the botm of the grdn is my

seshl Pas. it's got los of flaws.

I did pirnt sum of thos Flaws.

My Fafrt Flawr is a pase

and I put sum Ponses in.

My Special Place
The bottom of my garden is my special place. It's got lots of flowers. I did plant some of those flowers. My favourite flower is a pansy and I put some pansies in.

Figure 2.2 'My Seshl Pas' by Laura aged 6;7 years.

consistent and clear for her age. She also has learned her letters and the sounds they make. By reflecting on her speech production, she can map her letter knowledge on to what she feels in terms of her articulation and what she hears herself and others say. Laura's consistent articulation allows her to take a word and segment it into bits that she recognizes as sounds of letters. She can thus convey meaning through print in an unconventional but logical way. This is typical of the alphabetic stage of literacy development and should be a firm foundation for her future literacy skills. Figure 2.3 shows Laura's spontaneous writing on the same topic at the age of 13 and how she has developed into a competent writer.

Various studies have applied speech analysis skills to spelling and found similarities between speech and spelling development (Clarke-Klein and

---

My Special Place

My special place is my bedroom.

Why is it Special?

My bedroom is special because it is a place that can be my own. Everything in there I can use. I like being there because I've personalized it to suit me e.g. There are posters of my favourite bands and actors (such as Green Day), lots of photos of my friends, family and my dog and I've stuck my sketches and drawings on the wall. I can also do whatever I want in there like write, draw, read, play my electric guitar, listen to my favourite music and so on. I can also do my favourite thing in my room, sleep! I feel safe when I'm in my bedroom and it is also somewhere I can think about anything and just be alone. My bedroom is the only room on the top floor so it is separate from the rest of the house. I also like it because my dog sleeps on my bed and he is my only pet so he is really special.

Things in my room which make it special for me

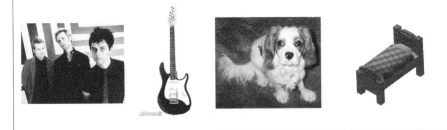

Figure 2.3 An extract from 'My Special Place' by Laura aged 13;4 years.

Hodson, 1995; McCormick, 1995; Stackhouse and Wells, 1993; Treiman, 1993). Clear and consistent speech production is an important skill for young children to have when starting school. Without it, they are disadvantaged when rehearsing words for spelling or when learning new vocabulary. When asked how many syllables there are in a word, children typically repeat it, segment it out loud or sub-vocally (whispered), and then count the beats on their fingers. If they are not able to produce the right number of syllables in the word or if they cannot say the word in the same way on more than one occasion, they cannot begin to get the spelling correct. When trying to spell a long word, one 12-year-old boy with speech and dyslexic difficulties said exasperatedly: "If I can't say it, I can't split it up!"

This is clearly the case in children with persisting speech difficulties. Michael had dyspraxia of speech, an inconsistent production of multisyllabic words and particular difficulties producing clusters/blends. When trying to spell a long word, he attempted to segment it into its bits first but then transcribed each of his attempts. The result was rather dramatic:

Target	*Spelling*
UMBRELLA	\<rberherrelrarlsrllles\>
CIGARETTE	\<satersatarhaelerar\>

In his spelling of UMBRELLA, Michael has dropped the first unstressed syllable ('um') from his spelling and is trying to write the first stressed syllable 'br', which he cannot pronounce. This takes up at least half of the spelling attempt. He is also aware that the word includes more than one letter 'l'! When spelling CIGARETTE, he wrote down the beginning sound ('sa') and end sound ('ter') of the word twice before losing it completely (\<haelerar\>).

Given that children with such persisting speech difficulties are at risk of associated literacy problems, it would be helpful to know as early as possible which children are not going to resolve their difficulties before the age of 5 years and therefore be vulnerable at the start of school and in more formal literacy instruction. Adopting a psycholinguistic approach to identification can help.

Predicting literacy performance: a longitudinal study

A number of studies have attempted to identify predictors of literacy outcome in children with speech and language difficulties. These studies have had interesting but sometimes conflicting results. Some report that syntax performance is a particularly good predictor of literacy outcome (e.g. Bishop and Adams, 1990; Magnusson and Naucler, 1990), whereas others have emphasized aspects of speech production as being the strongest predictor (e.g. Bird, Bishop and Freeman, 1995; Larivee and Catts, 1999; Webster and Plante, 1992). Combined speech and language problems may also put children at risk of literacy difficulties (Leitao, Hogben and Fletcher, 1997). However, what all these studies have in common is the fact that phonological awareness skills are particularly difficult for children with speech, language and literacy problems.

The basic premise of our own longitudinal study (Nathan et al., 2004a) was that the skills necessary for successful phonological awareness and literacy development arise from an intact speech processing system, as depicted in Figure 2.1 above. The hypothesis was that, compared with matched controls, children with specific speech difficulties would have a deficit at one or more points in the speech-processing system and that this deficit (or cluster of deficits) would not only manifest in speech difficulty, but also affect performance on phonological awareness and later literacy tasks.

Forty-seven children with primary speech difficulties and forty-seven normally developing controls matched on age, IQ, gender and education were assessed on a range of speech, language and phonological awareness tasks at three points in time (T1, T2 and T3) at ages around 4;6 (T1), 5;8 (T2) and 6;8 (T3) years. At the end of the study (T3), the children with speech difficulties were divided into two groups on the basis of reading and spelling development: typical (i.e. within the normal range) and delayed. Their concurrent and past speech and language-processing skills were examined for predictors of literacy outcome to establish whether any of the speech-processing tasks could predict children's emerging literacy skills, and if so, how early this could be done. Table 2.2 shows the tests which differentiated between typical and delayed readers at T3.

Table 2.2 Skills at times T1, T2 and T3 that differentiated typical from delayed readers/spellers at T3

Chronological age (years)	Tests
4;6 (T1)	None
5;8 (T2)	Speech input: auditory discrimination Speech output Grammar Phonological awareness: alliteration fluency Letter names
6;8 (T3)	Speech output Grammar Phonological awareness: phoneme deletion + completion Letter names

Four things are apparent about the skills that differentiated children with typical versus delayed literacy development at T3 (6;8 years). First, in children as young as 4 years of age, there were no unique predictors of literacy outcome at 6;8. Performance on speech output, grammar and auditory lexical decision (the child says whether or not words are correctly pronounced) narrowly missed being significant signs of future literacy problems. It was only at ages 5;8 and 6;8 that the typical and delayed reading/spelling groups could be differentiated statistically. Second, although phonological awareness skill is a predictor of literacy outcome from the age of 5 years, it is specifically the ability to segment at the sound (phoneme) level that is important, for example the production of as many words as possible beginning with a given sound (alliteration fluency), saying words without a specified sound (phoneme deletion) or adding a sound to a gap left in a word (phoneme completion). At no point was rhyme skill a unique predictor of literacy outcome, a finding that replicates others in the literature (see Chapter 4 in this volume). Third, as is well established, we found that letter knowledge was an essential skill for literacy to develop (see Laura's writing in Figure 2.2 above). Fourth, there is no single skill or difficulty that predicts a child's literacy outcome. At both 5 and 6 years of age, children draw on a variety of speech, language, phonological-awareness and letter-knowledge skills when learning to read and spell.

If we re-examine the data from our longitudinal study and this time divide the group of children with speech difficulties into those who did and did not resolve their speech difficulties by T3, we now get predictors of speech outcome at an age as young as 4;6, these being:

- speech output (severity of difficulties);
- speech input (auditory discrimination)
- expressive language (retelling a story).

The severity of speech output difficulties, problems with speech input (auditory discrimination) and accompanying language delay cluster together to predict poor speech outcome at around 6;8 years. This is a useful finding given that children whose speech difficulties persist beyond the age of 5;6 years are likely to have associated literacy problems (Bird, Bishop and Freeman, 1995; Bishop and Adams, 1990).

As Table 2.2 and the list above indicate, it was the children who had both speech and language problems, rather than speech problems alone, who were most at risk of both persisting speech difficulties and associated phonological awareness and literacy problems at 6;8 years. These children had more pervasive speech-processing problems involving both speech input and output processes as well as the storage of lexical representations (see Figure 2.1 above). They had more severe difficulties in speech production and had poor letter knowledge.

Spelling was a particular problem for the group of children with speech difficulties in our longitudinal study. At T3, the control children had broken through to the alphabetic stage of spelling development, whereas the children with speech difficulties were still showing signs of errors typical of the logographic/whole-word approach to spelling. Because all the children took part in the national Statutory Assessment Tests (SATs) of literacy and maths, we were able to examine their spelling skills further (Nathan et al., 2004b).

Statutory Assessment Tests

At the time of our longitudinal study, all children in the UK completed tests of reading, reading comprehension, spelling, writing and maths at school around the age of 7 years. We were therefore able to examine the educational attainment of children diagnosed earlier with speech difficulties (at around the age of 4 years) compared with matched normally developing controls. In addition, we could subgroup the children into those whose speech problems had resolved by the time the SATs were administered (when they were around 7 years of age) and those whose problems persisted, and then compare performance between these two subgroups.

Thirty-nine children from the original group of children with speech difficulties, and 35 matched controls, took part in this study. Table 2.3 shows the SATs performance of these children compared with controls. There were more children scoring below average performance (level 2) in the speech-disordered group than in the control group, particularly in spelling and reading comprehension (a finding replicated by Leitao and Fletcher, 2004; see also Chapter 7 in this volume).

Table 2.3 Percentage of children with speech difficulties compared with controls at each level of the Statutory Assessment Tests (level 2 being average for each age)

| | **% Speech-disordered group** | | | | **% Controls** | | | |
	Below 1	1	2*	3	Below 1	1	2*	3
Reading	8.6	28.6	48.5	8.6	0	11.8	64.7	8.8
Reading comprehension	40	0	40	20	14.3	5.7	45.6	34.3
Spelling	36.8	28.9	29	5.3	11.4	14.3	51.4	22.9
Writing	5.3	23.7	68.4	2.6	0	14.3	74.3	11.4
Maths	2.7	16.2	64.8	16.2	0	0	68.7	31.4

*Some tests are given three categories (a, b, c) at level 2. For this analysis, the categories have been merged.
Data from Nathan et al. (2004b).

Only 11 of the 39 children in the speech-disordered group had resolved their speech difficulties by the age of 7 years. Table 2.4 shows the performance of children with persisting versus resolved speech difficulties compared with the matched controls. The children with persisting speech difficulties performed significantly less well than controls on all of the tests but were particularly poor at spelling. The children who had resolved their difficulties performed significantly better than the children who had persisting speech difficulties on all tests and as well as controls on everything except spelling.

In summary, the implications of this study are that children with a history of speech difficulties generally perform less well than controls on SATs. However, children who resolve their speech difficulties before the age of 6 years tend to perform as well as controls across most aspects of the curriculum, even though many still underachieve when spelling. This suggests that an underlying speech-processing difficulty persists. A characteristic of developmental speech difficulties is that, just like the children themselves,

Table 2.4 Percentage of children scoring at level 2 (average performance) on Statutory Assessment Tests in each of three groups: normally developing controls, children with persisting speech difficulties and children whose speech difficulties have resolved

	Controls	Persisting speech difficulties	Resolved speech difficulties
Maths	100	74.1*	100
Reading	83.3	53.8*	88.9
Reading comprehension	76	48*	90
Writing	84	66.7*	81.8
Spelling	72	25.9*	54.5*

*Significantly poorer performance than matched controls.
Data from Nathan et al. (2004b).

they change over time. The unfolding nature of speech difficulties needs to be recognized; even though the overt speech difficulty appears to have 'resolved', problems in other domains, such as spelling, may persist.

The unfolding nature of speech and spelling difficulties

Group studies of adolescents with a childhood history of speech and language difficulties suggest that they are still likely to underperform on national attainment tests compared with IQ-matched controls (Snowling, Bishop and Stothard, 2000; Stothard et al., 1998).

Longitudinal case studies illustrate how speech difficulties can persist and impact on spelling in particular. Stackhouse (1992) describes a boy at four points in time: preschool and at aged 8, 14 and 18 years of age. Danny had been referred to speech and language therapy when he was two and a half years old as both his mother and health visitor were concerned that Danny was 'not talking'. His expressive vocabulary comprised a small number of single words (e.g. NO, MUMMY, LOOK), and he was not joining words together as would be expected at this age. He was, however, very communicative through gesture, he played well, and he appeared to have age appropriate comprehension. Indeed, at the age of 5;5 years, his verbal comprehension was at the 6 year level. He had no hearing problems, and all milestones apart from speech had been passed appropriately. Although there were no obvious physical difficulties, he could be clumsy, had some early feeding difficulties and was slow establishing handedness. Other members of the family also had delayed laterality and were described as having 'minor speech problems' and 'terrible spelling'.

By 4 years of age, Danny talked a lot but was very difficult to understand. He used mainly 'b' and 'd' at the beginnings of words. He did not use any fricatives ('f', 'v', 's', 'sh') or affricates ('ch', 'j') and could not produce 'k' or 'g' at all. This means he would use one pronunciation for many words (e.g. "dee" for TEA, KEY, SEA and SHE), and the listener would be reliant on context to understand his meaning. Danny also left off the endings of words, which made his speech sound non-fluent.

At 8 years of age, Danny was able to produce sounds in isolation but had difficulties sequencing them in words. He found it very difficult to produce a longer word in the same way on consecutive occasions: BUTTER-CUP, for example, was pronounced "buttertup", "bukertup", "butterpuk" and "bukerpup". At school, teachers commented on his untidy writing and disorganized presentation of work. Although he quite enjoyed looking at books and recognized familiar words, he could not crack the code when presented with new material. He was not able to apply letter–sound rules, and his reading was not developing as quickly as expected given his overall ability. He was still functioning in the logographic stage of literacy development, and his spelling appeared illogical.

By 14 years of age, Danny could be understood in everyday conversation. However, speech errors persisted in longer words, for example SYSTEMATIC was pronounced as "sinsemakit" and BIBLIOGRAPHY as "biglegrafefi". He would sometimes avoid words he knew he could not pronounce. At other times, word-finding difficulties prevented him producing a word accurately. Testing at this time confirmed that Danny was a boy of above-average intelligence whose reading and spelling skills were below the age-appropriate level. His reading had progressed more than his spelling, and he was now reading for pleasure. Spelling showed signs of specific segmentation difficulties: for example, MYSTERIOUS was spelt as <mistreriles> and CALCULATOR as <catltulater>. Although he usually knew how many syllables were in a word, he had difficulty working out which sound combinations were within the syllable. This segmentation difficulty was compounded by his inconsistent speech-production attempts.

At 17 years of age, Danny's speech was mainly intelligible although described as 'mumbley', and speech errors were still evident. Intrusive sounds sometimes crept in, SPAGHETTI, for example, being pronounced "spleghetti", and the programming of longer words proved difficult, such as HIPPOPOTAMUS pronounced as "hitopotanus" and CHRYSANTHEMUM as "chrysanfefum". His reading comprehension was superior to his reading aloud, at which he had an age equivalent of 12.4 years. Spelling was still difficult, particularly on articulatorily complex words – FAMILIAR was spelt as <ferminiler> and AMATEUR as <amiayture> – but Danny now had a spelling age of 12.6 years. Although he could perform tasks of rhyme and sound identification at the beginning or end of words, more advanced phonological awareness tasks such as spoonerisms (transposing the onsets of two given words, e.g. SUNNY DAY to "dunny say") were problematic for him. His written work at this age was imaginative, interesting and tidier, although it took him longer than his peers to produce a piece of written work, which was a problem for him in assignments and examinations. He still needed help organizing ideas in sentences and would produce more than one draft in attempting to get it right. The following is an extract from one of his essays:

> Imagine that you are in the fifth year of your secondary school, the end of the school year and perhaps school life is drawing near . . . . So questions rush to your head while you speaking to your careers adviser . . . . Perhaps one of the questions you might of asked in the careers room was 'What about if I want to do just practical you know no written work?'

Danny's above-average intelligence has helped him to compensate for his pervasive speech-processing difficulties. He can use his good verbal comprehension to make use of context when reading, but this does not help him to decode unfamiliar words in isolation. Danny's inconsistent speech production prevents him from using articulatory rehearsal to hold a word in memory while he segments it into its bits in order to allocate the appropriate letters. For spelling, he is therefore reliant on having learned the word and is not good on new or complex words. Danny's positive attitude and insight into his difficulties have clearly stood him in good stead. In his twenties, he successfully completed a college course in a trade that kept him in employment. His main hobby was sailing, which he took up on a school trip. In spite of opposition from his tutors because of his persisting speech difficulties evident in complex words, he persisted with his training to be a sailing instructor and came back for a short course of speech therapy specifically to work on the necessary vocabulary.

Danny's case illustrates the unfolding nature of speech and literacy difficulties through the school years and into adulthood. They do not go away: the level of difficulty may change, but the characteristics remain the same.

Conclusions

This chapter has attempted to explain why children with persisting speech difficulties are at risk of literacy problems and, in particular, why they have trouble with spelling. A psycholinguistic perspective helps to understand the nature of speech difficulties, how to investigate and manage them, and why they impact on literacy development. Viewed from this perspective, phonological awareness is the product of a child's speech-processing skills and not a separate entity, as often presented. Without normal speech input, output and clearly stored lexical representations, children cannot experiment with spoken language and perform the phonological awareness tasks necessary to connect spoken and written language (Figure 2.4).

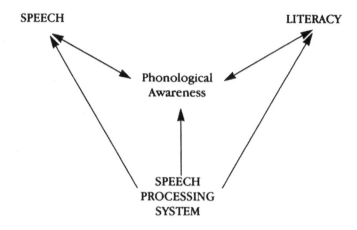

Figure 2.4 Phonological awareness – connecting speech and literacy development (from Stackhouse and Wells, 1997).

Children who do not have an intact speech-processing system have an unstable foundation on which to superimpose literacy teaching and need additional support to use strengths they may have to develop phonological awareness skills. A focus on the training of professionals and carers in the early years is essential to ensure not only that children with specific difficulties are recognized and treated, but also that all children receive support with their spoken language development in readiness for the start of school and more formal literacy instruction (see Chapter 14 in this volume). Intervention strategies are particularly important in areas of social disadvantage where spoken language skills can be delayed across the pre-school population, particularly in boys (Locke, Ginsborg and Peers, 2002). Once at school, children with delayed spoken and written language can benefit from intensive and explicit sound-linkage work (see Chapter 9 in this volume), coupled where necessary with targeted speech and language work (see Nathan and Simpson, 2001, for a good case example of intervention). Where possible, this should be carried out within a collaborative framework in which teachers, speech and language therapists, psychologists and assistants share a common terminology, beliefs and goals (Popple and Wellington, 2001). Add to this supportive home and school environments and the active involvement of the child in his or her own intervention programme, and a successful outcome is more likely. When Danny was asked at 14 years of age what advice he would give to others, he stated (Stackhouse, 1992, p. 97):

> If you have any problems to see a therapist, to always try and write letters. Enjoy it. Do not take it as thing you never get out of it 'cause if you try you will'.

CHAPTER 3
The dyslexic brain[1]

W.A. LISHMAN

Practitioners who work with pupils with reading difficulties (teachers and other professionals) confront problems in a number of areas, in particular with regard to matters of definition, early diagnosis and the rival merits of different approaches to remediation. Theories about causation can equally be at variance with one another. Studies of developmental dyslexia proceed in various domains – the cognitive, the behavioural and the biological – often in conjunction with one another.

This last, the biological approach to developmental dyslexia, has been increasingly pursued in recent years. As new techniques for investigating the brain have been discovered, they have yielded intriguing findings in relation to dyslexia and show promise of bringing greater clarity to the subject. This is especially true of the remarkable techniques of 'brain imaging', which will be described in some detail in this chapter. As a result, it is necessary for practitioners in the field to have a basic understanding of brain structure and function in order to understand contemporary views of the causes, consequences and treatments of dyslexia and related disorders.

A principal merit of the biological approach is that it can side-step the difficulties inherent in studying symptoms in a vacuum, so to speak, without some 'objective' index against which to judge the situation. This is especially true of *behavioural* symptoms, which can tend to be elusive and to have a number of possible causes. Hence the advantage to be gained by seeking out ties, whenever possible, to their biological roots, which, if

[1]This chapter is based upon the Marjorie Lishman Memorial Lecture, delivered in honour of my wife at the request of her colleagues in May 2002. Marjorie established the Royal Society of Arts Diploma Course in Specific Learning Difficulties in Bexley Education Authority in 1989, enabling successive cohorts of teachers to acquire expertise in the diagnosis and treatment of children with dyslexia and allied disorders. Material is also incorporated from an editorial published by the author in the Journal of Neurology, Neurosurgery and Psychiatry, 2003, volume 74, pages 1603–1605.

found, can provide the firmest of all objective indications of what may be afoot. In the absence of such ties, one can remain forever uncertain.

For example, are reading difficulties a reflection of nature or nurture, i.e. built in from the start to unusual patterns of brain functioning, or are they the product of the environment? Or are both sets of factors operative? Does dyslexia represent a distinct disorder, or is it merely the tail end of a normal distribution? Where may the cut-off point lie? Medicine has often been plagued by exactly the same questions until the biological underpinnings of a given disorder have been clarified.

So this is the central theme of this chapter – is there a biological basis in the brain for developmental dyslexia, and are we coming closer to identifying it? Let us consider further how this has operated in the field of medicine. Tuberculosis, once the scourge of the population, was long considered to be a 'social disease', of a very obscure nature, until the tubercle bacillus was discovered in 1882. Parkinson's disease was at one time thought to be a neurosis, resulting from emotional conflict, until distinctive changes in the midbrain were highlighted. And it is only within the lifetimes of many of us that we have seen a profound change in our understanding of dementia in the elderly – from viewing it as no more than 'senility', the result of growing old, to realizing that it mainly represents Alzheimer's disease with a distinctive pathological basis in the brain.

Could such conceptual changes ever apply to developmental dyslexia? This chapter will outline some recent discoveries about 'the dyslexic brain' that may be leading us in just that direction. First, however, it may be useful to revise, very briefly, certain aspects of brain anatomy and physiology in relation to reading.

Brain anatomy and physiology

The two cerebral hemispheres, the left and the right, look remarkably similar to each other but in fact have some important differences in function. In particular, the left hemisphere is specialized for language in the great majority of people. It is the left-handers among us who may sometimes prove anomalous in this regard, with language represented in the right hemisphere (some 15 per cent) or bilaterally (a further 15 per cent).

The cerebral cortex has grown dramatically with evolution so that the older, more primitive parts of the brain have become buried beneath it. Its surface is wrinkled and fissured so as to increase the surface area. The fissures are known as 'sulci' and the bulges between as 'gyri'. The outer 2 mm of the cortex consist of grey matter containing nerve cells ('neurones'), which number some 15 000 per cubic millimetre.

Neurones communicate with one another by transmitting information along their many fine 'dendritic' processes. This transmission is by a combination of chemical and electrical processes, all occurring in thousandths of a second. Messages are sent to more distant parts of the brain, and indeed to other parts of the body, via long processes derived from the neurones, known as axons. These are often congregated as bundles of nerve fibres to form the various 'tracts' of the brain. An important and very large bundle of fibres (the corpus callosum) connects the right and left hemispheres of the brain with each other.

In each hemisphere a broad division is made into the four major lobes – frontal, parietal, occipital and temporal (Figure 3.1). These are demarcated from one another by the major fissures of each hemisphere – the Sylvian and Rolandic fissures. Different areas of the cortex are specialized for various functions – vision, hearing, somatosensory inflow (i.e. touch, pressure and position in space), and motor output for movement (Figure 3.1). The primary receiving area for hearing appears in Figure 3.1 to be much smaller than is actually the case as much of it is buried deep within the Sylvian fissure. Similarly, the primary receiving area for vision extends on to the inner (medial) surface of the occipital lobe.

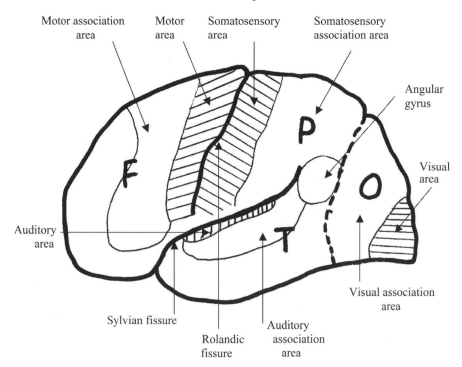

Figure 3.1 Subdivisions of the cerebral cortex. F, frontal lobe; P, parietal lobe; O, occipital lobe; T, temporal lobe; ▤ , primary cortical areas for sensation and movement.

Each of these specialized centres has its 'association area' adjacent to it. The association areas are essential for building up information about what has been perceived, giving it meaning and allowing a connection with other centres. A stimulus coming into the visual area, for example, is greatly enhanced by the visual association cortex, allowing us to evaluate what the stimulus means and to relate it to past experience. For example, if we see a ball in flight, the visual association cortex notes the size, roundness, colour and movement of the object, and allows us to realize that it is indeed a moving ball. Transmissions to the motor association cortex, and thence to the motor area itself, may indeed enable us to catch it! Pay special note to the region of the 'angular gyrus'. This is uniquely placed to integrate information from vision, hearing and other sensory impressions. All of the major sensory association areas abut on to it. Not surprisingly, it is important in reading and writing, as discussed further below.

Figure 3.2 indicates that an enormous amount of the cortex of the left hemisphere is involved with language, and within this language cortex certain areas have specialized functions.

Wernicke's area in the left temporal lobe is situated within the auditory association cortex near the back of the primary receiving area for sounds in general, and is highly specialized for the detection of language signals.

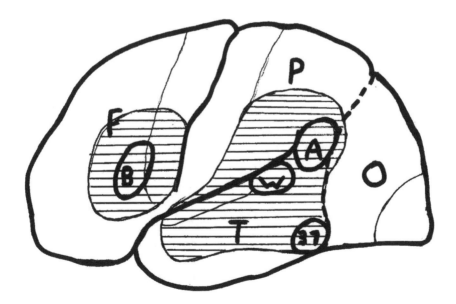

Figure 3.2 Cortical areas involved with language in the left hemisphere. A, angular gyrus; B, Broca's area; F, frontal lobe; O, occipital lobe; P, parietal lobe; T, temporal lobe; W, Wernicke's area; 37, area BA 37; ▨ , cortical areas involved with language.

It holds the records for phonemes and the phoneme sequences that make up words. It is exquisitely adept at recognizing these particular sounds, no matter what the pitch, accent or speed of the speech, and at distinguishing language from background noise. It also links the words to meaning. When Wernicke's area is damaged, for example after a stroke, the language input cannot be properly classified and recognized, and meaning cannot be accurately ascribed to it.

Broca's area in the frontal lobe is closely connected to Wernicke's area by a dense strand of nerve fibres – the arcuate fasciculus. This area is responsible for producing fluent speech, as well as for assembling words according to syntax (grammatical rules) in order to transmit meaning. When the area is damaged, the output of speech is slow and hesitant, with faulty grammar.

The *angular gyrus* is a special case. It lies, as we see, at the junction of hearing, touch and vision, and allows complex linkages between them. It therefore has special relevance to written language and acts with Wernicke's area to give meaning to language that is visually perceived. In effect, the angular gyrus maps visual images of printed words on to the phonological structures of language. When the area is damaged, the patient can no longer read and write. He or she can, however, still speak and understand spoken speech.

Area BA 37 is far more important than such a name suggests. As we shall see later on, this is the area that appears to give access to our 'word dictionaries' and allows us to select the appropriate word to match a given perceived object.

Although aspects of brain organization have been understood for many years, we were limited in our attempts to study it properly until around the 1970s. Up until then, it was necessary, for any thorough examination, to wait until the person had died. We now have a wide range of 'brain-imaging' techniques for studying the brain in the living person, and these have revolutionized brain research. Importantly, virtually all of these techniques have now been applied to developmental dyslexia.

Brain investigations and dyslexia

Structural brain investigations

Galaburda and his colleagues were among the first to focus attention on structural brain changes in dyslexia (Galaburda, 1992; Galaburda and Kemper, 1979; Galaburda et al., 1985; Humphreys, Kaufmann and Galaburda, 1990). Their work involved an in-depth series of autopsy studies on a small number of individuals with dyslexia, seven in all, who had died early from various causes. The planum temporale is an area lying on the upper surface of the temporal lobes, deep within the Sylvian fissure, and is closely associated with language. The left planum is usually considerably larger than the right. Taken together, these studies revealed a consistent lack of asymmetry in the size of the planum temporale of the two hemispheres – specifically, the right planum was larger than is usually the case. In addition, the same group reported areas of 'cortical dysplasia' (disruptions of the normal layering of neurones in the cortex), along with numerous 'ectopias' (abnormal nests of nerve cells, sometimes called 'brain warts'). Such changes were found particularly in the left hemisphere and within the language areas of the brain. The conclusions the researchers came to were that the abnormalities in the planum temporale could reflect the familial predisposition to dyslexia, and the dysplasias and ectopias the effect of additional factors disturbing the brain development of the fetus during pregnancy.

Arguably, brain imaging with magnetic resonance imaging (MRI) has provided the most accurate structural images of the brain available to date. It relies on the capacity of powerful magnetic fields to disturb the orientation of the hydrogen nuclei in the water of the brain. Bursts of radiofrequency impulses are then applied to disturb the nuclei further, and the electrical signals produced are analysed by computer. In this way, it is possible to visualize the distribution of water throughout the brain, and hence its structure. The use of this technique initially seemed to confirm the planum temporale abnormalities. In particular, a study by Larsen et al. (1990) of 19 adolescents with dyslexia showed a close relationship between this feature and measures of phonological dysfunction. Other MRI investigations have, however, been less consistent, and this particular area of research has turned out in the end to be rather disappointing. Moreover, brain imaging has not been able to clarify the issue of brain dysplasias and ectopias because such changes are visible only under the microscope.

More recently, Eliez et al. (2000) scanned the brains of 16 men with dyslexia (aged 18–40 years) and 14 controls (all right-handed) and took careful measurements of brain volume in different regions. The temporal lobes proved to be smaller in the men with dyslexia, significantly so on the left. The difference here was substantial, with a 12 per cent reduction in size. On separately assessing the grey and white matter – quite easily done with MRI – it was the grey matter, and not the white, that accounted for the reduction. This, of course, is the superficial layer of the cortex containing the neurones, in contrast to the underlying white matter, which contains the axonal fibres proceeding to other parts of the brain.

So it would seem from this study that the left temporal lobe may be significantly smaller in men with dyslexia, principally due to a decrease in grey matter. Eliez et al. suggest that such grey matter reductions might account for some of the findings we shall be examining below – for example, the impaired activation noted in the left temporal lobe of readers with dyslexia when scans are carried out during reading activities. Such a regional decrease in neuronal number could also conceivably contribute directly to the reading difficulties observed in dyslexia. It would presumably reflect developmental anomalies during the intrauterine period of life, when the major migration of neurones into the cerebral cortex takes place.

So far, however, Eliez et al.'s findings do not appear to have been replicated in other samples. Instead, volume reductions have been observed on MRI in frontal lobe regions bilaterally and in the right cerebellar anterior lobe among children (mean age 11;4) with dyslexia (Eckert et al., 2003). Moreover the extent of reductions in these areas was significantly correlated with reading, spelling and language measures related to dyslexia.

Functional brain imaging

'Functional imaging' involves imaging the brain while a task is carried out, in order to visualize the changes in cerebral blood flow and metabolism that occur during performance of the task.

Cerebral blood flow

One of the first attempts to study dyslexia in this way was reported by Flowers, Wood and Naylor (1991), who administered what they labelled a 'spelling task' to 83 adults with a well-documented childhood history of dyslexia and to controls. Participants had to listen to a list of spoken words and signal (by lifting a finger) whenever a word contained exactly four letters. While the test was in progress, brain blood flow was measured by over eight brain regions on the left and eight on the right of the brain. Normal readers from the sample showed peak left temporal blood flow in the Wernicke region, and the accuracy of performance on the task was related to the amount of flow in Wernicke's region. In contrast, those who had been reading-disabled in childhood showed a poor response in Wernicke's area and, interestingly, a shift to a more posterior focus in the temporoparietal region. The worse the childhood disability had been, the greater was the posterior focus.

Various possibilities were considered to account for this result. It might possibly reflect different reading strategies employed by the readers with dyslexia, as a result of problems with the functioning of Wernicke's area in childhood, or it might reflect abnormal patterns of connectivity in their brains. Axons that would normally have been destined for Wernicke's region during brain development might have ended up at targets more posteriorly in the brain.

Phonological studies

A marked advance in understanding of the 'dyslexic brain' came with the advent of positron emission tomography (PET) scanning. PET scanning involves the injection of a tiny dose of a radioactive chemical, which is taken up by the brain. Positrons (positively charged electrons) are emitted from the chemical, and their presence can be detected by counters arranged around the head. A computer is then used to build up pictures of the distribution of radioactivity within the brain. The scans essentially show which parts of the brain have been most active in taking up the radioactive chemical. The scan can then be repeated some minutes later while the participant performs a given task; by subtracting the first scan from the second, it is possible to see which brain regions have increased or decreased their activity during performance of the task.

Paulesu et al. (1996) at the Institute of Neurology in London used the PET technique to obtain a more detailed picture of the brain areas involved in language processing. Specifically, they administered tasks that made particular demands on phonological processes, i.e. the language processes that are, according to behavioural evidence, impaired in developmental dyslexia (see Chapter 1 in this volume). Paulesu et al.'s participants were five right-handed men with a clear history of developmental dyslexia who were now 'compensated' to the extent that they had successfully completed higher education. Four were university students or postgraduates. They were compared with right-handed controls matched for age and educational level.

While the scans were carried out, participants were given two tasks (on separate occasions). The first was a rhyming task, in which pairs of letters were presented on a screen and the participants had to signal (by moving a joystick) to indicate whether or not the letters rhymed with each other (e.g. *BG* versus *BL*). This involves 'segmented phonology' because each letter name must be segmented into its consonant and vowel to determine whether rhyming has occurred. The second was a short-term phonological memory task. Here, the subjects were shown six consonants at 1 second intervals (e.g. *S K G R T N*); then, after a 2 second gap, they were shown another (e.g. *K*). They had to signal whether or not it had been present before. These tasks were so simple that the adults with dyslexia performed as well as the controls even though they were significantly impaired on more demanding phonological tasks (e.g. spoonerisms) and also significantly worse on standard reading and spelling tests.

On the rhyming task, the controls activated the language areas of the left hemisphere extensively – from Wernicke's area posteriorly to Broca's area anteriorly, as well as the tissues of the insula in between. They also activated the cerebellar hemispheres bilaterally. In contrast, the participants with dyslexia activated a very restricted area, in fact Broca's area alone.

There was no activation of Wernicke's area, and none in the insula. The cerebellum was barely activated at all. On the short-term phonological memory task, the controls activated much the same regions as in the rhyming task. The participants with dyslexia activated Wernicke's area normally, but Broca's area only weakly, and there was no activation in the region between these two.

Paulesu et al. (1996) concluded that, when performing phonological tasks, readers with dyslexia (even those who ultimately achieve high levels of reading skill) activate severely restricted areas of the brain: the rhyming task activated Broca's area but not Wernicke's area, whereas the memory task activated Wernicke's area but Broca's area only weakly. There was thus a failure to activate the posterior and anterior brain areas in concert with one another. In particular, neither task activated the brain region (the insula) that lies between the posterior and anterior language areas of the brain. It is therefore not surprising that readers with dyslexia experience difficulty associating between the different 'codes' required for reading skills. Normal reading requires one to map the codes for the sound of the heard word, the sight of the written word and the articulation of the spoken word one upon another. If there is indeed an impaired connection between the posterior and anterior language areas of the brain, it is not hard to see why children with dyslexia have difficulties in achieving fluent reading.

Following on from this, Shaywitz et al. (1998) used functional MRI to assess phonological skills in dyslexia. Functional MRI consists of a series of very rapidly repeated mini-scans that are designed to be sensitive to changes in the amount of oxygen in the blood. When a task is performed, it is possible to see which parts of the brain have become active and have thus taken extra oxygen from the blood. The absence of radiation hazard with this technique allows a much larger number of participants (including children and adolescents) to be tested, and the greater resolution of MRI allows numerous brain areas to be examined individually.

In the study by Shaywitz et al. (1998), 29 people with developmental dyslexia (aged 16–54 years) were compared with 32 controls (aged 18–63). Again, the focus of attention was on phonological processing, and this was examined by devising a hierarchical series of tests that made progressively greater demands on phonological functions. First, a baseline task was employed against which later tasks could be compared. The baseline task consisted of a simple line orientation test that involved visuospatial analysis alone. Further tasks were then incorporated. The first was of letter case judgement (e.g. are *bBbb* and *bbBb* the same as or different from one another?) – a task requiring orthographic but not phonological processing. The second was a simple rhyming task, much as that employed in Paulesu et al.'s study – for example, do the letters *T* and *V* rhyme or not? The third was a more demanding phonological task in which non-words (such as *leat* and *jete*) had to be analysed before deciding whether or not they rhymed.

In all of these tests, the subject had to signal yes or no by pressing a response button. The serial MRI scans were then examined (after subtracting those produced by the baseline task), to see which brain regions showed a systematic increase in activation as the phonological demands increased. The results were clear. The controls showed a systematic increase in activation in several posterior areas of the cortex as the phonological demands of the task increased – namely in Wernicke's area, the angular gyrus, the primary visual cortex and, less impressively, the visual association cortex. The participants with dyslexia failed to show such an effect. The anterior brain regions, however, showed something different. Here, the individuals with dyslexia, compared with the controls, showed an *overactivation* in response to phonological tasks – in Broca's area and in the adjacent inferior frontal cortex. The fact that these two effects were opposite in direction made it unlikely that the results merely reflected an increased effort on the part of those with dyslexia.

Another finding reported by Shaywitz et al. (1998), albeit little commented upon in the paper, related to some interesting differences between the hemispheres. In two crucial language areas of the brain (the angular gyrus and area BA 37), the controls showed greater activations in the left hemisphere than the right, as would be expected, but the readers with dyslexia showed precisely the reverse, with greater activations in the right hemisphere than the left. We shall see later that magnetoencephalography (MEG) has raised this issue of hemispheric anomalies again.

Shaywitz et al. concluded that readers with dyslexia demonstrate a functional disruption in an extensive system in the posterior cerebral cortex, encompassing both visual and language regions. In particular, this reflects an imperfectly functioning system for segmenting words into their phonological constituents. They noted that the disrupted system included the angular gyrus, which is pivotal in mapping the visual images of print on to the phonological structures of language, and suggested that the results supported the critical role of impaired phonological analysis in developmental dyslexia.

We should not be dismayed that these MRI findings fail to mirror Paulesu et al.'s (1996) PET scan findings exactly. Much can depend on the precise techniques used, both to image the brain and to exercise its functioning, as well as on the nature of the samples of dyslexic cases studied – Shaywitz et al.'s sample covered a wider age range than Paulesu et al.'s, and the subjects were on the whole more severely affected. The important areas of agreement between the studies are that both show differences between readers with dyslexia and controls when the brain is imaged during the performance of phonological tasks, and that both concur in indicating that both posterior and anterior language areas function abnormally.

Word recognition

A further series of studies has dealt with tests of word recognition. Although somewhat removed from the totality of skills involved in reading, this concentration on a single aspect of the reading process has again shown interesting differences between readers with dyslexia and non-impaired readers. Brunswick et al. (1999) used PET scans to monitor the brain activity produced when adults with dyslexia read aloud a series of words presented at 1 second intervals, one at a time on a screen. All of the words were phonologically simple. There were six adults with dyslexia, all university students with documented childhood histories of reading impairment requiring special tuition, and six controls matched for age, IQ and educational attainment. They were from the same universities as those with dyslexia.

During the reading of a word, all participants activated their visual cortex, the left temporoparietal receptive language areas and the articulatory cortex of Broca's area. However, the readers with dyslexia differed from the controls in several respects. They showed *increased* activation in Broca's area (much as in Shaywitz et al.'s functional MRI study) and *decreased* activation in three regions – the cerebellum, the caudate nucleus deep within the hemisphere, and area BA 37 low down in the posterior part of the left temporal lobe.

The cerebellum has been incriminated on certain evidence as functioning abnormally in readers with dyslexia (Fawcett and Nicolson, 1999; Fawcett, Nicolson and Dean, 1996; Nicolson and Fawcett, 1990). The finding of reduced activation in area BA 37 is, however, also of special interest. This was one of the areas highlighted in Shaywitz et al.'s study as showing anomalous *right* hemisphere activation on functional MRI. It is an area that has been of particular interest to neurologists for a considerable time in that it appears to play a critical role in the retrieval of the names of words and objects. If it is damaged, for example after a stroke, the patient cannot find the name for a presented object but is clearly aware of the identity of the object, can recognize its name and can easily demonstrate its use. This condition is termed 'word-selection anomia'. There seems, in effect, to be an isolated difficulty in gaining access to the storehouse of word names – the so-called 'word dictionary' that each individual possesses (Benson, 1979). Any impairment in the functioning of area BA 37 would clearly contribute to the reading difficulties of individuals with dyslexia.

Reading difficulties in other languages

Steps have also been taken to explore brain imaging in readers with dyslexia who speak languages other than English. This is an important issue. All of the work described so far was carried out on English-speaking subjects, and English is notorious for the complexity and inconsistency with which sounds are represented in written language. How far would these brain imaging findings hold up in readers with dyslexia from other countries?

English has a so-called 'deep orthography' in that 1120 graphemes (letters or letter combinations) are used to represent 40 sounds (phonemes) (Paulesu et al., 2000). French and Danish are similar (Grigorenko, 2001). Italian, in contrast, has a 'shallow orthography' in that 33 graphemes suffice for the 25 phonemes of the language. Spanish and German are similar in this respect. Moreover, the prevalence of dyslexia across different languages appears to be related to the depth or shallowness of their orthographies. An important question, therefore, is how universal are the emerging findings about brain functioning in dyslexia?

In a pioneering study, Paulesu et al. (2001) compared English, French and Italian adults with dyslexia with controls from the same countries. There were 24 readers with dyslexia and 24 controls from each country, matched for age and IQ. All had achieved tertiary education. In all three countries, the adults with dyslexia were equivalently impaired in relation to their controls on reading and phonological tasks. The same experimental paradigm as described just above was carried out – namely PET scanning during single-word reading. The readers with dyslexia from all three countries showed equivalent reductions in activation of the key brain regions already known to occur in English-speaking readers with dyslexia. Paulesu et al. (2001) concluded that a phonological processing deficit appeared to be responsible for literacy problems in both deep and shallow orthographies, and that there appeared to be a universal basis in brain dysfunction for dyslexia in all three languages. With shallow orthographies (such as Italian), the impact is understandably less, and dyslexia is rarer, whereas learning to read in a deep orthography (such as English or French) stands to aggravate the literacy impairments of otherwise mild cases of dyslexia.

Magnetoencephalography (MEG)

MEG is a recent development for monitoring the electrical activity generated within the brain. The electroencephalogram has long been used to detect such electrical signals, for example in the diagnosis of epilepsy. But MEG aims to detect not the electrical signals themselves, but the minute magnetic fields that are the by-products of the electrical activity. This has an advantage in that the magnetic flux is not reduced or distorted by passage through the tissues of the brain, skull and scalp. Localization can therefore be very accurate, no matter how deeply within the brain the activity is taking place. In addition, the magnetic changes can be charted over extremely brief periods of time, measured in thousandths of a second after the presentation of a stimulus. MEG is thus unique in its ability to monitor both *where* brain activity is occurring, and exactly *when* it occurs after stimulus presentation. MEG is a complicated procedure. Detection coils are positioned around the head and must be kept at extremely low temperatures in the superconducting range. In addition, the examination room must be carefully shielded to protect the apparatus from fluctuations in the magnetic fields of the environment. Few such systems are available, yet even this technique has been applied to dyslexia.

Simos et al. (2000) used MEG to study 10 children with dyslexia (mean age 12;6 years) and eight age-matched normal readers as controls who participated in a word-reading task. The words were exposed on a screen for 1 second at a time, at intervals of 3–4 seconds, and the children had to respond by hand when certain target words were recognized. While the test was in progress, MEG was used to monitor the sources of electrical activity in the brain for the first second after each word stimulus was presented. The brain areas examined included the posterior parts of the superior and middle temporal gyri (including Wernicke's area), the supramarginal gyri, the angular gyri and the basal temporal cortex (on the underside of the brain) in both the left and right hemispheres. The procedure was then repeated using spoken instead of printed words.

The results were very interesting. The basal temporal cortex of the left hemisphere was activated first in all subjects (within 200 milliseconds), representing the pre-lexical analysis of print. Normal readers then activated the *left* temporoparietal language regions of the brain (within 300 milliseconds), whereas the children with dyslexia primarily activated the corresponding regions in the *right* hemisphere. Only one of the 10 children with dyslexia showed reliable left temporoparietal activity, and this was delayed and weak in comparison with the right-sided activity. In contrast to this, the findings on spoken word presentations were substantially normal in the readers with dyslexia, indicating that their unusual patterns of brain activation were specific to reading.

Simos et al. (2000) therefore concluded that there are marked and consistent differences in the patterns of brain activation between young readers with dyslexia and normal readers during the first half-second after reading the printed word. They suggested that the consistency of their findings might have reflected the testing of *children*, i.e. at a stage before compensatory alternative reading strategies had become well established.

The general conclusion was that the reading difficulties of children with dyslexia might be associated with aberrant patterns of functional connectivity between the basal temporal cortex (involved in the pre-lexical analysis of print) and the key language areas of the left temporoparietal cortex (involved in phonological analysis and assembly). Finally, Simos et al. offered the suggestion that the technique of MEG showed promise as a tool for evaluating possible changes in brain function resulting from educational strategies targeted at the core phonological deficits of dyslexia.

Studies of remediation

This last aspiration has in fact been put into practice. Simos et al. (2002) have now reported repeat MEG studies on eight children with dyslexia (mean age 11;4 years) after an 8 week period of therapy. This consisted of approximately 80 hours of one-to-one instruction focused on the development of phonological and decoding skills. On this occasion, Simos et al. employed a visual rhyming task in conjunction with the MEG recordings.

Before the intervention, all of the children with dyslexia had, as before, shown little or no activation in the left temporoparietal regions, in sharp contrast to the controls, and the predominant activity had been in the homologous regions of the right hemisphere. After treatment, all showed dramatic changes in regional activation profiles: activation in the left superior temporal gyrus now exceeded that on the right, with non-significant trends in the same direction for the supramarginal and angular gyri. All children showed significant gains in reading skills, and a strong correlation was observed between the improvement in response accuracy on the rhyming task and the degree of increased activation in the left superior temporal gyrus. There were, however, indications that the restoration towards normality was incomplete in that the time to the peak development of left superior temporal gyrus activity was longer in the treated dyslexic children than among the normal reading controls (800 and 600 milliseconds respectively).

Temple et al. (2003) have similarly reported a move towards the normalization of functional MRI scans in 20 children with dyslexia after an intensive 8 week course of therapy. This group of workers had previously shown that, in children with dyslexia (aged 8–12 years), there were identifiable deficits in left temporoparietal activity on functional MRI in comparison to controls (Temple et al., 2001). Indeed, while performing a visual phonological rhyming task, the children with dyslexia showed virtually no temporoparietal activation whatsoever. Left inferior frontal regions were activated well, albeit in a somewhat more anterior location than in the controls.

A subsample of these children was then re-examined after treatment, tests consisting of a computerized battery of exercises (*Fast For Word Language*) including practice in auditory discrimination, phoneme identification and language comprehension (Temple et al., 2003). Identical tasks and imaging procedures were used before and after therapy. Following treatment, the left temporoparietal cortex showed activation when this had not been present before, and the left frontal activation had moved more posteriorly to the area seen in controls. Moreover, significant correlations could be observed between the magnitude of increased left temporoparietal activation and improvements on certain measures of language ability and phonological awareness. Other brain regions, not active in controls, also showed activation after treatment; these included right hemisphere areas homologous to the language areas on the left. This may have reflected compensatory processes. It was also clear that the new left temporoparietal activation was in a region near to, but not identical with, the focus seen in normal-reading controls, indicating that the return towards normality was as yet incomplete. More could scarcely be expected after so brief an intervention.

These studies combine to show that the anomalies in brain activation characteristic of dyslexia are already present at a young age, during the period of literacy acquisition, and that they are amenable to amelioration in considerable degree with appropriately targeted therapy. That this is so is a tribute to the plasticity inherent in the human brain.

Summary and conclusions

The main findings from these brain-imaging studies seem to provide compelling evidence for the existence of a biological basis in the brain for developmental dyslexia. First, Eliez et al. (2000) found that the left temporal lobe was significantly reduced in size in their adult dyslexic cases, due principally to a reduction in its grey matter content. If confirmed, this will be an important finding, setting the stage for many of the functional brain deficits that have also emerged in dyslexic subjects. In contrast, Eckert et al. (2003) found volume reductions in frontal and cerebellar areas among dyslexic children.

With regard to functional imaging, certain patterns of brain dysfunction have been clearly demonstrated in readers with dyslexia. When *phonological analysis* has been the object of study, the language areas of the brain, including Wernicke's and Broca's areas, have been found to function abnormally. These are the areas highly specialized for phonological analysis and transformation. Evidence has sometimes been forthcoming of a seeming disconnection between the posterior (receptive) areas for language, and the anterior (motor) areas responsible for language output. Disproportions have sometimes been detected, with diminished activity in the posterior language brain regions and a peculiar overactivity in those situated anteriorly. The angular gyrus, the part of the brain strategically situated to have special relevance to written language, has also proved to be underactive in dyslexia.

A conclusion common to all of these phonological studies is that phonological processes, such as segmentation and assembly, fail to activate the brain in an entirely normal manner and with optimal efficiency. The problem clearly persists even in 'compensated' dyslexics who have moved on from their childhood difficulties to higher education.

Where *word recognition* has been investigated, additional parts of the brain are found to function poorly. These include area BA 37, towards the back of the left inferior temporal gyrus, known to play an important role in selecting the names of words and objects, i.e. for gaining access to our personal 'word dictionaries'. The person with dyslexia may thus be additionally disadvantaged by a global word-recognition problem. Findings from MEG indicate that, in tests of word recognition on readers with dyslexia, the relevant information may initially be shunted to the right instead of the left hemisphere of the brain, this occurring within milliseconds after exposure to the printed word. The information may ultimately gain access to the language areas in the left hemisphere, but presumably by a circuitous and inefficient route. Finally, brain imaging in children, before and after an intensive period of therapy, has shown that this appears to be followed by a change in brain functioning towards normality in some considerable degree.

Origin and causes

What can be the origin of the brain changes that have been observed in dyslexia? The answer is unlikely to be simple, especially since they involve brain function so widely. The obvious contender lies with genetics, which is known to be a powerful influence in developmental dyslexia. The problems may thus be 'built in' from birth, or more accurately from the time in fetal development when the brain is being formed and organized.

This may not, however, be the whole answer. The brain continues to develop well after birth, through childhood and some would say adolescence as well. It also becomes 'fine-tuned' in relation to environmental influences. Those connections which are activated appropriately become strengthened and endure, whereas others that turn out to be redundant are pruned and discarded. When the child becomes involved with language, such modifications no doubt affect the language systems of the brain to a substantial degree. In addition to this, minor trauma, infections and a host of other adverse influences can disturb the maturation of the brain during early postnatal life. Thus, both genetic and environmental influences (including social processes and educational inputs) may contribute in varying degrees to the final shaping of the dyslexic brain.

Here, we may touch on another large issue, namely whether the brain dysfunction may have somewhat different determinants in different individuals. There is evidence from other avenues of research of a range of problems other than those within the realm of phonology in dyslexic individuals – for example, work on transmission defects in the magnocellular sensory pathways (Galaburda and Livingstone, 1993), on complex visual processing difficulties (Stein and Walsh, 1997) and on problems with high-speed auditory discrimination (Tallal, Miller and Fitch, 1993). Many children with dyslexia appear to show abnormal cerebellar function (Fawcett and Nicolson, 1999; Fawcett, Nicolson and Dean, 1996; Nicolson and Fawcett, 1990). All of these have been incriminated in contributing to dyslexia. So how can we reconcile these different approaches to understanding 'the cause' of dyslexia? There may, of course, be a number of causes, each producing its own definitive stamp. And, just conceivably, the patterns of brain dysfunction observed in dyslexia could represent a 'final common path' derived from a variety of adverse influences. A great deal of further work will be needed before we can attempt to decide such issues.

Implications

This assembly of evidence appears to be valid and to reflect the disturbance of important brain processes in dyslexic individuals. It is impressive, not least because it highlights dysfunctions in areas where one would expect to find them – in brain regions known to be involved with language generally and with phonological processes in particular. In word-recognition tests, area BA 37 is highlighted – the part of the brain involved in the retrieval of names of words and objects. Such dysfunctions appear to be present from an early age, at least from the period of learning to read, yet they have proved to be amenable in some degree to modification with training. This reinforces the importance of identifying vulnerable children at the earliest opportunity and engaging them in appropriate remediation.

So we appear to gain strong and compelling evidence for the idea that developmental dyslexia is a valid entity with a basis in unusual brain functioning, and not merely some false construct derived from a skewed appreciation of the concerns of middle-class society. Furthermore, some evidence has been forthcoming that the patterns of brain dysfunction may transcend the vagaries peculiar to different language systems. So far, they seem to be remarkably similar in people with dyslexia from different countries – to apply equivalently to English and French with their complex 'deep orthographies', and to Italian with its transparent and shallow orthography.

But we should not be entirely complacent about these findings. As always when dealing with brain research, we have to guard against uncritical enthusiasm. Most of the studies discussed have been performed during the past decade and are pioneering in the sense that they are using very new technologies to extend the boundaries of knowledge. Many have relied on a small number of subjects, not least because brain imaging is extremely expensive. The various findings will need to be replicated several-fold before we accept them in their entirety.

Moreover, there are still some discrepancies between one study and another with respect to matters of detail. Much probably hinges on precise details of the experimental set-up employed, but it may also rest in part on the selection of the dyslexic subjects examined. It is possible, for example, that there are subclasses of dyslexia, or differences in brain functioning that develop as the person with dyslexia matures. Here, the findings of Shaywitz et al. (2003), of differences between 'persistent' and 'compensated' poor readers, may be a case in point. Shaywitz et al. were able, in a prospective longitudinal study, to detect contrasting patterns of brain activation in two groups of young adults who had had reading problems in childhood, compared with those who had persistent and continuing problems with reading and those whose childhood reading problems had partially resolved. We must therefore keep in mind that all studies to date have reported on group comparisons rather than data from individual people. Considerable variation from one dyslexic individual to another may yet be obscured within these overall group results.

When reading this evidence for the biological basis of dyslexia, practitioners may rightly ask whether it tells us anything about the best way to proceed in efforts to help treat such individuals. That debate would appear to remain wide open. The only hint received so far is that those parts of the brain concerned with phonological processes are the most clearly dysfunctional in dyslexia. This would suggest that phonological difficulties are fundamental to *most* people with dyslexia and that phonological approaches to remediation are extremely important. Indeed, the concentration in teaching on the rehearsal of phonological skills is given a large measure of scientific respectability.

Acknowledgements

Special thanks go to Mrs Claire Stevens and her colleagues at Bexley Local Education Authority, and to Dr Barbara Gil-Rodriguez and Professor Valerie Cowie for valuable advice on the manuscript.

CHAPTER 4

The prediction and screening of children's reading difficulties

VALERIE MUTER

Our knowledge and understanding of how children learn to read and how this process can go wrong has grown enormously over the past 20 years, not least because of research that takes what might be termed a 'predictor' approach. Predictors are skills or abilities that contribute to individual differences in reading attainment and that are definable, measurable and potentially modifiable through teaching. In the case of very young children, a knowledge of such predictors indicates the cognitive skills that children need to have in place to enable them to learn to read effectively. These measures are also helpful because they are tools that enable us to predict, albeit with some degree of error, which children will find reading easy and which children may find it difficult. This chapter considers the predictors of reading achievement and the characteristics of reading difficulties before proceeding to discuss the screening and assessment of children's phonological skills.

Predictors of reading achievement

Most predictor research takes the form of correlational studies that examine the relationship between predictor abilities and reading outcomes. The research is usually conducted longitudinally – i.e. children are seen and assessed at a given point in time (time 1) on tasks that are thought to measure predictors of subsequent reading progress and are then reassessed some time later (time 2). Performance on the time 1 predictor measures is then correlated with performance on reading tests at time 2 to determine the predictors of reading skills. Once these have been established, they may form the basis for screening populations of preschool or primary school children. Alternatively, measures of the predictors might be used in the diagnostic assessments of children whose histories suggest that they are 'at risk', for example children who have been delayed in their early speech development, or where there are other family members with literacy problems. If a child shows a significant difficulty in a predictor skill that is known to be closely related to reading progress, this provides important clues on how to remediate the problem.

Typically developing phonological awareness

Research with normally developing readers and those with reading problems (including dyslexia) has shown that the phonological processing skills are powerful predictors of later reading ability. The most extensively studied of these phonological abilities is *phonological awareness* – sensitivity to, and the capacity to manipulate, the speech sound segments of words. There are a number of tasks that can be employed to assess phonological awareness, which include:

- detecting and producing rhyming responses, for example, which word is the odd one out (i.e. non-rhyming) word in the sequence CAT, PAT, FAN? (Bradley and Bryant, 1983);
- blending syllables or phonemes in words, such as joining 'c-a-t' to make the word "cat" (Perfetti et al., 1987);
- segmenting syllables or phonemes in words, by for instance having the child tap, count or identify the constituent syllables and/or phonemes, for example tapping three times to indicate the separate phonemes in the word CAT (Liberman et al., 1974);
- manipulating phonemes in words, such as deleting, adding, substituting or transposing phonemes within words – for example "cat" without the 'c' says "at" (Bruce, 1964).

Phonological awareness tasks vary considerably in difficulty. Children as young as 3 and 4 years of age are able to demonstrate skills of syllable-blending and segmentation and some aspects of rhyming (e.g. a knowledge of nursery rhymes). Other skills, such as deleting phonemes in words, do not emerge until much later in development and usually depend on children being exposed to printed material (initially alphabet letters and later reading books). There may be an intermediate stage during which children demonstrate an ability to segment and blend onsets (initial consonant/s) and rimes (the succeeding vowel and final consonant) within words (Treiman, 1985); in the word TRIP, for example, the onset is 'tr' and the rime 'ip'. Figure 4.1 depicts the developmental progression of phonological awareness skill and relates it both to chronological age and experience of print during the first three years of learning to read.

Large-scale longitudinal research has convincingly demonstrated that measures of phonological awareness are robust predictors of reading

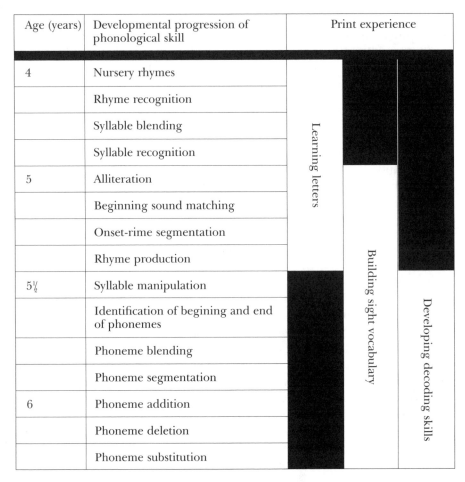

Age (years)	Developmental progression of phonological skill	Print experience
4	Nursery rhymes	
	Rhyme recognition	
	Syllable blending	
	Syllable recognition	
5	Alliteration	
	Beginning sound matching	
	Onset-rime segmentation	
	Rhyme production	
5½	Syllable manipulation	
	Identification of begining and end of phonemes	
	Phoneme blending	
	Phoneme segmentation	
6	Phoneme addition	
	Phoneme deletion	
	Phoneme substitution	

Figure 4.1 The developmental progression of phonological awareness skill (from Muter, 2003).

ability in normal populations throughout the primary school years (Muter et al., 1998; 2004; Wagner, Torgesen and Rashotte, 1994; Wagner et al., 1997). In both our studies, we found that measures of phoneme awareness (tasks requiring the segmentation or manipulation of phonemes within words) were more powerful predictors of early reading achievement than measures of rhyming. Indeed, tests of phoneme awareness given at age 5 and 6 have been demonstrated to be significant long-term predictors of reading skill. Muter and Snowling (1998) found that children's scores on a phoneme-deletion task administered at ages 5 and 6 significantly predicted reading outcome when they were aged 9–10 years of age. Findings such as this point to the considerable stability and robustness of phonological awareness measures as predictors of reading success and failure.

Letter knowledge

In the early years, phonological awareness interacts with children's emerging *letter knowledge* acquisition in order to promote literacy skill development. Ease of learning letter identities is acknowledged to be a very powerful predictor of reading achievement during the first 2 years at school (Byrne et al., 1997; Muter et al., 1998). In our study, we found that not only did phonological awareness (or segmentation) and letter knowledge make separate contributions to the first year of learning to read, but there was also a significant contribution from the product term 'letter knowledge – phonological segmentation' that reflected the interaction between these two component skills. It seems, therefore, that in order to progress in reading, children need to forge meaningful connections between their developing phonological skills and their appreciation of print – what Hatcher, Hulme and Ellis (1994) referred to as *phonological linkage*. It is not simply having adequate phonological awareness and letter knowledge that permits good progress in learning to read. Instead, both of these factors are important, and they act in an interactive fashion. In essence, phonological abilities combine with letter knowledge acquisition to enable young readers to acquire the *alphabetic principle*, i.e. the realization that particular sound sequences are systematically associated with printed letters.

According to Byrne (1998), three conditions need to be met for children to acquire the alphabetic principle. First, they need to have been taught the letters of the alphabet. Second, they require a minimal level of phonological segmentation skill that enables them to split words into sounds. Third, children need to connect or link their emerging speech sound sensitivity with their experience of print.

Verbal memory

It seems obvious that learning to read will involve memory processes in one form or another (see Chapter 8 in this volume), and parents and teachers talk a great deal about children's ability to remember new words that they have come across in their reading books or on their spelling lists. Moreover, it has been well documented that short-term verbal memory is closely related to level of reading skill, whether the materials to be remembered are digits and letters (Katz, Healy and Shankweiler, 1983), words (Brady, Shankweiler and Mann, 1983) or sentences (Mann, Liberman and Shankweiler, 1980). However, the role of verbal short-term memory in reading development is not well understood. It is not entirely clear whether verbal memory span is an important predictor of reading skill, independent of and separate from children's phonological abilities. Hansen and Bowey

(1994) found, in their correlational study of 7-year-olds, that both phonological analysis and verbal working memory contributed separately and uniquely to three reading measures. Other studies have, however, found that short-term verbal memory does not significantly predict reading skills after controlling for the children's level of phonological skill (Rohl and Pratt, 1995; Wagner, Torgesen and Rashotte, 1994).

There are other memory-related tasks beyond the use of verbal span tests that have been proposed as predictors of reading achievement. Gathercole and Baddeley (1989) suggested that measures of phonological *working memory* may have more relevance to reading processes than verbal memory span measures. They developed a measure of phonological working memory, namely a non-word repetition task, that required children to listen to and repeat nonsense words such as GLISTOW, TRUMPETINE, CONTRAMPONIST and DEFERMICATION, items taken from the *Children's Nonword Repetition Test* (*CNRep*; Gathercole and Baddeley, 1996). In a 3-year longitudinal study, Gathercole, Baddeley and Willis (1991) demonstrated that children's non-word repetition ability was closely related to their reading ability during their second year of learning to read. Some authors have, however, disputed whether non-word repetition tasks are 'pure' measures of phonological working memory. Snowling, Chiat and Hulme (1991) have suggested that non-word repetition tasks are complex measures that certainly contain a memory component but that also tap into children's phonological segmentation skills and their ability to articulate sequences of speech sounds. Metsala (1999) would agree with this view: in a cross-sectional study of children aged 3–5 years, she found that both verbal short-term memory span and phonemic awareness skill contributed to children's performance on a non-word repetition task.

Naming speed

There has recently been increased interest in *naming speed tasks* as predictors of reading achievement. The naming speed task, developed by Denckla and Rudel (1976), requires children to name series of letters, digits, coloured patches or common objects while being strictly timed with a stopwatch. A large body of evidence has accrued that has demonstrated a strong predictive relationship between naming speed and later reading skill (see Wolf and O'Brien, 2001, for a review). Having said that, it would seem that the association between naming speed and reading is not as consistent or as robust in normal populations as is the association between phonological awareness and reading skill. Wagner et al. (1997) found that individual differences in naming speed initially influenced subsequent individual differences in word-level reading, but that these influences faded with development. A naming speed deficit may, however, be a robust characteristic in impaired readers across development. One study by Wolf (1982) investigated the relationship between naming speed and reading in 64 children aged 6 to 11 years (32 average readers and 32 severely impaired readers). The naming speed tasks differentiated average from impaired readers throughout this age range; indeed, the naming speed tasks proved to be the best predictor of reading group membership.

It is not entirely clear what naming speed tasks are essentially measuring and by what mechanisms they influence learning to read. There are currently two views on this issue. First, naming speed might be just another indicator of the quality of children's phonological representations – i.e. the specificity with which they can encode the speech attributes of words (Wagner et al., 1997). It is harder, and it takes longer, to 'find' a word in long-term verbal memory during a naming speed task if it is represented in a 'fuzzy' or incomplete way. Expressed more technically, naming speed tasks appear to tap into children's ability to access their phonological representations in long-term memory; incomplete or coarsened phonological representations are more difficult to access so that the child's speed of recalling even these highly familiar names is impaired.

The alternative account views rapid-naming deficits as an impairment of a timing mechanism (Wolf and Bowers, 1999) that is independent of the phonological skills children bring to bear on the reading process. Indeed, Wolf (1997, p. 85) has suggested that naming speed is 'appropriately depicted as a complex, rapid integration of many cognitive, perceptual and linguistic processes'. If children are slow to name symbols such as letters or digits, they will be slow to automate their reading processes, which will ultimately affect their fluency of reading. This automatization process may be particularly critical in helping children to acquire and retain letter patterns in exception (or irregularly constructed) words (Manis, Seidenberg and Doi, 1999).

It seems likely that we are some way from clarifying what exactly naming-speed tasks measure and specifically how and why they relate to learning how to read. Compton et al. (2002) studied the contribution of two different versions of a naming speed task to word-level reading skills. They concluded that a variety of different explanations were incapable of fully explaining the relationship between naming speed and reading, and that 'the underlying processes that relate naming speed to word reading are very complex and in need of further study' (Compton et al., 2002, p. 365).

Speech rate

A further measure that has a predictive relationship with reading is that of *speech rate*. This refers to the speed with which a specified word or words can be spoken, for example reciting the same word over and over again and seeing how long it takes in seconds to say the word 10 times. Hulme and Roodenrys (1995) have suggested that speech rate provides evidence of the speed and efficiency with which phonological representations in long-term memory can be activated. McDougall et al. (1994) and Muter and Snowling (1998) showed that speech rate not only was a significant predictor of reading skill among primary school children, but also made a greater contribution to individual differences in reading than did verbal memory span.

To what extent phonological awareness and phonological memory skills are inextricably linked within the reading process and to what extent they function independently remains an issue in need of some clarification. It may be a question of whether one looks at the phonology–memory association from a structural or processing perspective. From a structural viewpoint, tests of phonological awareness, verbal memory, naming speed and speech rate are seen to be tapping the specificity of underlying phonological representations of words, and it is the quality or 'fine-grainedness' of these representations that in turn affects children's ability to learn to read. From a more process-orientated view, naming speed, measures of working memory and speech rate may be seen as tapping speed and efficiency of access to phonological representations in the memory store, which is separate from phonological analysis although still within the phonological domain.

Phonological deficits in children with dyslexia

Research into normal reading development has shown that phonological abilities are powerful predictors of reading success. In particular, it is argued that it is the status of the child's underlying phonological representations that critically determines the ease with which he or she learns to read (Snowling, 2000). Given that this is true of children with a wide range of reading skills, is it the case that those who are recognized as dyslexic are deficient in phonological skills (see Chapter 1 in this volume)? Research with children with dyslexia has shown that they exhibit selective deficits (relative to normal readers) in tasks that assess:

- phonological awareness, particularly the ability to segment and manipulate phonemes within words;
- short-term verbal memory span, including recalling number or word sequences, and lengthy sentences;
- non-word repetition accuracy;
- naming speed, whether with letters, numbers or objects;
- speech rate.

As discussed above, the conditions that need to be met in normally developing children to enable them to acquire the alphabetic principle are letter knowledge acquisition, phoneme awareness and the ability to link these. All of these skills are slow to develop in children with dyslexia, with the result that they have difficulty in learning to read using phonological strategies. Indeed, it is estimated that the vast majority of dyslexic children have problems mapping alphabetic symbols to speech sounds: 83 per cent in Vellutino and Scanlon's (1991) analysis of hundreds of impaired readers. One direct way of tapping the level of phonic reading skill in dyslexic children is to ask them to attempt to read nonsense words that cannot be recognized from previous experience or accessed through semantic clues. These words can only be read if the child is able to apply sound-to-letter correspondence rules in a systematic way. Indeed, there is a great deal of evidence that dyslexic children have considerable difficulty in reading non-words such as FUP, TWEPS and SOLTIP (Rack, Snowling and Olson, 1992; Van Ijzendoorn and Bus, 1994).

The role of wider language skills in learning to read

The foregoing discussion is likely to give the reader the impression that only phonologically related abilities function as predictors of reading skill in normally developing readers and dyslexic children. However, other language skills, such as *grammatical awareness* and *vocabulary knowledge*, are also known to predict reading achievement, particularly when children have moved beyond the acquisition of the alphabetic principle. Children's understanding of syntax has been shown to predict reading comprehension skills in young readers (Bowey, 1986; Tunmer, 1989). Indeed, our own research with beginning readers has demonstrated a dissociation, with early phoneme awareness (but not grammatical awareness) being a significant predictor of reading accuracy at age 6, whereas grammatical awareness (but not phoneme awareness) is a predictor of reading comprehension at the same age (Muter et al., 2004).

This apparent dissociation does not appear to be sustained into later childhood. In fact, children's awareness of grammar (including syntax) begins to impact on not just reading comprehension, but also reading accuracy from around 8 years onwards. Muter and Snowling (1998) found that children's awareness of grammatical inflections was a significant concurrent contributor to reading accuracy skill in 9-year-olds. Tunmer and Chapman (1998) have suggested that children often combine incomplete phoneme–grapheme information with their knowledge of sentence constraints in order to identify unfamiliar words. Nation and Snowling (1998a) took this a step further by suggesting that the extent to which children can use sentence context to facilitate word recognition depends on their level of verbal skill. Indeed, these authors have proposed that some children with dyslexia, with poor phonological but good verbal skills, could use their advanced spoken vocabulary, in tandem with the surrounding context provided in prose reading material, to aid word identification. This 'contextual facilitation effect' provides a powerful compensatory resource for the older, verbally bright child with dyslexia.

Children from families with a history of dyslexia

The interrelationship between phonological and language skills is particularly strongly highlighted in research on children who are genetically at risk of dyslexia. It has long been recognized that dyslexia is a phenomenon that 'runs in families'. If a person with dyslexia becomes a parent, the chance that a son will be dyslexic is 35–40 per cent, whereas that for a daughter 20 per cent. Phonological awareness skills have been demonstrated to be highly heritable, so it is not surprising that dyslexia is as a strongly inherited trait.

A number of studies have compared the reading outcomes of children from dyslexic families with those of children from families in which there is no known history of dyslexia. Children are typically recruited for these longitudinal studies at the age of 2–3 years, long before it is known whether they will have reading difficulties. A number of studies have shown that children from at-risk families who go on themselves to become dyslexic perform significantly worse than both controls and non-affected at-risk children on a wide range of phonological and language measures (Gallagher, Frith and Snowling, 2000; Scarborough, 1990, 1991; Snowling, Gallagher and Frith, 2003). What is particularly interesting is that the at-risk affected children exhibit problems at 2–4 years of age on a wide range of language skills including:

- receptive and expressive vocabulary;
- use of grammar;
- narrative skills.

Later on, at age 6 years, the deficits are most obvious on tests of phonological ability and reading. The fact that different language skills have differing predictive power according to the age at which they are assessed is an important consideration when devising screening instruments. A series of tests relevant for 3-year-olds may have a very different language content, beyond that of difficulty level, from those devised for 6–8-year-olds.

Gallagher, Frith and Snowling (2000) noted that the at-risk children who were making the best progress were those with better vocabulary and expressive language skills. This differential degree of impairment was even more evident when this same group of children was followed up at age 8 (Snowling, Gallagher and Frith, 2003). Thus, the at-risk children who had good oral language skills were able to draw on these by way of compensation for their phonological processing difficulties. In so doing, they managed to avoid more severe reading difficulties, although mild problems, particularly in spelling and speed of reading, invariably remained.

The finding that most reading problems have their origin in preschool spoken language deficits means that early identification, intervention and even prevention have now become very real possibilities. Whether a disorder such as dyslexia manifests itself as a reading difficulty very much depends on the complex interaction of the at-risk children's deficient language processes with the learning environment to which they are exposed. Thus, being genetically at risk for dyslexia may not inevitably result in persistent reading difficulties or long-term educational failure, provided early identification and intervention take place.

Screening for children at risk of reading difficulties

The goal of a screening instrument is to use the prediction methodology to identify children who are failing to learn to read so that suitable intervention programmes can be set in place. One seemingly obvious way to do this might be to ask teachers to identify which children in their class seem to be 'getting off to a slow start' or are 'making poor progress'. This would appear to be a plausible, hands-on and cost-effective means of identifying at-risk poor readers since it draws on the observations and knowledge of teachers who are already familiar with the child. Unfortunately, the prediction rates for this method are disappointingly low. In a review of teacher prediction rates conducted by Flynn (2000), these ranged from 15 to 41 per cent. We shall see shortly that screening test prediction rates can be as high as 80–90 per cent.

Flynn discusses a number of reasons for low teacher prediction rates. First, teachers may be reluctant to predict failure in young children at a time of rapid and unpredictable growth spurts; with so much individual variation in children's rate of progress, this is an understandable reservation. Second, teacher training does not typically include instruction in the theoretical and scientific underpinning of reading development. Thus, teachers may be poorly equipped to identify the skills that have relevance for how children learn to read. Instead, they may base their criteria of 'at-risk' status on general developmental observations rather than validated predictors of reading success. This is neither a good strategy for effective decision making (Flynn and Rahbar, 1993) nor of assistance in devising teaching strategies to promote reading success. Notwithstanding this,

Flynn goes on to argue a case for the greater involvement of the class teacher. It is after all the teacher who will ultimately be the deliverer of intervention support programmes and who will have a great deal of say in the child's day-to-day educational management, which will of course significantly affect outcome. Before we consider how teachers might be helped to improve their ability to identify at-risk poor readers, let us look in more depth at the use of standardized (i.e. norm-based) screening instruments.

The earlier part of this chapter highlighted the importance of prediction studies that tell us about the knowledge and skills children bring to bear on the task of learning to read. In particular, we have looked at the predictive relationship between children's phonological abilities and their later progress in learning to read. We might propose, therefore, that phonological awareness measures, generated from sufficiently large samples of children, could provide norms for the purposes of screening children, or against which individual 'slow' readers might be compared.

Whether, however, these research studies can suggest a strategy for reliably identifying those specific children who go on to have severe and persisting reading problems that necessitate special needs intervention is a rather complex issue. When considering individual children, it is not always possible to conclude confidently that a child who obtains a low score on a measure of phonological awareness will necessarily go on to have significant and persisting reading difficulties. Indeed, in terms of individual prediction, two errors are possible. First, there is the error of neglect (a false negative), i.e. failing to identify an 'at-risk' child and therefore preventing the child having access to reading intervention that might prevent reading failure. In a review of studies that attempted to predict later reading status from phonological awareness skill in kindergarten, Scarborough (1998) found that, on average, 22 per cent of children who later developed a reading disability were not initially classified as 'at risk' on the basis of their kindergarten phonological awareness scores. The converse is that of the error of identification (false-positive errors) in which children are labelled as 'at risk' but then go on to have normal or above-average reading skills. This could be seen as 'stigmatizing' because of the expectation of parents and teachers that the child's development will be slow. Scarborough (1998) found that, on average, 45 per cent of children meeting the at-risk criteria in terms of their phonological awareness scores in kindergarten did not in fact become disabled readers.

Bradley and Bryant (1985) have suggested that a phonological awareness test on its own might not be a particularly effective way of predicting persisting reading problems. In their (1985) longitudinal study of early readers, only 30 per cent of those children who initially produced good sound categorization scores went on to become exceptionally good readers. Of greater relevance to the identification issue is the finding that just 28 per cent of those who initially produced poor sound-categorization scores became exceptionally poor readers.

If a single phonological awareness measure is inadequate for predicting individual outcome in learning to read, can the sensitivity rating of a screening instrument (i.e. the proportion of correctly identified poor readers) be increased if we use more than one predictor measure? More recent studies that have used a number of independent predictors have indeed reported higher sensitivity ratings. Such studies have typically employed one or more phonological awareness measures, together with measures of short-term verbal memory, rapid naming or even both.

In a German predictor study conducted by Schneider and Naslund (1993), sensitivity was reported as 48 per cent, based on a combination of phoneme awareness and rapid-naming measures. Even more impressively, Badian (1994) used three reading-related measures to predict accurately the problems of 14 out of 15 poor readers. These measures were syllable-counting, rapid object naming and a test of orthographic processing (the latter task requiring the children to match sequences of letters or numbers from an array of similar stimuli). A high sensitivity rating such as this may, however, occur at the cost of a relatively high number of false alarms or false positives, depending on where the cut-off point for group inclusion is placed. In Badian's study, 10 out of 24 children did not develop later reading difficulties as predicted.

It is possible to improve prediction by including a large number of predictor measures that cover a wide range of potential contributors to reading skill. However, this practice of adopting a large number of predictors in order to achieve higher prediction rates also has its disadvantages. Using a large number of independent predictors will provide an almost perfect or even a perfect prediction (Elbro, Borstrom and Petersen, 1998). Beyond the practical limitations of time and cost, this is not in itself desirable, either theoretically or methodologically. From a statistical point of view, prediction is best when each measure is strongly correlated with the outcome measure of reading but uncorrelated with the other measures (Tabachnick and Fidell, 1989). What this means is that each of the predictor measures should correlate highly with the reading outcome measure, but the predictor measures should have very low correlations with each other so that we can ensure that they are indeed separate and independent, not redundant, measures. Thus, the goal of any screening test is to select the fewest independent measures necessary to provide a good prediction of reading outcome where each measure predicts a substantial and independent segment of the variability in reading outcome.

Screening instruments for identifying young at-risk poor readers

There are a number of tests that have employed phonological awareness measures as screening instruments for children in preschool or year 1 of primary school. One of the first screening tests was the *Test of Awareness of Language Segments* (*TALS*; Sawyer, 1987). This can be used as a screen for children in the 5–7 year age range but is also recommended for diagnostic use with older children who are already exhibiting delayed reading development. In this test, children are required to segment language, first from sentences to words, then from words to syllables and finally from words to sounds. Torgesen and Bryant's *Test of Phonological Awareness* (*TOPA*; Torgesen and Bryant, 1994) is a group-administered test in which children use pictorial material to demonstrate their ability to identify initial sounds (preschool version) or end sounds (elementary version) within words. Predictive validation studies have shown that preschoolers' TALS or TOPA scores significantly predict reading skill through to the third grade (Sawyer, 1987; Torgesen and Bryant, 1994).

The above instruments have adopted one single measure of phonological skill to predict, and to screen, reading success or failure. This may in itself be inadvisable bearing in mind the observation of Bradley and Bryant (1985) and the error rate findings in Scarborough's review (1998). At the other extreme, however, some authors have produced screening tests that contain a very large number of measures. Although these may well ensure long-term overall predictive validity, they fail to meet the criteria of parsimony and economy that were discussed earlier. The *Dyslexia Early Screening Test* (*DEST*; Nicolson and Fawcett, 1996) aims to screen and to assess dyslexia from the age of 5. The DEST consists of 10 subtests: bead-threading, postural stability, digit span, phonological discrimination, shape-copying, naming digits, naming letters, rhyme detection and alliteration, sound order and the rapid naming of pictures. Given the wide range of skills and abilities covered, it is possible that the DEST might be better at identifying children who have general developmental immaturities that could predispose them to educational failure, rather than more specific problems of dyslexia.

Nicolson and Fawcett (1996) claim that, with an appropriate cut-off point, the DEST given at age 5 can predict later reading failure with 90 per cent accuracy. They do not, however, discuss which subtests, or combination of subtests, account for that high success rate. As we shall see later, it is possible to achieve 90 per cent predictive accuracy in terms of determining which children eventually become good or poor readers using just two or three measures given at age 5. It seems possible that the DEST subtests that carry the greatest power in terms of predictive validity are those assessing letter knowledge and phonological skill, and to a lesser extent naming speed and short-term verbal memory. Other subtests that form part of this battery, and that assess visuomotor skills, may be useful for detecting co-occurring difficulties or more generalized developmental problems. Indeed, in a recent study that assessed the ability of the DEST to predict future literacy skills in 4-year-old boys, the only subtests that significantly predicted reading outcome were the sound order and rapid-naming tasks (Simpson and Everatt, in press); these two subtests, taken together with letter-name knowledge, were better predictors of reading ability than was the global score taken from the DEST.

Development of a screening instrument: research evidence

A number of years ago, my colleagues and I developed a multi-measure screening and early diagnostic instrument that met the objectives and criteria discussed in the earlier part of this chapter (Muter, Hulme and Snowling, 1997). First, we wanted to devise a theoretically motivated assessment that would move beyond the sensitivity limitations of a single measure screening instrument. Second, we wanted to include phonological awareness tests that were representative of the skills that young children bring to bear on their earliest reading experiences. We selected two measures of children's ability to segment words into syllables or phonemes – a test of syllable and phoneme completion, and a test of beginning and end phoneme deletion. Although we would argue that current evidence favours segmentation over rhyming as the better predictor of beginning literacy (MacMillan, 2002), rhyming skill may have a bearing on later stages of learning to read, in particular on children's ability to adopt analogical strategies (Duncan, Seymour and Hill, 1997). We therefore included tests of onset-rime awareness. In view of strong evidence of the paramount importance of letter knowledge acquisition in early reading development, it was important to add a test of letter knowledge and finally, to tap children's phonological memory processes, a test of speech rate. The *Phonological Abilities Test* (*PAT*; Muter, Hulme and Snowling, 1997) comprises four phonological awareness subtests (Rhyme Detection, Rhyme Production, Word Completion – Syllables and Phonemes, Beginning and End Phoneme Deletion), a speech rate test (timed repeating of the word BUTTERCUP), and a test of letter knowledge.

The test was standardized on 826 children aged 4–7 years, and norms were provided in 6 month age bands between 5 and 7 years (and in a 12 month age band for the 4-year-olds). When given in full, the PAT takes approximately 25–30 minutes to administer, each subtest varying in administration time from around 3 minutes (Letter Knowledge and Speech Rate) to up to about 8 minutes (Beginning and End Phoneme Deletion). The individual subtests have good internal and test–retest reliability.

A criterion-related validation study demonstrated that the PAT total score and measures derived from individual subtests had strong relationships with reading. Correlations between the PAT subtests and a concurrently administered standardized reading test (*British Abilities Scales Reading Test*; Elliott, Murray and Pearson, 1983) varied from 0.41 to 0.66; the measures that had the highest correlation with concurrent reading were the Phoneme Deletion and Letter Knowledge subtests. The predictive validity of the PAT has been demonstrated in a sample of 90 UK children studied longitudinally during their first 2 years at school (Muter et al., 2004). Here we are looking at the capacity of the PAT to predict reading skill into the future, a critical issue bearing in mind that we want to use it for the purposes of prediction and early identification. We administered the PAT to rising 5-year-olds who had had only very minimal exposure to formal reading instruction. The measures of Letter Knowledge, Phoneme Completion and Phoneme Deletion (Beginning and End Sounds) accounted for 52 per cent of the variance in the children's reading skills 1 year later. These measures together predicted, with 90 per cent accuracy, whether the children could be categorized as good or poor readers 1 year later, and these can therefore be used effectively as a short form of the test (Muter, 2003).

The PAT has also been found to be useful for screening children from multilingual backgrounds. Muter and Diethelm (2001) assessed 55 such children who were being educated in English at an international school. The Phoneme Completion, Phoneme Deletion (Beginning and End Sounds) and Letter Knowledge subtests of the PAT were good concurrent and longitudinal predictors of reading achievement for the sample as a whole and also when split into language of origin. Just under half the children in the sample had English as a mother tongue. Of the non-English mother-tongue sample, half the children were French-speaking while the remainder spoke languages as varying as Japanese, Spanish, Turkish and Russian. Again, the accuracy of the PAT Letter Knowledge and Phonological Segmentation tests in predicting later good versus poor readers (of English) was in the region of 90 per cent. The findings of this study suggest that instruments like the PAT, which have been developed with English mother-tongue children, may be useful more generally for identifying children from widely varying linguistic and cultural backgrounds who will have problems learning to read in English.

How screening data can be used

The information from screening procedures may be processed and used in a number of ways. A school may adopt the policy of selecting and focusing on an agreed percentage of the class (e.g. 10–20 per cent) who achieve the lowest scores on the screening measures. The children in this identified 'at-risk' group might then be closely monitored for a period of one or two terms. Those who went on to make improved progress might be discharged from the 'at-risk' list, whereas those who continued to have problems would be targeted for learning support. The aim would then be to set up one-to-one or small-group intervention groups that would specifically train the skills that the screening procedure had identified as being below age-appropriate levels.

Beyond their screening role, tests (such as the PAT) may also be administered to older children who are already experiencing reading problems and for whom a diagnostic phonological profile is required. The PAT, for example, may be used diagnostically with children up to 7 or 8 years of age. Information from the PAT used in this way may help to determine the following:

- The level of phonological skill in norm-referenced terms, specifically, is the child's developmental level of phonological ability in keeping with his or her chronological age and the expectation of the class?
- The pattern of phonological strength and weakness. Some children may be uniformly weak at all phonological subskills, whereas others may be strong at one sort of phonological ability but weak at others.
- Where and at what level to begin phonological training. Do all phonological skills, or just subskills within the phonological domain, need to be trained? Does the child need to commence with simple rhyming and syllable-level training, or does he or she have rudimentary rhyming and syllable awareness that may enable the teacher to commence training at the level of onset-rime or even the phoneme?
- Progress during the course of phonological training by repeating the subtests at suitable regular intervals and charting the rates of change in the test scores over time.

Phonological assessment in diagnosis and management

The following single-case study illustrates how tests (in this example the PAT) might be used diagnostically and as a prescription tool for teaching. Andrew, aged 7;11, had a *Wechsler Intelligence Scale for Children* (*WISC III*; Wechsler, 1992) verbal IQ of 101 and could thus be regarded as being of average ability. He scored at barely the 6-year level on a standardized test of single-word reading (*Wechsler Objective Reading Dimensions,WORD*; Rust, Golombok and Trickey, 1993), and he was unable to read any non-words from the *Graded Nonword Reading Test* (Snowling, Stothard and McLean 1996). On the PAT, it is possible to make reference not only to the norms (given in centiles), but also to the graphically represented PAT Profile

(Figure 4.2). Andrew's scores on the Rhyme Detection, Rhyme Production, Phoneme Completion, Phoneme Deletion and Letter Knowledge subtests were all at or under the 10th centile, i.e. well below average. He had no difficulty with Syllable Completion (50th centile) or with Speech Rate (75th centile).

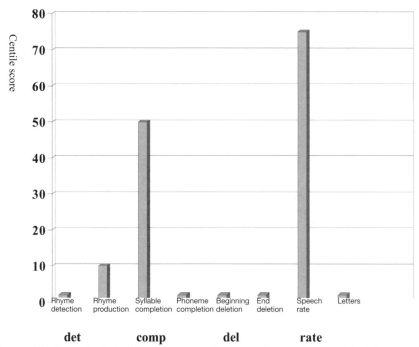

Figure 4.2 Phonological Abilities Test profile for Andrew, a 7-year-old with phonological difficulties.

Andrew clearly had rather specific problems. Although his basic phonological processing was average for his age, as evidenced by his normal-range performance on tests of Speech Rate and Syllable Completion, he nonetheless experienced great difficulty in metalinguistic tests tapping phonological awareness. He was unable to detect or produce rhyme, which suggests that his awareness of onset-rime boundaries was underdeveloped, and he could not explicitly manipulate phonemes within words, hence his inability to delete beginning or end phonemes from words. Andrew's pattern of difficulty, taken together with his marked reading under- achievement and his lack of decoding ability, is clearly indicative of a specific difficulty that has the hallmarks of dyslexia.

Andrew's profile has direct implications for a management plan. He needs to embark on a systematic literacy training programme that emphasizes phonological awareness and related skills (see Chapter 9 in this volume). Of the phonological abilities in which Andrew is deficient, rhyming is the ability that appears earliest in the developmental progression of phonological skills (see Figure 4.1 above). It is therefore recommended that this be trained first. Later on, Andrew needs to work on his phonological manipulation skills through exercises that teach him to add, delete, substitute or transpose phonemes within words. Andrew also needs to be trained in his letter knowledge, with a teaching approach that emphasizes the multisensory learning (feeling, writing and naming) of both letter names and sounds and in which there is the opportunity for much practice and reinforcement.

When Andrew has developed phoneme awareness, and when he knows all his letters, he should be exposed to 'linkage' exercises that help him to make important connections between his improving speech sound sensitivity and his experience of print. After Andrew has worked through a programme such as this, he should be ready to embark on a structured phonic-based programme that teaches him about grapheme-to-phoneme consistencies and about sequential decoding skill.

Screening and diagnosis of older children

As reading develops, the performance of phonological awareness tasks typically improves and therefore more sensitive measures are needed for older children if their underlying difficulties are to be detected. One such phonological test battery suitable for children aged 6 years to 14;11 is the *Phonological Assessment Battery* (*PhAB*; Frederickson, Frith and Reason, 1997). This test consists of nine subtests, of which three tap phonological awareness: Alliteration, Rhyme and Spoonerisms. In addition, there are two naming-speed tasks (Digit- and Object-naming), a test of Non-word Reading and three Fluency tests (Rhyme, Alliteration and Semantic). Criterion-related validation studies have confirmed that the PhAB tests show significant correlations with a standardized reading measure, the *Neale Analysis of Reading Ability* (*NARA*; Neale, 1989). Moreover, the validity of the PhAB was demonstrated by comparing children with significant reading underachievement with those in the standardization sample; the specific reading-disabled group obtained significantly lower scores on the PhAB subtests, with the notable exception of all three fluency tasks.

The *Comprehensive Test of Phonological Processing* (*CTOPP*; Wagner, Torgesen and Rashotte, 1999) was developed in the USA. This test assesses phonological awareness, phonological memory and rapid naming. There are two versions of the test, one developed for the 5–6 year age range (which can be used for early screening), and the other developed for use with older individuals, from 7 to 24 years of age. In the 5–6 year age range, there are three core phonological awareness subtests: Elision (deletion of a specified phoneme in a single-syllable word), Blending Words (joining sounds together to form single-syllable and multi-syllabic words) and Sound Matching (asking the child to choose, from an array of pictures, the word that begins with the same sound as the target word). For the older age group, only Blending Words and Elision are core phonological subtests, but there is a wide range of supplementary tests that include segmenting real and non-words, and phoneme reversal. The CTOPP also includes a Memory for Digits Task, a Non-word Repetition Test and two sets of naming tests (Colour and Object Naming for the 5–6 year age group, and Letter and Digit Naming for the older age group). The CTOPP was normed on 1656 individuals across the USA according to a stratified sampling procedure that ensured it represented the population as a whole. Validation studies have shown that the subtests of the CTOPP correlate significantly with reading tests administered 1 year later, the phonological awareness tests demonstrating somewhat higher correlations than the memory or naming tests.

Prediction and screening: outstanding issues

Although prediction-based screening instruments are now increasingly being used to identify at-risk poor readers, there are still a number of outstanding issues that need to be addressed. First, the age at which children should be screened for reading difficulties is an important concern. Phonological skills are less stable in young children, a factor that can impair their predictive relationship to later reading skill. Consequently, it may be advisable not to attempt the large-scale screening of very young children (below the age of 5), but instead to concentrate screening and early identification around the first year of formal schooling. Second, there is a need to adopt increasingly refined measures of phonological abilities that are sensitive to the core deficit in reading disorder. Part of this refinement process will stem from determining the relative importance of some phonological skills above others (e.g. rhyming versus segmentation) in predicting literacy success. Third, we need to include measures that reflect the interaction of phonological awareness skills with other reading-related abilities, in particular letter-knowledge acquisition. One way to do this might be to include a dynamic measure, such as the active learning of a specific word or word set as part of the assessment; for example seeing whether the child could use his or her available phonological skills to 'sound out', learn and retain a presented word.

An effective screening instrument aims primarily to identify children at risk of reading failure, but it may be possible for it to do more than this. Through studying the pattern of the child's relative strengths and weaknesses in reading-related skills, we may provide both a prescription for amelioration of the deficits while at the same time highlighting specific compensatory resources that the child can use. It will therefore be important to include other language-related tasks, such as verbal memory, semantic and syntactic tasks. Indeed, the PhAB has a measure of semantic fluency. An important reason for bringing in syntactic and semantic measures is because these types of linguistic knowledge may be predictive of the child's capacity to compensate for a core phonological weakness. Also, deficiencies in broader language skills may, in some children, have an impact on subsequent reading development, particularly when children read prose material in context and when they need to understand and recall what they have read (see Chapter 7 in this volume).

Finally, we may want to develop screening instruments that draw more on teacher observations and that ultimately involve the classroom teacher to a greater degree in order to ensure his or her continued commitment to monitoring and helping the at-risk child. This brings us back to where we started, looking at how teachers might use their knowledge and expertise to identify poor readers. Flynn (2000) explored this possibility by developing a teacher rating scale that was designed to mirror the skills covered in an already established kindergarten screening test (*Literacy Screening Battery*, LSB). This test comprised measures of vocabulary, syntax, alphabetic sounds, phoneme segmentation, form-copying and visual discrimination. These same skills were adapted into a series of scales on which the teachers rated the individual children's performance from 1 to 10. Flynn compared this skill-based teacher-rating instrument with simply asking teachers to predict whether a given child was likely to become a poor reader, looking at a sample of 2000 kindergarten children. Use of the rating instrument increased the accuracy of predicting later reading skill by 34 per cent. Thus, involving teachers in at-risk screening is an effective way forward, provided they are given access to validated and objective instruments on which to base their decisions.

In addition, there is no reason why teachers should not use a standardized screening test in conjunction with rating scales, to assess and to target at-risk children. For example, it may be appropriate for the school's learning support teacher to administer the standardized screening test while the class teacher completes a rating scale on a whole-class or selected sub-sample basis. This spreads the testing and rating load across school personnel, and, because two teachers are involved in evaluating each child, the reliability of the screening procedure is likely to be increased accordingly. Moreover, resources permitting, early intervention and even prevention of reading failure become realistic and achievable goals.

CHAPTER 5

Assessing speech and language skills in the school-age child

HILARY GARDNER

It is well understood that there is a reciprocal relationship between the development of oral language and learning to read (Catts, 1993; Snowling, 2000; Stackhouse and Wells, 1997). Good oral language skills enable children to deal with written language. Being able to read means in turn that children are exposed to a greater range of language styles, genres, vocabulary and structural forms. Inevitably, when there are difficulties or delays in the development of oral language, problems with the development of literacy often follow (see Chapter 7 in this volume).

Bishop and Snowling (2004) describe the growing recognition of the commonalities between dyslexia and specific language impairment (SLI), with around 50 per cent of children with dyslexia meeting the criteria for SLI. Bishop, however, also cautions that evidence from neurobiological and genetic investigations suggests that dyslexia and SLI should not simply be categorized together. The diversity of difficulty that children display must certainly lead practitioners in the field to the same conclusion. It is essential to find out at what level and in what area of functioning any linguistic weakness lies. Assessment can be diagnostic in that it may reveal a more global language disorder of which reading and writing difficulties are a part. There may alternatively be subtle, residual difficulties that remain when an earlier language delay appears to have resolved and are reflected in a child's literacy development. Having an accurate profile of any child's needs will mean that any intervention can then be targeted appropriately.

There are therefore valid reasons for allocating time to the assessment of children's speech and language, both within the school setting and through outside agencies. This chapter will start by describing essential background information that can be gathered in a case history. A range of informal and standardized assessments will then be described whose use can help to compile a communicative and linguistic profile. These will include:

- the collection of spontaneous speech and language samples in the classroom;
- the use of observational checklists;

and the use of standardized tests that:

- provide a profile of a wide range of language skills;
- target more specific areas such as grammar and word knowledge;
- assess children's competence 'above the sentence' level, for example with narrative skills;
- investigate speech-sound skills.

To aid the description of these, the cases of two children with language impairments, one of primary school age (Danny, aged 10 years) and one of secondary school age (Andrew, aged 15) will be used to provide illustrative examples of their language skills and performance on a number of assessment procedures.

The assessment process

Children can have global language difficulties or a profile of strengths and weaknesses in the development of different areas of oral language skill. Children with a specific language impairment have, by definition, a discrepancy between their language and their non-verbal intelligence, the latter falling within normal limits. The balance between a child's understanding (receptive language skill) and spoken language (expressive skills) is a fundamental area for investigation. This basic dichotomy can be broken down further into various components dealing with semantic and grammatical development at the sound, word and sentence levels. Several assessment procedures cover these various receptive and expressive language skills. Some areas of language development may be more significant than others for the development of literacy, although other skills may be compensatory (see Chapter 1 in this volume).

The assessment process is very much a collaborative exercise between teachers and other professionals. The role of the class teacher in this process should never be underestimated, contributing a range of information from assessments in all areas of the curriculum. In secondary school, tracing a child's language needs across the wider curriculum is far harder than it is in the primary classroom. With staff changes for each subject, efficient coordination of the available information is essential.

The teacher's contribution is complemented by information from a variety of professional and other sources such as:

- speech and language therapists;
- educational psychologists;
- specialist support staff;
- the school medical service;
- the child and his or her family.

The case history

Both past and present information can be gathered from the family and added to the description of the child's progress in school. Specific areas to be considered in a case history include the following:

- A history of slow language and/or speech development is very common in children with literacy difficulties, even if the problem appears to have resolved. Parents may not have considered it worth mentioning that their child was once referred to speech and language therapy, perhaps before the age of 3 years.
- A history of 'glue ear' and a subsequent implantation of grommets may well be an indicator of past fluctuating hearing loss. This can be a factor in speech/language delay (Shriberg et al., 2000a, 2000b).
- A positive family history of speech, language and literacy difficulties can be significant. There is often only anecdotal evidence of a familial problem. In earlier generations, dyslexia often went unrecognized and unsupported. Parents may recall their own poor school performance, especially in literacy, but they may never have received a diagnosis. Longitudinal research on families with a history of dyslexia shows that even those siblings who appear to be reading well have a weaker profile of language skills compared with a control group from non-affected families (Snowling, Gallagher and Frith, 2003) .
- Poor fine and gross motor skills may be part of a coordination difficulty such as dyspraxia. This developmental problem can also affect articulation for speech and co-exist with literacy difficulties.

Danny's case history

Danny, aged 10 years, was referred to speech and language therapy at 3 years of age with very little speech and having been unresponsive to a preschool setting. He proved to have very low levels of auditory comprehension, and this continued to be his main area of difficulty. He came from a family of four with two academically able older brothers, but his younger brother also had language and communication difficulties. Danny's speech developed clearly, but he used a lot of 'jargon' (made-up words) that he fitted to the appropriate intonation, rather like much younger children may do. As his language skills have increased, this pattern has faded except when he has difficulty recalling new vocabulary. He writes quite effectively by using simple repetitive sentence forms with straightforward grammar. He has also learnt some phonic spelling skills but has to work hard at retaining more complex spellings. The discrepancy between Danny's language and other skills is obvious from his score in the British School Attainment Test system, in which his work was rated at only level 1 in literacy (i.e. well below the target level) but at level 3 in maths and science, which is within the low-average range expected for his age group.

The educational psychologist carried out a simple standardized assessment of Danny's non-verbal skills, the Coloured Progressive Matrices (Raven, 1984), in which he scored above average (110), confirming that he does not have a global cognitive delay. Danny is still quite passive in the classroom and is easily overwhelmed by too much talk, needing reassurance at all times. Socially, he can be quite isolated from his peers as the classroom banter moves too fast for him.

Andrew's case history

Specific language impairments can affect children's academic performance throughout their school career. Take Andrew, 15 years old and in mainstream secondary school with support. He was first referred to speech and language therapy at 2 years of age and entered specialist language provision at age 5. He has a history of fluctuating hearing loss with upper respiratory tract infections, which resolved at about 6–7 years. Andrew had some significant speech difficulties as a young child. These have resolved except for minor elements such as THR and SPR said as "fr", but Andrew is still difficult to understand owing to his jerky, gruff speech (see Chapter 2 in this volume). His family history revealed an uncle with significant language and literacy difficulties.

Information from the educational psychologist suggests that Andrew's non-verbal intelligence is in the average to above-average range, and Andrew is now managing level 4 across the curriculum (level 5 and above is the expectancy at secondary level in the British School Attainment Tests). He is predicted a low grade (E/F) in an English language General Certificate School Examination (GCSE), which children take when they are 16 years old. Andrew's comprehension of grammar and vocabulary have always been better than his expressive skills. In conversation, he uses minimal language with one-word responses where possible and has little confidence in himself.

Assessing language skills within the classroom

Speaking and listening are now very much embedded in the British school curriculum, and the assessment of oracy skills within the classroom can make a very valuable contribution to a child's language profile. Speech and language therapists have for some time been encouraged to use class-room-based assessments as well as more formal approaches (Nelson, 1989), and collaborative working is very important. Within the English national curriculum, for example in handbooks on speaking and listening (Qualifications and Curriculum Authority, 1999, 2003), oral language skills are divided into four main areas:

- speaking for different audiences;
- listening and responding;
- discussion and group interaction;
- drama activities.

Within these areas lie pointers for some key grammatical and social developments. Let us take story-telling as an example. It is said that children aged 5–6 years of age (year 1) should be able to use 'time connectives used to organise the recount: WHEN, THEN, AFTER, NEXT, FIRST', and should be able to use 'elaboration to mark detail', e.g. 'The monkeys were swinging across the cage on the branches and ropes' (Qualifications and Curriculum Authority, 2003, p. 23). The use of complex language forms is highlighted in the following school year in the 'Group Discussion and Interaction section'. One example is the use of the language that expresses possibility, for example IF, MAY, MIGHT, COULD, PERHAPS, at the ages of 7–8 years (Qualifications and Curriculum Authority, 2003).

It is not necessary to carry out lengthy testing in order to gain an impression of a child's language skills. A very short sample of language can tell us a lot about a child's oral language and can be passed on to other professionals for further formal and informal testing. Let's look at Danny (D) at age 10, describing a three-card story sequence to an adult (A), which shows a woman first preparing to wrap a parcel, then wrapping it and finally showing the finished product:

D: The lady was going to . . . build a thing.
A: She's building it?
D: And he put the paper . . . in, over there and he just doing it and it's all done.
A: What do you call it when you wrap something up?
D: . . . paper present.

This short extract shows so many of Danny's difficulties in expressing his ideas verbally. On the plus side, he can use some differentiation for events in the past, and he can also sequence ideas with 'and'. However, the sequence of tenses is muddled, and his word choice is vague and inaccurate. There is a lack of grammatical structure to support his ideas. The intonation of his last utterance suggests that he is saying a complete phrase or sentence-like construction, yet these words do not hang together as a unit. One can see how this might affect creative writing as well as effective communication.

Word learning and retrieval difficulties have resulted in inaccurate word selection, for example the use of "building" for WRAPPING. Danny has confused a knowledge of prepositions (IN, OVER THERE) and pronouns ("he" used for LADY, despite the therapist's model of "she" in her turn). Danny uses predominantly the masculine form in his talk, although he can comprehend gender words appropriately. "Thing" is used when he is struggling to find a word. The specific word was retrieved only after a prompt when the therapist asked him, "What is it we wrap?", to which he replied "present". This response to cueing is one way of helping Danny to access what he knows. Later in this chapter, we shall see how Danny did on a similar but standardized assessment.

What this extract does not tell us is that Danny's greatest area of difficulty actually lies with language comprehension. In the classroom situation, he is quickly overwhelmed by the amount of verbal input and becomes passive and inattentive. This is unlike his conversational style, where he tries very hard to comprehend the speaker and to maintain his turn-taking appropriately, covering up poor comprehension through lively interjections. Careful observation can tell us about the effect of poor comprehension on his interaction, and it is noticeable that Danny, owing to his language difficulties, is focused on formulating his ideas and not on tuning in to the adult. He fails to attend to the adult's interjection or realize that there is a request for clarification – "She's building it?" – because of this focus. Bishop and Adams (1989) discuss the difficulty of assessment using naturalistic conversation. Narrative can be a useful alternative if carried out in an informal but controlled way (Botting, 2002).

Andrew, at 15 years of age, shows a more sophisticated development of narrative and sequence with some of the simple sequential markers that have been mentioned above. When asked to retell a story in his own words he wrote:

> <One day there were 3 boys and 2 girls to find treasure of gold in the tornado wall of clouds. 3 boys are Liam, Ash and Mike, 2 girls are Alice and Kate. If there was to go the next town to the island of Rift City. The next morning he said 'hey, Alice wake up. We are going to Rift City and meet my brother Jack'>

From the evidence of this sequence, there are a number of areas that warrant further investigation. Andrew has retold the main elements of a story well, but his underlying comprehension of the original narrative may be weak and revealed by his omissions. The tale contains less inference and abstract thought than might be expected from a child of his age. On the positive side, Andrew has begun to show the development of the story style or 'genre'. He can link some complex ideas and use some good vocabulary from the original he has heard. It would be interesting to assess whether he can explain the meaning of the words he has used. He also shows difficulty with using the appropriate grammatical forms to communicate his intended meaning accurately. Although the use of reported speech is good stylistically, a lack of coherence in the use of nouns and pronouns mean that the listener does not know who is the 'speaker' in the story. There is also a lack of coherence in tense usage. In order to help Andrew, it would therefore be useful to assess receptive and expressive word knowledge, and grammatical and inferential comprehension and use. It will then be possible to see where omissions are due to poor understanding and where they are part of an expressive (output) problem.

Informal assessment can be followed up in specific areas of the curriculum.

How a child learns new target topic vocabulary can be an indicator of language problems. A child with word-finding difficulties may acquire the concepts associated with a word such as electrical CIRCUIT, for example, but never be able to recall the key word itself. Wellington and Wellington (2002) describe how the metaphorical derivation of much science vocabulary, for example the concept of a magnetic FIELD, makes understanding and acquiring new concepts difficult. A child with syntactic formulation difficulties may not be able to describe the concept adequately but may do better when allowed visual representations. For example, Danny accurately draws and then tries to describe a simple switch diagram with words and gesture as follows: "It goes round and that's going. Not joining, off safe." He cannot name what he has drawn even though the word CIRCUIT was used by the teacher when setting up the task.

Poor comprehension and expressive syntactic skills often affect word-learning and reading. Children cannot predict what word or word type might fill a slot in a sentence despite the fact that they may have managed to decode the majority of the words as individual items. To judge whether a child has specific problems with sentence structure, it is possible to see whether he or she can make judgements about grammaticality. This can occur quite naturally within the classroom when considering sentences the children have written themselves. When Danny is asked to judge whether a sentence is 'right', he will respond according to the sense he can impose on it despite the poor grammatical form. For example, when listening to the inaccurate sentence ANNA PUT THE DOLL THE TOY IN THE DOLL HOUSE (from Nelson and Stojanovik, 2002), he stated that this sentence was correct and made sense despite the superfluous object phrase.

Observation checklists

There are a number of observational checklists that can be used by teachers to help to decide whether the language difficulty warrants further assessment by other professionals. Most of these ask questions about how children cope in everyday situations when communicating, for example how much they speak to their peers and/or adults at home and in school, and how they cope in social and educational contexts. There may be questions about the amount and appropriateness of their conversation and how reliant they are on others.

Checklists for teachers

The *AFASIC Checklists* are produced by a charity for language-impaired children. There are two checklists designed specifically for teachers who work with reception-age (4–5 years) and primary-age (6–10 years) children. The former emphasizes what the child can do in the first year at school and includes questions about milestones in grammar, sound production, comprehension and expression. The checklist for the older age group identifies problematic areas in communication and cognitive processes such as sequencing. For example, in the Response to Sound section, items include:

- Cannot imitate a simple handclap rhythm.
- Has difficulty in screening out irrelevant sound.

In the Grammar section are:

- Does not change word order to form questions.
- Omits word endings.

Other available checklists involve interviewing parents or carers: the *Pragmatics Profile of Everyday Communication Skills in Children* (Dewart and Summers, 1988), for example, looks at the child's pattern of communication and language use.

Specialist diagnostic checklists

The *Children's Communication Checklist* (CCC-2) targets the age range 4–16 years and aims to screen children for specific language impairment and pragmatic and autistic-spectrum difficulties. Children who are on the mild end of the autistic spectrum may have superficially fluent language but are often socially inappropriate in their talk and behaviour. An over-literal interpretation of language may mean that they have reasonable mechanical early literacy skills but cannot deal with the more subtle nuances of idiomatic and figurative language.

The checklist is a quite thorough, 70-item schedule that is designed primarily for use by speech and language therapists, psychologists and paediatricians, although teachers and carers may be asked to make a contribution either by judging the validity of a statement or by rating the frequency of a particular behaviour as 'less than twice a week', 'once or twice a day' or 'several times a day'. Positive and negative statements include the following:

- S/he is left out of joint activities by other children.
- Can be hard to tell if s/he is talking about something real or make believe.
- Makes good use of gesture to get his/her meaning across.

A critical differential score for language and pragmatic skills is derived from this rating, which discriminates between children on the autistic spectrum and those with a language impairment.

Danny was assessed on the CCC-2 at 10 years of age. His behaviours include some that a child with pragmatic difficulties and/or lying on the autistic spectrum might exhibit. For example, his penchant for using dialogue learned from film characters is often found in such children, as is his lack of flexibility when adapting to unexpected situations. However, his score on the CCC-2 shows that he does not have many such behaviours, nor do they occur routinely. It is likely that the underlying causal factors are different, and Danny's overall score shows that he falls into the 'specific language impaired' category. It is hardly surprising that a child with poor oral comprehension will be worried in a new environment as any prior preparatory discussion may have been poorly understood or missed all together. Danny's good memory for dialogue from cartoons and films is built on his liking for these media and compensates for his inability to generate language creatively himself. He also uses this dialogue appropriately in play. Nathan (2002) has written about children with speech difficulties and their performance on the CCC. They were found to score less well than controls in aspects of social communication, including those of conversational coherence and use of conversational context.

Standardized language assessments

Profiling language skills

Appropriately targeted language assessments should reveal a child's specific pattern of strengths and weaknesses, and provide an insight into how oral and written language difficulties might be connected. There are a number of standardized assessments that can be used to draw up a child's language profile. The assessments described below look at both receptive and expressive skills, including word-level knowledge and naming, syntactic comprehension and formulation, inferential and above-sentence level comprehension and expression through narrative. Used annually, these tests can help to track progress in discrete areas of language and give an overall language score.

Assessment of Comprehension and Expression

This assessment battery (*ACE*; Adams et al., 2001) was standardized in England and covers the age range 6–11 years. As well as containing the areas of functioning listed above, there is a subtest that targets non-literal language in which expressions such as CAVE IN, BOXED IN and GET OVER SOMETHING are presented with a range of literal and non-literal interpretations to choose from. This type of language can be especially hard for children with SLI. Each subtest yields a standard score, and the whole test gives a clear profile of these discrete language skills as well as an overall level in relation to peer performance.

Danny completed the ACE when he was 10 years old. Table 5.1 presents his scores, and Figure 5.1 illustrates his profile. It can be seen clearly that it is one of severe global language disorder with few skills that reach into the low-average range. Danny's performance shows what enormous difficulties a child with SLI can have in coping in class:

- *Sentence Comprehension* was very poor as Danny struggles with word order, tenses, prepositions and other complex constructions. His performance lay at the first centile: 99 out of 100 children would do better than him.
- *Inferential Comprehension* performance was better. This test taps conceptual knowledge. It is based on a picture of a BURGLARY and is not totally reliant on precise grammatical comprehension. It asks questions that go beyond what can be seen, for example "What clues will the police find about who broke in?" and "Why would someone steal something?" Danny scored on the 37th centile (low-average range).
- *Naming* from coloured pictures presented a huge problem for Danny. He scored at the lowest level (1st centile); there is a discussion of his errors in a later section on this skill.
- *Syntactic Formulation* tasks involve answering questions or completing sentences to describe a coloured picture. Various syntactic structures are modelled by the tester. One item shows a fat man holding an umbrella and a thin lady with flowers. When a postmodifying clause was modelled – "The girl who's holding the flowers is thin and . . ." – Danny

said, "holding, the man . . . is blue". Vital syntactic constituents are omitted and others transposed, giving him a percentile rank of 2.

- *Semantic Decisions* were also on the 1st centile. Here, Danny had to choose a simile for a given word in a selection with semantic and phonetic distractors as well as the true response. Examples of his responses are also given later, in the section on word knowledge.
- In the subtest of *Non-literal Comprehension*, expressions such as CAVE IN and GET OVER SOMETHING are presented with a choice of literal and non-literal interpretations to choose from.

Table 5.1 Danny's scores on the Assessment of Comprehension and Expression (ACE; Adams et al., 2001) at 10 years of age

ACE 6–11 subtests	Raw score	Standard score	Percentile rank
Sentence Comprehension	12	3	1
Inferential Comprehension	8	8	25
Naming	1	3	1
Syntactic Formulation	13	4	2
Semantic Decisions	2	3	1
Non-literal Comprehension	2	3	1
Narrative Propositions	12	5	25
Narrative Syntax/Discourse	5	8	37
Overall score			11

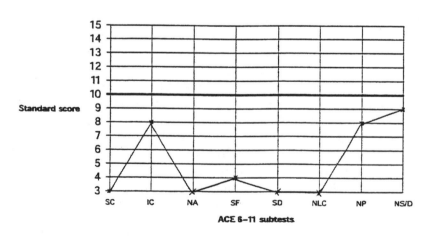

Figure 5.1 Subtest profiling chart for Danny at 10 years of age on the Assessment of Comprehension and Expression (adapted from Adams et al., 2001, with kind permission of NFER-Nelson). SC, Sentence Comprehension; IC, Inferential Comprehension; NA, Naming; SF, Syntactic Formulation; SD, Semantic Decisions; NLC, Non-Literal Comprehension; NP, Narrative Propositions; NS/D, Narrative Syntax/Discourse.

- *Narrative Propositions and Narrative Syntax/Discourse* skills are derived from retelling a story. Danny's narrative was surprisingly strong in both the number of ideas he included (where correct grammar is not important) and the range of constructions he used. This was despite his poor syntactic comprehension and performance on sentence formulation when he was asked to put a word in a sentence and scored very poorly. We have described before how Danny has the ability to memorize chunks of dialogue. Here, where the story was told to him, Danny used this ability to help retell the story. His account is given later in the section on narrative skills.

It can be seen from the above that the task demands of the different assessments affect a child's performance, and how a professional interpretation of these tests is very important. Danny's overall 'language score', a summation of all the subtests, puts him on the 11th centile for his age group, but this does not make transparent the magnitude of his difficulties in some areas.

Clinical Evaluation of Language Fundamentals

As the ACE standardization only goes as far as 11 years, Andrew's profile will be discussed in terms of the *Clinical Evaluation of Language Fundamentals (CELF-III*; Semel, Wiig and Secord, 2000). This is a test that has an English and an American standardization and has been popular for a number of years. It is a useful assessment in that it has a preschool version (age 3;0–6;11 years) and a school-age test that can be used on children from 6 to 16 years. This assessment gives a composite score for three comprehension subtests and three expressive subtests. There are additional subtests such as Narrative Comprehension, which is assessed through listening to paragraphs (appropriate for different age groups) rather than retelling a story spoken by the tester, as in the ACE. Comprehension was a comparative strength for Andrew, with a set of scores between the 19th and 42nd centiles (average to low-average) for the following:

- *Following Directions* – managing such items as "Point to the white squares while you point to the little white triangles."
- *Sorting Word Classes* – involving opposites and synonyms.
- *Understanding Semantic Relationships* – in which two (or more) pieces of information had to be integrated and the correct paraphrase selected from a choice of four similar items; for example:

  "Carla found the kitten in the front garden of the house behind the school. The kitten was:

  a) in front of the school,
  b) in front of the house,

c) behind the school,
d) behind the house."

In contrast, Andrew's expressive language skills were weaker; scores lying between the 3rd and 10th centile ranks. There are three subtests:

- *Formulating Sentences* – requires the incorporation of a given word such as AFTER, OF OR HOWEVER (pictures are provided to support creativity). For example, given 'WHENEVER . . . UNTIL', Andrew said, "Whenever this place is full until the stage falls."
- *Sentence Assembly* – requires meaningful sentences to be made from a group of written words, for example THE BOY, THE RACE, TO WIN, GOING, ISN'T. Acceptable forms were "The boy isn't going to win the race" and "Isn't the boy going to win the race?"
- *Recalling Sentences* – requires the child to repeat sentences of increasing complexity. Andrew found all these difficult, with many paraphrases that showed he had retained the meaning but not the structure. He typically omitted word endings when under pressure and made many restarts in his formulation. For example, to the item "THE BOY WHO DIDN'T TURN UP FOR PRACTICE WASN'T ALLOWED TO PLAY FOR THE TEAM UNTIL A WEEK LATER", Andrew responded, "That boy didn't get football and, cos he . . . allow, he play later . . . week".

Tests of discrete language skills

There are tests that look at one particular area of functioning, such as receptive or expressive syntax or semantics. These focus on the single-word level, sentence level and above-sentence level. Those mentioned here are widely available and can be used to reinforce and expand on findings from other profiles that have highlighted significant areas of difficulty.

Single-word level

British Picture Vocabulary Scales

In the *British Picture Vocabulary Scales Test* (*BPVS-II*; Dunn et al., 1997), the child has to pick out one of four pictures that most accurately represents a word spoken by the examiner. For example, the tester says "wrist" and the child has to select the correct picture from the following sequence: WRIST, THUMB, NECK, SHOULDER; or the tester says "eagle" and the choice of pictures presented is NEST, EAGLE, HATCHED CHICK, CAGED BIRD. The stimulus words are graded in difficulty, and the test is stopped as soon as the child gets 6 out of 8 presented words incorrect. The derived assessment scores are said to correlate closely with verbal IQ skills as measured in standardized intelligence tests, such as the *Wechsler Intelligence Scale for Children* (*WISC*; Wechsler, 1992).

There are also tests that look more closely at children's vocabulary knowledge, retrieval and organization. When children with language difficulties are asked to generate lists on a topic such as TRANSPORT or PETS, it often appears that there is little semantic or categorical grouping. Their word knowledge seems to be stored randomly, with little of the networked organization that is typical of children with normal language development. Good vocabulary knowledge is strongly associated with good literacy development in later stages (Nathan et al., 2004a).

Test of Wordfinding

The *Test of Wordfinding* (*TWF-2*; German, 2000) has an American standardization on children in the age range 4–12;11 years. It includes grammatically significant items such as tense forms as well as polysyllabic and compound words. The text has supplementary analyses that look at the child's response to phonemic and other cues to aid in differential diagnosis. There is also a version for adolescents and adults – the *Test for Adolescent/Adult Wordfinding* (German, 1989) – which can be used for ages from 18 to 80!

The tests give a useful picture of the development of an older child's semantic development in terms of speed and accuracy. Tasks tap into conceptual, higher-order categorization in the mental lexicon (word store) as well as the confrontation naming of individual items from different word groups. Subtests include picture-naming for objects and actions (which are generally less well recalled). Reaction times are measured for subtests on sentence completion, supplying a name following a description and category naming. Children with word-finding difficulties often have long latencies when struggling to retrieve items, even if they eventually do so accurately.

Test of Word Knowledge

This test (Wiig and Secord, 1992) can be used with children from 5 to 18 years of age and is therefore very useful right up to school-leaving age. It looks at aspects of expressive semantic skill but also has a section on understanding word meaning. Subtests include the assessment of single-word recognition and higher-order skills such as figurative usage and sorting by semantic categories. Children with language difficulties are often perceptually driven and will sort items by shape, colour or other visual attributes rather than by any collective function.

Looking at Danny's and Andrew's word knowledge and retrieval, we find they both struggle but in slightly different ways. Danny failed to produce a measurable performance on the TWF-2 as he found all the sections very difficult. On the CELF III, Danny found it hard to generate spontaneously a list of ANIMALS in the minute allowed. He came up with only four – "cat, bird, shark, pig" – whereas Andrew gave a more organized response, moving from wild to domestic categories – "elephant, lion, tiger, cat, dog, rabbit, mouse . . ." – naming over a dozen items. On a less familiar topic, however, Andrew could not name items quickly or move easily from one category to another. He gave only four TYPES OF WORK PEOPLE DO in a minute: "supermarket manager, shop owner, paper-news reporter, officer". Over 10 suggestions would be a reasonable score for his age.

Danny's word knowledge has been shown to be stronger in conceptual understanding than in his ability to name items, but he lacks precision. On the ACE naming test, he gave the following answers:

MICROSCOPE	"you can see what it is – it's disgusting"
AXE	"cut that thing, you go like that [gesture]"
PYRAMID	"a secret place, maybe there's a mummy"
EQUATOR	"the world".

Danny's responses on the Semantic Decisions subtest of the ACE, in which he had to choose a simile for a presented word from a choice of four (written and spoken) words, suggest that he might find it easier to relate to, retrieve or retain words by sound rather than meaning. Danny frequently chose a similarly sounding distracter item rather than the word with similar meaning, for example:

BRAVE	"kind, fearless, grave, afraid"
ERROR	"correction, mess, arrow, mistake".

In contrast, Andrew tended not to use phonological routes to access word knowledge; instead, the opposite was often true. He frequently substituted or retrieved a word of similar category. When asked, for example, to find a simile for LISTEN, he pointed to <speak> rather than <hear> in the following sequence of written words: <speak, hear, glitter, watch>.

Sentence level

Test for Reception of Grammar

The *Test for Reception of Grammar* (*TROG*; Bishop, 1983) and the more recent restandardized and extended edition *TROG-2* (Bishop, 2003) look at comprehension of a range of syntactic structures. These progress from simple declaratives through to passives and complex embedded clauses. This assessment is applicable to a wide age range of 6–16 years, with an adult sample also included.

The child is asked to point to one of four similar pictures in response to a spoken sentence. Andrew, at 15 years, fails at a complex level with items such as the 'postmodified subject'. For example, given "THE ELE-PHANT PUSHING THE BOY IS BIG" he must choose from four pictures:

1. A little boy pushing a big elephant
2. A little elephant pushing a big boy
3. A big boy pushing a little elephant
4. A big elephant pushing a little boy.

Andrew chose number three, in which the boy rather than the elephant is big.

He also had problems with more unusual constructions such as NEITHER THE GIRL NOR THE DOG IS SITTING. He passed 16 out of 20 blocks, giving him an age equivalent of 10;10 years, a standard score of 90 and a 25th centile rank.

The revised version, TROG-2, has additional items that test whether it is simply lengthier sentences rather than grammatically complex constructions that cause problems. If longer sentences are failed, memory or auditory processing may be the explanation rather than language difficulties per se. Memory is not the problem for Danny, who can cope with the long but syntactically straightforward sentence THE BOY LOOKS AT THE CHAIR AND THE KNIFE. In contrast, he fails where the syntax is more complex, such as in the passive tense where the object being acted upon comes before the subject. Hence, THE COW IS CHASED BY THE GIRL will be understood as being the active form THE COW CHASED THE GIRL, in which the word order for a direct sentence (subject, verb, object) is followed. Danny scored very poorly on the original TROG as it targeted his weakest language skill. At 9 years of age, he passed only six blocks, which gave him an age equivalent of 4;6 years, a standard score of 66 and a percentile rank less than the 1st.

More specific tests that seek to probe particular grammatical skills include the following.

Rice–Wexler Test of Early Grammatical Impairment

This assessment (Rice and Wexler, 2001) has both a screening and a full version and is standardized on an American population (age range 3–8 years). It looks at the use of the past tense, third person singular and auxiliary verbs (e.g. BE, DO) as well as word-order errors in question forms and passives. The children are expected to repeat certain sentence forms after the examiner. Although much younger children may make errors in these constructions, persistent and particular patterns of difficulty can indicate a specific language impairment (Van der Lely, Rosen and McLelland, 1998; Van der Lely and Ullman, 2001).

Grammar and Phonology Screening Test

The *Grammar and Phonology Screening Test* (*GAPS*; Van der Lely et al., in press) has a British standardization on children between the ages of 3;6 and 6;6 years, and seeks to identify those children at risk of language and literacy difficulties at an early age. It has a sentence (and non-word) elicitation format and is designed to be carried out by any professional concerned about a child's language.

Test of Word and Grammatical Awareness

The *Test of Word and Grammatical Awareness* (*TOWGA*; Shaw, 2000) looks at the specific metalinguistic knowledge of the structure of language in 4–8-year-olds. There are six subtests that look at whether the child can recognize how many words there are in a sentence, repeat the first word in a sentence or listen for the presence or absence of a target word. The Correct/Incorrect Judgement subtest involves listening for grammatical errors such as THE CUP FALLED or THE CAT SLEEPING.

Above sentence level (discourse and narrative)

Above the single-word and sentence level, there are assessments that look at children's receptive and expressive abilities from the perspective of not only grammatical complexity and correctness, but also information content. It is important to know whether a child can construct a complete, complex sentence. It is, however, equally important to examine a child's ability to understand or produce a story or dialogue at a level above the grammar and vocabulary of a single sentence. Narrative sequences require sequenced sentences that show coherence in the use of pronouns and other anaphors, produce a cohesive story and have an overall identifiable theme. In recent years, there has been a growth in the range of assessments that look at children's narrative skills, in both comprehension and expression.

The Bus Story

This is a popular measure of basic narrative skill for children in the age range 3–8 years (Renfrew, 1995). This simple story-retelling test has been used in a number of longitudinal studies of speech and language difficulties (e.g. Conti-Ramsden and Botting, 1999; Nathan et al., 2004b) as it has been found to be a reliable indicator in younger children of later language and literacy abilities (Bishop and Adams, 1990). The child listens to a story about a 'naughty bus' while looking at the picture book of the story. He or she then is asked to retell the story from the pictures. The child's version of the story is scored for information content and grammatical complexity; the latter relying on mean length of utterance (MLU), which takes the average number of substantive words in the child's three longest sentences.

Other narrative assessments look more closely at the language used, for example the number and type of grammatical elements and structures. Such assessments are very useful for class teachers as they are easily related to the needs of the British National Curriculum, especially at lower primary levels. They provide targets for therapists and for class literacy work.

The Story subtest of the ACE

This is another story-retelling test (Adams et al., 2001). The child hears a story read by the tester, accompanied by pictures, and then has to retell it. The retold story is scored for discourse content, for example descriptions of the scene, the action or the characters' feelings. It is not necessary to use grammatically complete sentences to gain marks here as grammatical complexity is scored separately. Danny scored in the low-average range for discourse content through his lively re-enactment of the narrative, with plenty of characterful dialogue but little overall supporting structure. His narrative displayed difficulties similar to those of the sequence illustrated earlier in the chapter, but his good memory helped him to use more sophisticated language than he usually did. For example, he used the conditional "If you do find the treasure, I'll leave", which was not routinely apparent in his talk. Despite this, his grammatical score fell below the average for his peers (see Table 5.1 above). There is little complex structure but plenty of grammatical and word-level errors in the following extract from his response:

> "He found a food, 'This is – might be treasure' but no gets something. So he went to get the dress and he took it out and take it and he's got an idea to 'trat [sic] that terrapit [i.e. parrot] and off he went the tree."

Expression, Reception and Recall of Narrative Instrument

This 10 minute *Expression, Reception and Recall of Narrative Instrument (ERRNI)* has two story sequences based on common themes (FISHING and THE SEASIDE). Retesting is therefore possible without a practice effect. The test is suitable from 6 years to adulthood. There are comprehension questions as well as the story-retelling, which is scored for information and grammatical complexity.

Assessing the bilingual child

A growing proportion of the school population of English-speaking countries come from homes where English is not the predominant language. In Britain, the number of children from a minority ethnic background is expected to reach 1 in 5 by 2010 (DfES, 2003, cited in Mahon, Crutchley and Quinn, 2003). It is acknowledged that the development of two languages can in many respects enhance learning. However, a significant percentage of the bilingual population display problems with linguistic development across all the languages to which they are exposed. There has been a move to develop assessment instruments for these children, and Mahon, Crutchley and Quinn (2003) provide a useful overview of current issues. They point out the enormous difficulties involved in using tests that are culturally inappropriate because these can lead to an inaccurate interpretation of any results obtained. Specific instruments are being developed for some languages that are highly represented in Britain, for example Punjabi, Mirpuri and Urdu (Pert and Letts, 2003). There may, however, be a very high number of languages extant in any given population with whom teachers and other professionals are working. Assessment must therefore include information on a child's performance from a number of sources, including the home. Observation of a child's progress in light of the progress made by his or her peers from the same cultural background is essential.

Assessing speech output

Knowledge of a child's speech sound difficulties is essential when there is a history of delayed and disordered speech development as many but not all such children are at risk of literacy difficulty (Leitao and Fletcher, 2004; Nattan et al., 2004). Speech and language therapists often use the term 'phonological difficulty' to describe children's systematic use of speech sounds, including their errors. Speech and language therapists assess and analyse children's speech errors using single words and connected speech. Therapists must work out what regularities children have in their sound substitutions and omissions. For example, a child may omit most final sounds in words and/or substitute /t/ for /s/ and /p/ for /f/. In these examples, the friction involved is 'stopped', and this process will probably be noticeable in all sounds that require friction.

In most cases, these patterns are very consistent, and speech and language therapists provide programmes of work that target these 'processes' to help the child to reach the adult form, for example by teaching a sound or group of sounds with friction. Clusters of phonemes (e.g. ST, SPR and STS) can cause difficulties even when single phonemes have been appropriate for some time. Although most children's speech difficulties resolve before they are 6 years old, a significant proportion have persisting speech sound difficulties well into their primary years and beyond, and these children are most at risk of reading and spelling difficulties (see Chapter 2 in this volume). For the teacher, having access to a detailed assessment of children's speech patterns can lead to a greater understanding of the possible source of their written difficulties and how to remediate them. Poor speech can in itself lead to poor spelling as the child cannot access or rehearse the appropriate phoneme to link to the grapheme (Clark-Klein and Hodson, 1995; McCormick, 1995; Snowling and Stackhouse, 1983). A child may recognize /k/ when it is said to him, but when he says "tar" for CAR, that may well be what he writes.

Informal assessment of a child's speech skills

Residual speech difficulties can be very subtle, and a child may just be deemed to have 'lazy' speech with generally unclear diction, especially in longer utterances. Closer investigation may reveal particular difficulties with word endings ('swallowed up' as the child moves on to the next word), poor sequencing in polysyllables and difficulty recalling new words accurately. Poor fluency with stammering-like behaviours can also arise from difficulty in formulating spoken language.

These are the types of difficulty that are evident in Andrew's speech. Even at 15 years of age, he often repeats syllables or restarts phrases when trying to put a sentence together. Longer words are poorly articulated, especially in connected speech. For Danny, clarity of speech was not an issue. However, despite good non-word and new word repetition, he had a rapidly disintegrating memory trace for any such new word he had just said perfectly. For example, in the ACE narrative, the word PARROT ended up not only as "terrapit" but also as "poppet" and "poper", although he knew exactly what he was talking about. Constable (2001) describes how children with word-finding difficulties make such phonological 'groping' errors in their attempts at word retrieval, in some cases because of a difficulty in storing and/or accessing accurate motor speech programmes.

Informal assessments in class can look at speech sounds in simple and complex words without recourse to the phonetically balanced lists that speech and language therapists need to use. Nunes (2003) has produced a list of common polysyllabic words such as HOSPITAL, DIGITAL and SPAGHETTI. He describes significant patterns of error that differ between content and function words in children much older than those traditionally expected to have difficulty with speech sounds. Children such as Andrew can omit 'weak' syllables (such as in TOMATO said as "mato") or translocate sounds (e.g. "besteti" for SPAGHETTI). Trying new classroom topic vocabulary and novel names in stories can be an entertaining activity for any child and a good test of word repetition and ability to recall. Surnames can be a good 'non-word' repetition task as any included in a formal test. It certainly took Danny a term to recall his teacher's name accurately even though instant repetition was not a problem! Hesketh and Conti-Ramsden (2003) confirm that, in a population of children who are developing language slowly, non-word repetition can be a significant risk marker for specific language impairment.

Formal speech assessment

A speech and language therapy report may outline a child's simplification processes based on a phonetically balanced word list such as the following.

The South Tyneside Assessment of Phonology and the Phonological Assessment of Child Speech

The *South Tyneside Assessment of Phonology* (*STAP*; Armstrong and Ainley, 1988) and the *Phonological Assessment of Child Speech* (*PACS*; Grunwell, 1985) require children to name items in single and composite pictures. The therapist may then supplement this sample with words in connected speech because intelligibility may be reduced in such contexts, for example with sounds omitted between words. There are now an increasing number of formal assessments that give numerical scores and percentage ratings for intelligibility, which can prove useful as outcome measures.

Metaphon

Metaphon (Howell and Dean, 1991) is both a phonological assessment and a remediation programme that gives the percentage occurrence of certain types of commonly occurring error types in a sample of single words.

Diagnostic Evaluation of Articulation and Phonology

The *Diagnostic Evaluation of Articulation and Phonology* (*DEAP*; Dodd et al., 2002) is one of the only norm-referenced phonological assessments (age range 3;6–6;11 years). It also has norm reference for a Punjabi population. It starts with a diagnostic screen and has four specific assessments. These cover the accuracy and rate of articulatory 'oro-motor' movements; phonology in terms of the percentages of total phonemes, consonants and vowels that are correct; single-word versus connected speech; and inconsistency of use. The percentage correct ratings and qualitative data on articulatory skills and phonological patterns can be applied at any age.

The Articulatory Rate Subtest on the Phonological Abilities Test

A slow articulation rate may be a predictor of literacy development, and the Articulatory Rate subtest on the *Phonological Abilities Test* (*PAT*; Muter,

Hulme and Snowling, 1997) is a standardized assessment of this skill (see Chapter 4 in this volume). In this, the children (age range 5–8 years) are required to say the word BUTTERCUP as quickly as possible 10 times, and norms are given for comparison.

Articulatory rate may not, however, be the only important factor, particularly in young children. Williams and Stackhouse (2000) found that accuracy and consistency of repetition were generally more sensitive measures of younger (3–5 years old) children's articulatory proficiency than was the traditionally used rate of production. These measures have been incorporated into a revised edition of the *Nuffield Dyspraxia Programme III* (Williams et al., 2004), an assessment and intervention resource used by speech and language therapists.

Conclusions

Our understanding of the core spoken language skills that underlie the normal development of literacy is growing apace through further research and evidence-based practice. Some common assumptions have been put to the test. Although broad categories of disability exist, an individual profile of strengths and weaknesses is essential in order to maximize a child's potential across the curriculum. Informal, classroom-based and formal assessment can all contribute to this picture. Assessment measures that can be repeated and replicated help to track development and progress. To facilitate language development, individual education plans should incorporate oral as well as written targets, especially ones that can be integrated into the working day (see Nathan and Simpson, 2001; Popple and Wellington, 2001). There should be a balance between boosting a child's strengths to compensate for other areas of development, and setting realistic targets to strengthen weaker areas of functioning. In this way, although their underlying processing difficulties may never come up to the level of their peers, children can develop successful strategies for dealing with oral and written language in tandem.

Take the two children presented in this chapter. As Andrew nears school-leaving age, he has become quite a good phonic speller, with most regular patterns consolidated and some more complex words learnt visually. His oral language difficulties are still noticeable, but he is embarking on a life skills course at school and hopes to work within the family business on leaving school. Danny is soon to face the challenge of mainstream secondary school and is fortunate to be going on to a school with specialist language support where his progress will be tracked by both school and speech and language therapists in close collaboration.

Appendix 1: Assessment tests

Observation checklists

AFASIC Checklists, 2nd ed (1995) Wisbech: Learning Development Aids.
Bishop D (2003) Checklist of Communicative Competence. London: Psychological
Corporation.

Comprehensive language profiles

Adams C, Cooke R, Crutchley A, Hesketh A, Reeves D (2001) Assessment of
Comprehension and Expression: ACE. Windsor: NFER-Nelson.
Semel E, Wiig EH, Secord WA (2000) Clinical Evaluation of Language
Fundamentals: CELF-III. London: Psychological Corporation.

Narrative assessments

Bishop DVM (2003) Expression, Reception and Recall of Narrative Instrument:
ERRNI. London: Psychological Corporation.
Dewart H, Summers S (1988) Pragmatics Profile of Early Communication Skills in
Children. www.edit.wmin.ac.uk/psychology/pp/children/htm
Renfrew C (1995) Renfrew Bus Story: UK, 3rd edn. Bicester: Winslow Press.

Word-level knowledge

Dunn LM, Dunn LM, Whetton C, Burley J (1997) British Picture Vocabulary Scales
(II). Windsor: NFER-Nelson.
German DJ (1989) Test of Adolescent/Adult Word Finding: TAWF. London:
Psychological Corporation.
German DJ (2000) Test of Word Finding, 2nd edn: TWF. London: Psychological
Corporation.
Wiig EH, Secord WA (1992) Test of Word Knowledge: TOWK. London:
Psychological Corporation.

Grammatical level

Bishop DVM (2003) Test for Reception of Grammar: TROG2. London:
Psychological Corporation.
Rice ML, Wexler K (2001) Rice–Wexler Test of Early Grammatical Impairment.
London: Psychological Corporation.
Shaw R (2000) Test of Word and Grammatical Awareness: TOWGA. Windsor:
NFER-Nelson.
Van der Lely H, Herzog C, Froud K, Gardner H (in press) Grammar and Phonology
Screen: GAPS. London: University College London.

Speech-sound skills

Armstrong S, Ainley M (1988) South Tyneside Assessment of Phonology: STAP. Northumberland: STASS Publications.

Dodd B, Hua Z, Holm A, Ozanne A (2002) Diagnostic Evaluation of Articulation and Phonology: DEAP. London: Psychological Corporation.

Grunwell P (1985) Phonological Assessment of Child Speech: PACS. Windsor: NFER-Nelson.

Howell J, Dean E (1991) Metaphon Programme: Treating Phonological Disorders in Children: Metaphon, Theory to Practice. San Diego: Singular Publishing.

Muter V, Hulme C, Snowling M (1997) Phonological Abilities Test: PAT. London: Psychological Corporation.

Williams P, Stephens H (2004) Nuffield Centre Dyspraxia Programme III. Windsor: Miracle Factory.

CHAPTER 6

Assessing reading and spelling skills

NATA K. GOULANDRIS

Learning to read and spell is relatively effortless for most children in a classroom. However, the underlying linguistic and cognitive skills that are needed before learning can take place are numerous and complex. It is, therefore, not surprising that a number of children are unable to learn these skills in the normal way. A child whose progress in reading and spelling is slow by comparison to the others in the class, or even when compared with the child's ability in other areas of the curriculum, needs to be assessed.

Assessment is not simply a process of identification but is a vital prerequisite of effective teaching, enabling precise strengths and weaknesses to be pinpointed and thus provide appropriate learning experiences and instruction for that individual. By taking the time to assess a number of different components of reading and spelling skills, and considering these results alongside an assessment of phonological and spoken language skills (see Chapters 4 and 5 in this volume), the learning process can be facilitated as effectively as possible. Assessment has the following purposes:

- To determine whether an individual has reading and/or spelling difficulties and whether this child's literacy skills are significantly behind those of other children of the same age. Standardized tests help us to decide whether a child is only somewhat poorer or significantly below his or her peers (as a rule of thumb, a significant delay being more than 18 months behind the age-expected level if the child is less than 8 years old or 24 months or more from 8 years onwards).
- To undertake a detailed analysis of the individual's current literacy skills in order to construct a profile of the child's strengths and weaknesses.
- To establish a baseline for continuous monitoring.
- To determine the most effective type of remediation so that teaching

and learning can be coordinated, with teaching firmly based on an individual's cognitive and literacy profile.

In order, however, to assess literacy skills competently, we need to consider two questions. First, how do children who are *not* having difficulties, learn to read and spell? It is important to adopt a developmental model of reading and spelling so that we have, as a 'standard', the literacy skills of a typically developing reader. The more explicit and detailed the model, the easier it will be for us to pinpoint a child's difficulties in relation to children who are progressing along normal lines. Second, we need to ask whether the learner has the cognitive skills that are required to read and spell effectively. In short, what cognitive skills need to be developed in order to improve literacy in both the short and the long term?

The development of reading and spelling

The two different models of literacy discussed in this chapter provide alternative perspectives on the development of reading and spelling, giving insights into the way in which children's strategies shift with the passage of time and improving skills.

Frith (1985) has proposed three 'phases' of literacy development: logographic, alphabetic and orthographic. During the *logographic phase*, the child's word recognition is based on partial cues, often simple first-letter cues, and reading is consequently inaccurate because so little letter information is taken into account. Picture and contextual cues provide additional information, and for many beginners this may be the primary source of information about words. Spelling ability is rudimentary at this stage, consisting primarily of words learned by heart and recalled as a collection of arbitrary shapes.

The logographic phase is gradually superseded by the appearance of alphabetic strategies for spelling. The child who does not yet know the correct spelling relies on knowledge of a word's pronunciation to construct a spelling (Read, 1986; Treiman, 1993), and the *alphabetic stage* is marked by the realization that a particular speech sound can be represented by a specific letter: for example, the initial sound in the words SNAKE, SIT, SAND and SOME will be spelled with the letter <s>. Once this alphabetic principle has been grasped, the learner can begin to extrapolate information about the basic sound–letter mappings that form the basis of an alphabetic language – for example, the sound of 'b' is represented by the letter <b>, the sound of 'm' by the letter <m> and the sound of 'ks' by the letter <x>. The use of sound–letter correspondences is gradually extended to reading and propels beginners into a more independent reading style by enabling them to decode unfamiliar words.

Alphabetic readers are, however, restricted by their dependence on letter-by-letter decoding and are not yet aware that letter–sound rules may also be influenced by the position of the letter within a word. Their errors may include CITY ➤ "kitty", CENTRE ➤ "kenter", GEM ➤ "guem" (pronounced with a hard 'g' at the beginning rather than a 'j' sound) and similarly gym ➤ "guim". It is not until the commencement of the *orthographic phase* that the reader becomes conscious of other equally important linguistic features that are represented by the English spelling system. At this point, the reader recognizes that words can be subdivided into larger units such as common letter strings, for example <-ing>, <-tion>, <-ture>, prefixes such as <auto->, <hydro->, <pseudo-> and suffixes such as <-graph> and <-phobia>. Orthographic spelling is the final step of development and is characterized by a precise knowledge of word spellings.

Alternative interactive theories of learning to read (Ehri, 1985; Hulme, Snowling and Quinlan, 1991; Seidenberg and McClelland, 1989) throw some doubt on the rigid sequence of stage models, suggesting instead that the learning of whole-word spellings, sound–letter rules and spelling patterns may take place concurrently, with each type of information facilitating and promoting the development of the others. According to such models, learners continuously generalize information about spelling–sound mappings as they encounter new words. Since English is notorious for the unreliability of its spelling system, a beginner's initial attempts to understand such patterns are bound to be somewhat inaccurate, and many previous conclusions about letter–sound mappings will require adaptation.

To take a hypothetical example, Harry, aged 7 years, has read several early readers and has learned to recognize a number of words that are frequently repeated within these texts. Without realizing it, he has managed to detect some common patterns among the words he has already learned. For example, he perceives that MUM, MOUSE and MILK all begin with the same sound and has linked this information successfully with the letter sound "m". He is therefore able to predict quite reliably that other unfamiliar words that start with 'm' will begin with the same sound – "m". He has arrived at a similar conclusion for the letter 'c' based on his encounters with the words CAT, CATERPILLAR, CAN, COP and CUP but is bemused when he realizes that, in words such as CITY, ICE or BICYCLE, the letter 'c' represents an altogether different sound – "s". However, repeated exposure to the alternative sounds that the letter 'c' represents enables Harry to reformulate his understanding about the behaviour of the letter 'c' and the sounds that it can map. He will have to reconsider these conclusions later when he realizes that, in some cases, such as in the word EFFICIENT, the letters represent a different speech sound altogether – "sh".

Interactive models suggest that the beginner reader may not just learn isolated letter–sound patterns but may learn letter–sound mappings in the context of other letters. When Harry has come across more words containing the letter sequences <ci>, <ce>, <cy>, his experience of written language will enable him to incorporate additional information about the importance of letter position in phonological mapping, the possible influence of neighbouring letters and how often these alternatives occur. This implicit, but nonetheless extensive, knowledge of more complex letter–sound mappings will enable him to differentiate words that contain <ce> and those that contain <ca>. In this kind of model, there is therefore no distinction between the learning of whole words and the learning of spelling–sound rules. On the contrary, the understanding of letter–sound mappings is a consequence of the child's familiarity with words. In turn, a grasp of common sound–letter mappings enables the reader to recognize unfamiliar words more easily.

Both kinds of model have one fundamental similarity: they emphasize the importance of letter–sound mappings in the acquisition of literacy and stress that these serve as the framework upon which the more difficult and complex orthographic rules are based. According to the Frith model, a reader and speller needs to have alphabetic knowledge before the more complex orthographic knowledge can be learned. Frith's model of literacy development also highlights the fact that reading and spelling develop at different rates, each skill contributing to the evolution of the other; children first learn about sound–letter mappings through trying to figure out how to spell new words. Spelling therefore plays a particularly important role by helping children to uncover the fundamental relationship between the individual speech sounds in words and the letters used to represent them.

Requisites for reading and spelling

Stage models of literacy development make explicit that the learning of reading and spelling requires different sets of cognitive abilities at different points of the acquisition process. If the requisite cognitive resources are not available, literacy skills will not be able to proceed along normal lines. Early *logographic* reading can be achieved using the visual recognition skills normally needed for ordinary object-recognition tasks. Consequently, few children fail to achieve rudimentary word recognition, although they may mistake words that resemble each other. Linguistic and cognitive skills also play an important role in this early learning period as they permit an inexperienced reader to determine the approximate meaning conveyed by a particular text.

In contrast, attaining alphabetic skills requires an array of specialized phonological skills. Initially, *phonological awareness* (the ability to reflect on the structure of utterances rather than their meaning) enables a child to detect similar speech sounds in words and thus to map sound segments on to written language. However, learning to read in turn engenders more advanced types of phonological awareness as children become aware of and learn to manipulate different types of phonological unit, namely syllables, onsets, rimes and phonemes. An awareness of phonemes, the smallest units of speech sounds, which can change the meaning of a word (e.g. /p/and /b/ sounds in the words PIN and BIN), is a precursor of learning to read and develops as a result of repeated attempts to map speech units to written words when trying to spell.

Children whose phonological skills are weak will not realize that some words begin with the same phoneme and will consequently be unable to understand the 'alphabetic principle' that underlies written language. These readers will therefore have great difficulty learning about sound–letter mappings because they fail to appreciate the phonological characteristics of words. Both models concur that children who do not appreciate letter–sound mappings will have severe difficulties with some aspects of reading and spelling. This conclusion is supported by substantial research evidence demonstrating that individuals who have difficulty perceiving, comparing and identifying speech sounds in words, commonly referred to as phonological processing difficulties, are likely to have reading difficulties and extensive spelling problems (see Chapter 1 in this volume).

Reading and spelling deficits in children with developmental dyslexia

There are two basic profiles of developmental dyslexia with many gradations of severity: individuals with both reading and spelling problems and those whose difficulty lies primarily with spelling. The first and easier to identify are the learners with obvious reading and spelling difficulties. During the early school years, reading tends to be slow and inaccurate, and unfamiliar words cannot be decoded but must be guessed. Phonological processing difficulties usually lie at the root of these problems. Children with phonological problems have little sensitivity to the sound properties of language, do not learn letter–sound mappings as easily as phonologically competent children and therefore do not acquire decoding skills normally (see Chapter 2 in this volume). Writing in the early years of schooling is frequently indecipherable, as the illustration in Figure 6.1 demonstrates.

However, with exposure to print and specialist tuition, these children can often learn to read quite proficiently, especially if they have good visual memory to help them recognize words they have encountered frequently. The underlying problems with phonological processing may remain,

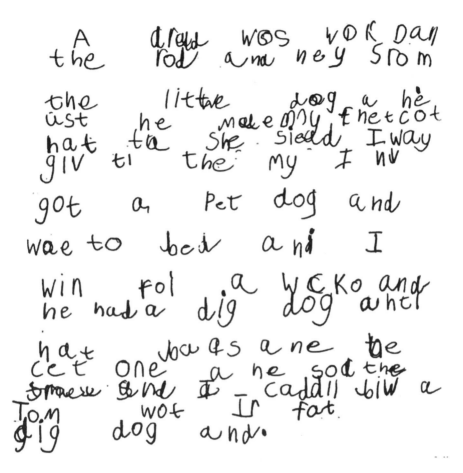

Figure 6.1 Example of handwriting from a child with specific learning difficulties.

although more difficult tasks are required to uncover them. Reading new words, decoding longer, orthographically complex words and spelling remain problematic for the majority (Snowling, Goulandris and Defty, 1996).

Children with the second profile typical of dyslexia, sometimes referred to as dysgraphic, appear to be competent readers but have inordinate difficulty with spelling. The underlying cognitive difficulties of this group are still not resolved. Many researchers have reported that children with dysgraphia continue to have underlying phonological deficits into adulthood, although these difficulties are only evident in more demanding phonological tasks such as spoonerisms or the repetition of polysyllabic, difficult-to-pronounce words and non-words (Bruck, 1992; Perin, 1983). Problems with decoding persist, although these are often masked by good compensatory strategies.

There is also a second type of poor speller whose difficulties do not appear to be accompanied by phonological deficits. These have been referred to as 'good readers/poor spellers' (Frith, 1980) or type B spellers (Frith, 1985). These individuals seem to have achieved reasonably good alphabetic skills when reading but are unable to recall the letter-by-letter sequences of words that do not conform to regular spelling patterns. When assessing these individuals, it is important to determine whether the person's difficulties encompass both reading and spelling, or whether they are restricted to spelling.

Assessing reading skills

Reading consists of three quite different components or subskills: word recognition, decoding and comprehension. Individuals with reading problems may have difficulties in only one or in several of these components. This chapter will discuss reading comprehension only when it contributes to word recognition and decoding since a detailed discussion of comprehension difficulties can be found in Chapter 7 in this volume.

A comprehensive assessment of reading can be undertaken using the following tests:

- a standardized single-word reading test;
- a standardized text-reading test;
- a test of non-word reading;
- a test of alphabet knowledge.

This battery of reading tests takes approximately half an hour to administer and can be undertaken in a single session or in several shorter ones, provided all the tests are administered with a month of each other

Assessing word recognition

The ability to recognize words quickly and accurately, also referred to as lexical processing, is a hallmark of skilled reading. It has been suggested that familiar words or lexical items are stored in a 'lexicon', or mental word store. New words can be added to the lexicon if a skilled reader supplies the word or if the learner identifies it using contextual cues. Alternatively, the reader can use phonological reading strategies to sound out the word and identify it – a strategy that enables the child to become a more independent learner.

Although some influential educators have argued that reading is primarily a 'psycholinguistic' process in which words are recognized through context (Goodman, 1967; Smith, 1971), there is convincing evidence that competent readers identify words at such a fast rate that they do not require the assistance of context to aid recognition. In contrast, many poor readers have difficulty establishing a reliable word-recognition system. These children need to use context to supply more information about the word they are trying to recognize.

The best way to assess word recognition is by using a single-word reading test that precludes the use of psycholinguistic, pictorial and contextual cues. Children will normally attempt to use all possible cues when trying to read, particularly if reading does not come easily to them (Nation and Snowling, 1998a). Hence, a number of children appear to read proficiently but are unable to recognize the same words if they are presented out of context. Although it is customary to encourage beginners to read by guessing the content of books in the early years, such a strategy is self-defeating when it remains the primary strategy beyond the early stages.

A standardized single-word reading test will provide information about children's performance in relation to their peers. (See Appendix 1 for a list of some currently available standardized single-word reading tests.) Obtaining a reading age is certainly an important component of the identification procedure but does not reveal the exact nature of a child's problems. The child's reading approach should be observed and all the incorrect responses recorded so that these can be examined and classified according to error type at a later stage.

When administering a single-word reading test, consideration should be given to the following questions:

- How does the child approach the task of reading single words?
- Are the words read easily and relatively quickly, or is each word identified slowly and laboriously?

The response to this question will indicate whether the word-recognition system is functioning adequately or whether the reader is having excessive difficulties identifying words out of context. Word attack skill should also be considered. For example:

- How does the reader attempt to identify unfamiliar words?
- Are the child's attempts to sound out unfamiliar words generally successful?
- If the reader is unsuccessful at sounding out words, at what stage in the process is the child having difficulty?: (i) in identifying the correct letter, (ii) in identifying the corresponding speech sound, (iii) in grouping the letters correctly, i.e. reading the word THEN as "th-e-n", or (iv) in blending the sounds?

Error analysis can provide further valuable information about the learner's reading strategies. Errors may be classified according to the following categories: visually similar, regularizations, unsuccessful sound attempts and refusals. Table 6.1 gives examples of each type of error.

Table 6.1 Examples of different types of reading error in single-word reading

Visually similar Few shared letters	Visually similar Many shared letters	Regularizations	Unsuccessful sound attempts	Partial phonologi- cal access
SAID ➤ she	CHAIN ➤ chin	PINT ➤ pinnt	CURIOSITY ➤	CONSCIENCE ➤ con
JUMP ➤ Jack	BEARD ➤ bread	COLONEL ➤	si ris ty	➤ consequence
COAT ➤ cut	USELESS ➤ unless	kol o nell	ABODES ➤	COMPEL ➤ com ➤
SHIP ➤ shout	THROUGH ➤	CHAOS ➤	ad bodeas	complete
	though	tcha oss		GENERALLY ➤ gen
		DOUGH ➤		➤ generate
		dow g h		TRANSPARENT ➤
				trans ➤ transport

Visually similar errors

Visually similar word errors indicate that the child is identifying the target as a word that resembles it but is unable to perceive the difference between the two spellings. Beginning readers often make visual errors in which the target and the response share a few letters, often only the initial letter, for example STOPPED read as "sat", AND read as "as" and HORSE read as "his". More advanced readers make visual errors in which the response resembles the target more closely, such as CHOIR read as "chair" or as "chore". The number of letters shared by the target and the response is a good measure of the amount of letter information used by the reader for word recognition (Stuart and Coltheart, 1988). Table 6.2 provides examples of these.

Table 6.2 Examples of visual reading errors according to number of letter cues taken into account

First-letter cue only	More than one letter cue	Minus one letter cue only
SIEGE ➤ spring	GLOVE ➤ gave	MATCH ➤ march
GLOBE ➤ jug	POLICE ➤ place	FLOOD ➤ food
SWORD ➤ shower	HATCH ➤ hut	PLAN ➤ plane
THIMBLE ➤ tapping	SIGN ➤ song	FELL ➤ felt
LEVER ➤ life	RUBBER ➤ robin	CEASED ➤ cased

Sound-based errors

There are two quite different types of sound-based error, the one type resulting from unsuccessful decoding, the other from the inappropriate use of decoding strategies on irregular words, such as ISLAND or COLONEL, whose pronunciation cannot be correctly arrived at using letter–sound correspondence rules.

Unsuccessful sound attempts occur when the reader tries to use letter–sound mappings, letter strings or other units to sound out words that could not be recognized automatically. Failure may occur because:

- parsing is inaccurate, for example THE read as "t-h-e" or LAUGH read as "l-a-u-g-h", with each letter sounded out as a separate speech sound;
- there is an incomplete or inaccurate knowledge of letter–sound rules;
- there are poor blending skills.

(A more detailed discussion of the subskills involved when using phonological processing is available in the section on non-word reading.)

Words are sometimes identified using a *partial decoding strategy* in which a segment (usually the beginning) of a word is sounded out and provides sufficient information for the retrieval of a word that shares a phonemic segment with the target but is in fact a different word (e.g. COLLECT ➤ "col; collar", SPORT ➤ "sp; Spain"). This type of error indicates that the reader has developed some decoding skills but is prone to guessing without taking meaning and the letter content of the rest of the word into account.

Regularization errors occur when irregular words are sounded out and pronounced as if they were regular words, for example FLOOD read as if it rhymed with "food" and HALF read as "hallf" with the /l/ sound pronounced.

A third type of error is to give *no response*. Beginners who have limited sight vocabulary and insufficient phonic skills to decode unfamiliar words frequently refuse to respond.

Other errors

Some errors do not fit into any of the previous categories because it is difficult to determine conclusively why a child has made a particular error. A certain amount of detective work may be needed and is warranted. The teacher may want to look for similar errors on other occasions in order to identify a common strategy. For example, if most words containing a 'final e' are read as if the vowels were short (e.g. HOPE read as "hop" or TUBE read as "tub"), the reader may need to be taught that a 'final e' lengthens the preceding vowel. On the other hand, the errors may be caused simply by a tendency to process words superficially and make visual errors. It is helpful to clear up this ambiguity.

Box 6.1 contains some guidelines for assessing word recognition.

Box 6.1 Checklist to determine a reading profile

READING PROFILE

Name: ....   Date: ....

School: ....   Chronological Age: ....

Class: ....

I. Word Recognition

1. Is word recognition   good .....   average .....   poor .....

2. Is there a predominance of refusals suggesting that the child has limited sight vocabulary and immature word attack skills?
   yes .....   no .....

3. Is there a predominance of visual errors indicating a tendency to identify words using partial cues?   yes ..... no .....
   Insert examples of errors and targets:
   ....

4. Are most words recognized on sight, or is the child sounding out the majority of words?
   % by sight? .....
   sounding out: often .....   never .....   excessive .....

5. Is there a predominance of sounding-out errors suggesting:
   (a) an excessive reliance on decoding   yes ..... no .....
   e.g. ....
   (b) unreliable decoding skills   yes ..... no .....
   e.g. ....
   (c) an inappropriate use of decoding on irregular words?   yes ..... no .....
   e.g. ....
   Insert examples of errors and targets:
   ....

6. Is speed of word recognition fast ..... acceptable ..... slow ..... extremely slow .....

II. Decoding

1. Letter knowledge   good .....   moderate .....   poor .....
   Letters to teach: ....

2. Letter sound knowledge: good .....   moderate .....   poor .....
   Letter–sound mappings to teach: ....

3. Application of letter–sound rules: good .....   moderate .....   poor .....
   Types of error: ....

4. Blending: good .....   moderate .....   poor .....
   Types of error: ....

5. Accessing correct word
   after blending: good ....   moderate ....   poor ....
   Errors:...

III. Comprehension

1. Use of context   good .....   average .....   poor .....

2. Reading for meaning using
   semantically appropriate guesses   good .....   average .....   poor ....

3. Self-correction   frequently ..... sometimes .....   not at all .....

4. Phrasing meaningful or
   disjointed and meaningless   meaningful .....   meaningless .....

5. Intonation   good .....   average .....   poor .....

6. Has the reader understood the
   text when asked pertinent
   questions?   Yes .....   No .....

7. Can the reader make reasoned
   inferences about the behaviour
   of the characters in the story or
   predict their future behaviour?   Yes .....   No .....

Assessing decoding skills

As already mentioned, decoding consists of a number of subskills:

- the ability to divide a word into its component speech sounds, for example HIM ➤ "h-i-m";
- the use of letter–sound conversion to translate each letter to the appropriate speech sound, for example ➤ "h", etc.;
- blending the speech sounds to form a word;
- identifying the correct word and its meaning.

Because of time constraints, it is rarely possible to test all these components separately, but by evaluating knowledge of letter names and letter sounds, and by administering a non-word reading test, it is possible to identify the locus of difficulties.

Letter naming

Letter-name knowledge has proven to be a remarkably good predictor of eventual reading and spelling attainment (see Chapter 4 in this volume). There are numerous reasons for this. First, children who learn letter names easily are more likely to have good phonological skills. Second, early readers can often use letter names to deduce which sound a letter represents (Treiman, Weatherston and Berch, 1994). The use of letter-name strategies is not always easy to detect but is evident when readers report that the sound of <Y> is "w" and the sound of the letters <F>, <M> and <N> is "e", an assumption arrived at by identifying the first phoneme of the letter name. Although, as indicated above, the letter-name strategy is sometimes unreliable, it gives children a good basis from which to derive sound–letter correspondences.

Two related tests can be used to assess letter knowledge. First, print each letter on a blank card. After shuffling the cards, ask the child to tell you the name of each letter. Then shuffle the pack again and ask the child to tell you the sound of each letter. Children who know few letter names will need instruction, as will children whose letter-name knowledge is quite good but who have not been able to extrapolate sounds from letter names.

Nonword reading

Nonword reading tests are used to determine how well readers can decode words they have never seen before. If we try to assess decoding ability using real words, it is not always possible to distinguish conclusively between word recognition and decoding strategies. When we use non-words on the other hand, there is no likelihood that the items will be familiar. These tests have proved extremely useful diagnostically despite some people's instinctive aversion to meaningless material.

Nonwords are letter strings that resemble English words, conforming to the sound and spelling structure of English, but do not make sense, for example SLINT, CRIDGE and DELINKERATOR. For most purposes, non-words can be derived from real words by changing one or more letters: PUMPKIN can be changed to LUMPKIN or LUMPGIT. Non-words can also be derived from irregular words with unusual spellings, such as ISLAND and COLONEL. These 'irregular' non-words can either be sounded out, grapheme by grapheme, i.e. read as "f-o-l-o-n-e-l", or pronounced by 'analogy', in the same way as the irregular word COLONEL ➤ "fernul". The use of non-words derived from irregular words enables us to monitor a reader's strategies with greater accuracy (see Chapter 11 in Stackhouse and Wells, 1997, for a further discussion of stimulus design).

Practitioners may wish to use a standardized test of non-word reading such as the *Graded Nonword Reading Test* (Snowling, Stothard and McLean, 1996). Alternatively, they may wish to compile their own: the non-words listed in Box 6.2 were originally used by Snowling, Stackhouse and Rack (1986). Each nonword should be printed on an index card. The first set should be presented in random order (shuffling the cards will do), followed by the remaining set, also in random order. The test should be discontinued if the child is not able to read at least five of the non-words in the first set. The following instructions should be given before presenting the test.

> "I am going to ask you to read some make-believe words. These make-believe words sound like words but they do not make sense. Even though they don't make sense, it is possible to read them. See how many of them you can read."

Record the child's pronunciation of each item so that error analysis can be undertaken later. Pronunciations arrived at either through the use of letter–sound rules or through lexical analogy with an irregular word are correct. For example, CHOVE can be pronounced so that it rhymes with "clove" (regular) or with "love" (irregular), and PETTUCE can be pronounced as "petyoos" (regular) or so that it rhymes with "lettuce", i.e. "petis" (irregular). Comparing the incidence of the two types of response (decoding and analogy) will give useful information about the strategies used when reading new words. Lexicalization errors in which the reader pronounces the non-word as if it were a real word also frequently occur, for example ISLANK read as "island" or KISCUIT read as "biscuit". An excessive use of lexicalization indicates reliance on a holistic visual strategy when reading non-words.

The number of non-words read correctly should be calculated first and the score compared with the mean for children in the comparable age group. Box 6.2 provides cut-off points for the Nonword Reading Test, which indicate whether scores are unduly low. In addition, it is often useful to count the number of phonemes correctly represented and to make a tally of the sounds that the child has found most difficult.

In order to identify the origin of the child's decoding difficulties, it is useful to examine his or her reading errors, looking for evidence of difficulty with one or more of the processes of parsing, sound–letter knowledge or blending. Parsing refers to the process by which the letters in a word are separated into units corresponding to speech sounds, so that sound–letter rules can be applied. Whereas one letter usually represents one speech sound or phoneme, some phonemes are represented by a grapheme consisting of two letters, i.e. <th> in the word WITH and <sh> and <ou> in SHOULD. When readers read the <oo> in PLOOD as two separate units, for example "o-o", or pronounce the <ea> grapheme in CREAD as "e-a", they

Box 6.2 A test for assessing non-word reading (from Snowling, Stackhouse and Rack, 1986)

Nonword Reading Test
Have the child read the following nonwords. Each nonword should be written on a separate card. Record reading responses in detail. Either a regular or an irregular pronunciation is acceptable, i.e. If FONGUE is pronounced as "fongew" (as in rhyming with FONDUE) it is regular whereas if is pronounced so that it rhymes with TONGUE, an analogy strategy has been used. ISLANK pronounced as "izlank" is regular but pronounced as "ilank" with no 'z' sound by analogy to ISLAND, is irregular.

One syllable	Two syllable
plood	louble
aund	hausage
wolt	soser
jint	pettuce
hign	kolice
pove	skeady
wamp	dever
cread	bitre
slove	islank
fongue	polonel
nowl	narine
swad	kiscuit
chove	
duede	
sworf	
jase	
freath	
warg	
choiy	

Control data

Nonwords read correctly

Reading age		One syllable	Two syllable
7 years*	Mean	9.5	3.6
	SD	3.6	2.9
	Range	3–16	0–9
10 years**	Mean	17.3	10.7
	SD	1.4	1.8
	Range	15–16	6–12

*A score below 3 on one syllable words falls significantly below the norm.
**A score below 13 on one syllable and 7 on two syllable words falls significantly below the norm.

need to be taught that some letter strings function as units and must be decoded as a unit.

Knowledge of letter–sound mappings can be very limited in children with reading difficulties. In severe cases, the child is unable to identify any new words or read any nonwords. Other children can produce the sound of the initial letter but can decode no further. As skill improves, the child may remain uncertain of some letter–sound mappings, especially the short vowel sounds, consonant and vowel digraphs (*sh*, *gh*, *ou*, *aw*, *ei*) blends (*bl*, *sw*, *shr*) and infrequent letters (*x* and *q*).

Blending presents a particular problem to children with severe short-term memory problems (see Chapter 8 in this volume). Such children are unable to recall the sounds they have just identified long enough to blend them together correctly. Other children may have articulatory problems that impede correct blending (see Chapter 2 in this volume). Blending errors may result from omissions (e.g. <PED> blended as "pe"), insertions (e.g. <PED> blended as "pedder"), substitutions, often due to a change of voicing or place of articulation (e.g. <PED> pronounced as "peg"), lexicalization (<PED> read as "bed" or "pet"), vowel changes (<PED> pronounced as "pud") or a combination of the above errors, for example <AUND> sounded out correctly but blended as "anud".

Assessing reading fluency

Speed and efficiency of reading

It is often useful, especially with older readers, to measure not only reading accuracy, but also reading speed. Many poor readers learn to read accurately but remain dysfluent, with a slow reading rate. A standardized test designed for this purpose is the *Test of Word Reading Efficiency* (*TOWRE*; Torgesen, Wagner and Rashotte, 1999). There are two subtests of the TOWRE, one tapping sight word reading efficiency and the other phonemic decoding efficiency. In both subtests, children are presented with a card containing lists of words (sight word reading) or non-words (phonemic decoding efficiency). The task is to read as many words as possible within a time limit of 45 seconds. A child who has good reading accuracy but poor reading efficiency may require help, especially practice, to automatize his or her reading skills.

Reading text

A comparison of reading accuracy and comprehension is of diagnostic significance because it enables us to determine whether a child has competent comprehension skills despite poor word recognition, or whether comprehension deficits are the main cause of reading backwardness. A child whose word recognition is excellent but comprehension limited will require very different remediation from a child who makes numerous reading errors but can nevertheless answer searching questions about the text, if the unfamiliar words are supplied.

There are a large number of different reading comprehension tests (see Chapter 7 in this volume). The *Neale Analysis of Reading Ability – Revised* (Neale et al., 1999) is particularly useful because it provides three reading ages: a reading accuracy age, a reading comprehension age and a reading rate age. The individual is asked to read a prose passage aloud and is told that questions about the passage will follow. The examiner supplies any word that cannot be recognized and makes corrections if the reader identifies a word incorrectly.

Once again, the tester should record every error for subsequent analysis and identification of strategies in use. To facilitate error analysis, Box 6.3 includes a list of important behaviours that should be monitored when assessing reading comprehension.

The importance of assessing the different types of reading strategy in tandem and evaluating the ease with which a reader can shift from one strategy to another as necessary cannot be overemphasized. However, skilled reading necessitates more than just knowing and being able to use different reading strategies: it also requires amalgamating these strategies so that 'reading for meaning' does not consist of guesswork alone but is guided by graphemic information. Even readers whose phonological skills remain poor into adulthood can be taught to read effectively and with comprehension if they are instructed to attend to sufficient graphemic information to ensure reasonable accuracy. In addition, it is essential to identify any discrepancies between reading accuracy and comprehension so that an accurate assessment can be made of the true nature of the reader's problems.

Sean, for example, had severe reading and spelling difficulties during his early and middle childhood. At 14 years of age, his reading scores were still several years below his chronological age, but his reading comprehension of text, as measured by the revised Neale Analysis of Reading Ability, was excellent. He was able to answer almost all the comprehension questions on the two most difficult passages. Nonetheless, Sean's word recognition remained inaccurate despite the availability of context. He misread SUSPICIOUS as "surprises", PURSUED as "pressured", THROUGH as "though" and NEGLECTED as "negligent". All of these errors showed a tendency to misidentify words as other visually similar words that began with similar sounds. His monitoring skills were also surprisingly weak since he did not

Box 6.3 Guidelines for the analysis of errors made in reading text

1. Word recognition errors (tick as applicable)
.... (a) Confuses visually similar words (SCHEME and SCHOOL)
.... (b) Substitutes phonologically similar words ("compare" for COMPASSION)
.... (c) Omission of short words especially function words (i.e. TO, OF)

2. Use of context and linguistic prediction
  Type of substitutions (insert examples of errors and target, e.g. IS read as "were")
  (a) Meaningful ....
      Meaningless ....
  (b) Grammatically correct ....
      Grammatically incorrect ....

3. Reading rate (tick as applicable)
.... Too slow (Difficult to integrate the meaning of the text at this rate)
.... Average (Reasonable speed enabling adequate comprehension and recall)
.... Too fast (Text read at a speed that precludes adequate comprehension and recall)

4. Type of word attack used for identifying unfamiliar words (tick as applicable)
.... (a) Use of letter–sound correspondences
.... (b) Use of analogy
.... (c) Use of context
.... (d) Use of pictorial clues

5. Monitoring skills and self-correction (tick as applicable)
  Immediate..........   Delayed..............   Does not occur...........

6. Ability to apply alternative reading strategies as needed and appropriate
.... (a) Word recognition
.... (b) Reading for meaning and use of context
      With letter cues..........   Without letter cues............
.... (c) Decoding

7. Intonation   Good .....   Average .....   Poor .....

8. Has the reader understood the text
  when asked pertinent questions?   Yes .....   No .....

9. Can the reader make reasoned
  inferences about the behaviour
  of the characters in the story or
  predict their future behaviour?   Yes .....   No .....

notice his errors or self-correct them except on one occasion. Word-attack skills were still poor and seriously impeded his identification of new words. As Sean was about to begin important examination studies that year (the General Certificate of Secondary Education, GCSE), his ability to cope with these exams was of concern. Although he was certainly bright enough to understand the content of his courses, he would have great difficulty identifying the many unfamiliar words he would encounter in his reading. Weekly support was therefore recommended, consisting of teaching Sean to:

- monitor his reading more successfully;
- make use of his excellent comprehension skills to aid word identification while paying attention to graphemic information;
- subdivide words into syllables and morphemes to help Sean to decode words more accurately.

Assessing spelling

Spelling can be assessed using a standardized spelling test (see Appendix 1 for some suggestions), a test comprising words of different syllable length (Box 6.4) and a sample of free writing. The standardized spelling test will furnish a spelling age and indicate the level of a child's attainment compared with that of other children of the same age. However, as our aim is to understand the strategies used, further error analysis will be needed.

Spelling errors should be evaluated at two levels:

- *phonological* – does the spelling sound like the word intended?
- *orthographic* – are the correct letters used?

When examining phonological spelling ability, errors can be classified as 'phonetic', 'semi-phonetic' or 'non-phonetic' according to how accurately the speech sounds are represented (Snowling, 1987).

Error analysis

Phonetic errors

Phonetic errors are spellings that contain all the speech sounds in the target word but are spelled incorrectly, for example KNOWLEDGE ➤ <nolej>, CROWDED ➤ <croudid> and SUITABLE ➤ <sootibol>.

Box 6.4 Diagnostic spelling test (after Snowling, 1985)

Test of Spelling by Syllable Length

Instructions Dictate the word, dictate the sentence or phrase containing the word, and then dictate the word again.

pet	A dog is a **pet**.	Spell the word 'pet'
lip	He bit his **lip**.	Spell the word 'lip'
cap	The little boy wore a **cap**.	Spell the word 'cap'
fish	She caught a **fish** in the pond.	Spell the word 'fish'
sack	A **sack** of potatoes.	Spell the word 'sack'
tent	Indians used to sleep in a **tent**.	Spell the word 'tent'
trap	The rabbit was caught in a **trap**.	Spell the word 'trap'
bump	Do not **bump** your head.	Spell the word 'bump'
nest	There were chicks in the **nest**.	Spell the word 'nest'
bank	The thieves robbed the **bank**.	Spell the word 'bank'
apple	An **apple** is a type of fruit.	Spell the word 'fruit'
puppy	A **puppy** is a baby dog.	Spell the word 'puppy'
packet	A **packet** of crisps.	Spell the word 'packet'
trumpet	To play the **trumpet**.	Spell the word 'trumpet'
kitten	A **kitten** is a baby cat.	Spell the word 'kitten'
traffic	There is a lot of **traffic** in the street.	Spell the word 'traffic'
collar	The **collar** of your shirt is dirty.	Spell the word 'collar'
tulip	A **tulip** is a type of flower.	Spell the word 'tulip'
polish	**Polish** your shoes.	Spell the word 'polish'
finger	He cut his **finger**.	Spell the word 'finger'
membership	**Membership** of a club.	Spell the word 'membership'
cigarette	To smoke a **cigarette**.	Spell the word 'cigarette'
catalogue	A **catalogue** from a toy shop.	Spell the word 'catalogue'
September	My birthday is in **September**.	Spell the word 'September'
adventure	An exciting **adventure**.	Spell the word 'adventure'
understand	Do you **understand**?	Spell the word 'understand'
contented	To be **contented** is to be happy.	Spell the word 'contented'
refreshment	A drink is a type of **refreshment**.	Spell the word 'refreshment'
instructed	The teacher **instructed** the children to behave.	Spell the word 'instructed'
umbrella	It is raining. You need an **umbrella**.	Spell the word 'umbrella'
mysterious	The haunted house was **mysterious**.	Spell the word 'mysterious'
machinery	The factory uses **machinery**.	Spell the word 'machinery'
politician	A **politician** works in politics.	Spell the word 'politician'
congratulate	I **congratulate** you on your fine work.	Spell the word 'congratulate'
geography	In **geography** we study other countries.	Spell the word 'geography '
magnificent	You have done a **magnificent** job.	Spell the word 'magnificent'
calculator	You need a **calculator** to do that sum.	Spell the word 'calculator'
discovery	The **discovery** of America.	Spell the word 'discovery'
radiator	Turn the **radiator** on. It is cold.	Spell the word 'radiator'
automatic	Do you have an **automatic** car?	Spell the word 'automatic'

Semi-phonetic errors

In semi-phonetic spelling, all or almost all of the consonant sounds are represented, for example DOG ➤ <dg> and ISLAND ➤ <ild>. The spelling is usually reasonably easy to identify in context, not all the component speech sounds are included. Most normally developing children make these errors in the early stages of spelling acquisition. Consequently, semi-phonetic errors have been referred to as 'normal immaturities' by Snowling (1985). Children with spelling difficulties are, however, likely to continue making these well beyond the age at which normal spellers have discontinued them.

Spellings should be assigned to this category if one or more of the following types of error are present:

- Vowel sounds are sometimes omitted, for example CUT ➤ <ct> and BALL ➤ <bl>, or are incorrect, as in CUT ➤ <cat> and BALL ➤ <bul>.
- Nasals ('n', 'm', 'ng'), which alter the sound of the vowel but are not a distinct phoneme, are omitted, for example TENT ➤ <tet>, BUMP ➤ <bup> and CONTENTED ➤ <coteted>.
- There is an omission of one of the letters in a consonant cluster, usually the second, as with TRAIN ➤ <tane> and DRESS ➤ <des>.
- There is an omission of unaccented syllables in longer polysyllabic words, for example AUTOGRAPH ➤ <orgraf> and UMBRELLA ➤ <umbrel>.

Non-phonetic spelling errors

Non-phonetic spellings, more commonly referred to as dysphonetic errors, do not sound like the target words, and readers would be unable to identify such spellings unless they knew which word the writer was attempting to spell. It is possible to examine dysphonetic spellings in more detail by counting the number of phonemes correctly represented in each attempt. This is a useful technique of error analysis that enables the tester to decide whether the speller consistently uses an appropriate letter for each phoneme (as opposed to grapheme) or whether only a few phonemes are accurately represented; for example, CATALOGUE spelt as <cang> scores 2 (1 each for the for the <c> and <a>) out of a possible score of 7 phonemes (c-a-t-a-l-o-g), whereas CALCULATOR spelt as <cala> scores 4 out of a possible 10 (k-a-l-c-y-u-l-a-t-e) or out of 11 if the child pronounces the final 'r' as well, as with an American or Scottish accent). The fewer phonemes represented in the written version, the more severe the spelling difficulty.

By sorting errors according to these categories, it is easier to establish whether a speller is having difficulties with the phonological or the orthographic component of spelling, or both. Table 6.3 shows some examples of each type of spelling error.

Table 6.3 Sample of spelling errors according to error categories (target in brackets)

Phonetic	Semi-phonetic	Non-phonetic
croudid (CROWDED)	grand (GROUND)	mbbst (MEMBERSHIP)
trafick (TRAFFIC)	polsh (POLISH)	aferch (ADVENTURE)
koler (COLLAR)	rowt (ROUTE)	insind (UNDERSTAND)
citon (KITTEN)	tap (TRAP)	cepint (CONTENTED)
tuch (TOUCH)	seet (STREET)	pepr (BUMP)
blud (BLOOD)	sad (SAND)	sgrk (CIGARETTE)
coam (COMB)	bup (BUMP)	goegagh (GEOGRAPHY)
ort (OUGHT)	back (BANK)	muore (MOTHER)
cigeret (CIGARETTE)	radater (RADIATOR)	calutur (CALCULATOR)
shuvel (SHOVEL)	content (CONTENTED)	prany (PEOPLE)

Spelling error analysis in practice

Nathan, aged 9 years, was asked to spell the words on the *Spelling by Syllable Length Spelling Test* shown in Box 6.4 above. He spelled 4 out of 10 of the one-syllable words correctly, making mainly semi-phonetic errors on these words, for example FISH ➤ <fis>, TRAP ➤ <trp>, BUMP ➤ <bup> and NEST ➤ <net>. He misspelled all the two-syllable words. Three of his errors were phonetic (<appll>, <pakit>, <citn>), one was semiphonetic (POLISH ➤ <polis>), and the remainder were dysphonetic (TRUMPET ➤ <tupt>; TRAFFIC ➤ <tapt>; COLLAR ➤ <cll>, TULIP ➤ <tllrnp> and FINGER ➤ <frgn>).

Although Nathan's spelling of TRUMPET was easily explainable in terms of normal immaturities, i.e. he omitted the vowels and the second letter in the cluster 'tr', his other non-phonetic spellings were more 'bizarre'. A phoneme count showed that approximately half of the phonemes were represented correctly, but Nathan inserted a number of extraneous letters in several words (FINGER ➤ <frgn> and TULIP ➤ <tllrnp>), which contributed to making all of the non-phonetic spellings impossible to identify.

Three conclusions can be arrived at from this analysis.

1. Nathan has attained reasonable competence in representing the basic sound–letter mapping of consonants in one-syllable words but is unsure of sounds that require two letters, for example 'sh'.
2. He is making many semi-phonetic errors and should be given some structured help with vowels, consonant clusters and nasals to enable him to pass through this stage. Although Nathan knows how to represent some vowels, he frequently omits them and needs further instruction. Similarly, he requires instruction on the spelling of consonant clusters,

such as 'st' and 'tr' , and on the need to represent nasals in written language. All these teaching points can be taught using word families and can be presented as games.

3. Nathan has serious difficulties with long words and with syllable segmentation. Although he could segment the one-syllable words quite efficiently, he had substantial difficulty when trying to encode two-syllable words. His performance on words of three syllables was very poor indeed, and he omitted one of the syllables on every single item. It might help Nathan to think of polysyllabic words as a collection of one-syllable words. Nathan should be able to learn to spell these reasonably well once he has learned how to segment words and has been taught to spell each syllable (i.e. TRUM-PET) as if it were a separate word.

Phonetic errors and orthographic difficulties

The spelling errors of many older children with spelling difficulties tend to be reasonably phonetic but incorrect. It is helpful to classify the source of these errors for assessment purposes and to provide guidance about the type of remediation needed:

- *Irregular words.* Words such as SHOVEL, THUMB, BEAUTIFUL and HONEST require word-specific knowledge and need to be taught using whole-word methods or mnemonics.
- *Vowel errors*, such as JAW ➤ <jor> and ROAD ➤ <rode>. It is always best to teach these words in the context of similar word families, for example JAW, DRAW, LAW, PAW, RAW, etc.
- *Derivational errors.* These stem from a lack of understanding that words derived from the same root are related in meaning and have similar spellings, for example AUTUMN and AUTUMNAL.

Allen, aged 12, made the following phonetic and semi-phonetic spelling errors on the words of increasing syllable length in Box 6.4: <appel>, <pupy>, <kiten>, <trafick>, <colar>, <tolip>, <palish>, <fingger>, <sigaret>, <katalog>, <advencher>, <radeater>, <deskavery> and <atamatick>. He never omitted syllables even on the four-syllable items and very rarely produced non-phonetic spellings. His pattern of spelling indicated that his appreciation of the sound structure of words was intact. However, his spelling errors showed that he found it very difficult to remember what spellings looked like, even when spelling easy words such as PUPPY and APPLE.

Second, it is evident that Allen has not been able to deduce certain common orthographic rules about the English spelling system, such as the fact that words of one syllable that end with the sound "ik" are spelled <ic> (COMIC, TRAFFIC, PANIC, etc.) or that most words beginning with the sound "k" begin with the letter <c>.

Allen will need to be taught a number of orthographic rules, along with being shown lists of words that share the same spelling pattern (see Chapter 10 in this volume). He should be helped to find a way of learning whole-word spellings so that he can begin to build up a written vocabulary of the words he often uses in his writing. It will also be important to teach Allen doubling and suffixing rules, which, although by no means infallible, will help him to make more informed guesses about spellings he cannot remember. Finally, he should be encouraged to use joined-up writing when practising writing the letter patterns he is being taught so that he can develop a tactile memory of the word spellings he finds so difficult to recall. Nathan, discussed above, will also need a similar type of instruction in due course when he has resolved his problems with correctly identifying the sound level of language.

Unassisted free writing

A sample of unassisted free writing is a particularly informative diagnostic instrument. Most children can produce quite acceptable spelling attempts by the age of 7 years. If a child aged 7 or over is still struggling to produce a short piece or is producing numerous non-phonetic spellings, so that it almost impossible to decipher what he or she is trying to say, spelling skills should be assessed.

The easiest way to obtain a sample of unassisted free writing is simply to ask a child to write about something that interests him or her for a specified amount of time, either 5 or 10 minutes. Poor spellers, however, often do not know what to write about because they detest writing. It is therefore more helpful to suggest a topic such as a popular story, television series or film, for example to tell the story of *Little Red Riding Hood*, *Batman* or *Harry Potter*. Younger children can be given a cartoon and asked to tell the story, adding any details they like. An error analysis of spelling should be performed in exactly the same way as has already been suggested for the spelling tests. In the case of free writing, the ability to communicate ideas and handwriting should also be examined. Writing speed should also be calculated as number of words per minute (see Chapter 11 in this volume). Further points to keep in mind when assessing free-writing are outlined in Box 6.5.

The story in Figure 6.1 (p. 103) was written as a retelling of a story depicted in a cartoon of a boy who sees a dog in a shop window, runs

Box 6.5 Guidelines for the analysis of free writing

Free writing

1. **Intelligibility**
   Easy to understand .....   Average ....   Difficult to understand .....

2. **If difficult to understand:**
   Can the writer read what has been written?   Yes .....   No .....

3. **Compared with the rest of the class, is this piece of writing?**
   Above average ....   Average .....   Below average .....

If below average, perform a detailed error analysis

4. **Errors:**
   Phonetic ....
   ....
   ....

   Semi-phonetic ....
   ....
   ....

   Non-phonetic ....
   ....
   ....

   Mainly phonetic .....   Partially phonetic .....   Non-phonetic ......

home to fetch his mother, brings her back to the shop so that they can buy the dog and returns home with it. Matthew, who was 9;10 years at the time of writing, wrote the following (with the author's interpretation in parentheses):

> A dreyd (boy) wos (was) wok (walking) Dan (down) the rod (road) and hey (he) srom (saw) the littwe (little) dog a(and) he ust (asked) he muemy (his mummy) thetcotd (he could) hat (have) ta (it??) she siead (said) Iway (I will) giv ti (it) the my I hv (have) got a pet dog and wae (went) to bed and I win (went) fol (for) a wcko (walk) and he had a dig dog ahtl (???) hat . . . .

It is clear that Matthew was still having inordinate difficulty producing writing that could be understood by others. Many of his non-phonetic errors were unintelligible and could only be deciphered because we knew the story content of the cartoon (e.g. BOY ⇀ <dreld>, SAW ⇀ <srom>, WALK ⇀

<wcko>, ASKED ➛ <ust>, COULD ➛ <cotd>, IT ➛ <ti> and WENT ➛ <wae>). There were also, however, one phonetic (GIVE ➛ <giv>) and two semi-phonetic (HAVE ➛ <hv> and ROAD ➛ <rod>) spellings. These show that Matthew could sometimes arrive at a good approximation of the speech sounds of the words. Moreover, he had a small vocabulary of words that he could sometimes spell correctly (I, GOT, PET, BED, AND, HE and HAD), and these could be used as a springboard for developing spelling and writing skills.

David was 14 years old at the time of writing the piece in Figure 6.2 and had a spelling age on the Graded Word Spelling Test (Vernon, 1977) of 9;8 years. This essay about his summer job, written in 10 minutes, shows that he had resolved most of his earlier problems with spelling by sound but was having residual problems at the orthographic level, for example <factery>, <ernt>, <controled>, <herd>, <stught> (STUFF), <wonted>, <aventully>, <dicided>, <whent>, <pirice> (PRICE), <bourt>, <of> (OFF) and

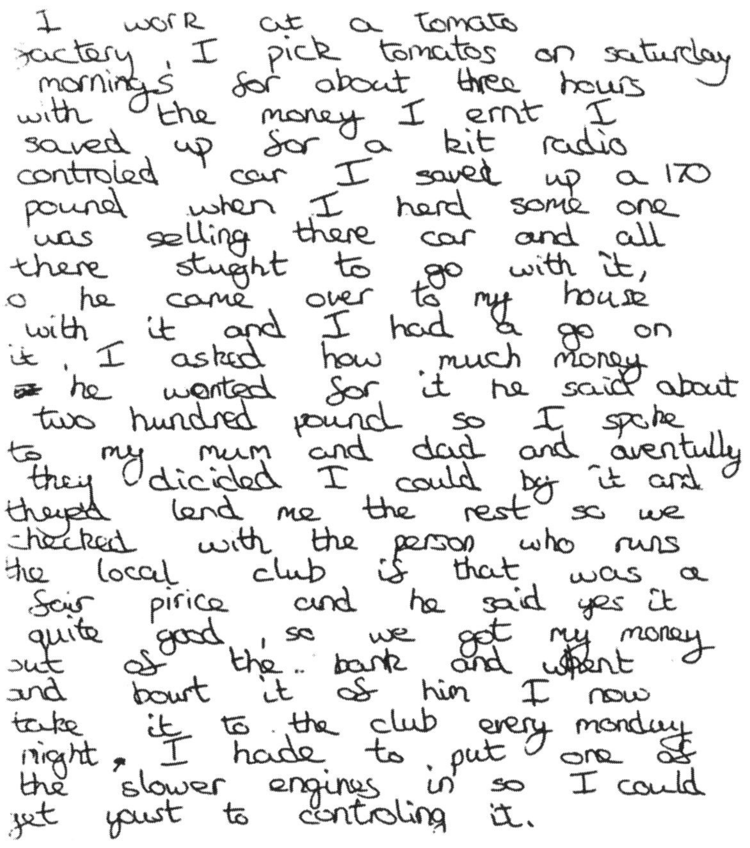
I work at a tomato
factery, I pick tomatos on saturday
mornings for about three hours
with the money I ernt I
saved up for a kit radio
controled car I saved up a 170
pound when I herd some one
was selling there car and all
there stught to go with it,
so he came over to my house
with it and I had a go on
it, I asked how much money
he wonted for it he said about
two hundred pound so I spoke
to my mum and dad and aventully
they dicided I could by it and
theyed lend me the rest so we
checked with the person who runs
the local club if that was a
fair pirice and he said yes it
quite good, so we got my money
out of the bank and whent
and bourt it of him I now
take it to the club every monday
night, I hade to put one of
the slower engines in so I could
get youst to controling it.

Figure 6.2 David's writing; aged 14 years.

<youst> (USED). It is apparent that David has particular difficulty with irregular words and with homophones (<there> for THEIR, <herd> for HEARD and <by> for BUY) and will need remediation that tackles these difficulties. Teaching should also include word families and alternative spelling patterns so that he acquires a firm grasp of orthographic regularities.

A case study of specific reading and spelling difficulty

To show how an assessment of reading and spelling can provide useful information about a child's current problems and indicate which areas are in most need of intervention, the case of Frances is presented. She was 8;8 years old when first assessed and had a reading age of 6;8 years on the British Ability Scales Test of Word Reading (Elliott, 1992). She was able to read a number of the easier words correctly, but her reliance on partial visual access made her reading inaccurate, for example:

IF	➔	"of"
WINDOW	➔	"windows"
MEN	➔	"man",
DIG	➔	"dog"
SPORT	➔	"spot".

On an experimental single word reading test in which she performed extremely poorly compared with readers with a reading age of 7 years, Frances made an assortment of visual errors, ranging from identifying words by first-letter cues only, to a few visual errors that closely resembled the target. Interestingly, the majority of her errors incorporated information about two letters, indicating that she was beginning to develop word-recognition skills that took letter information into account. None of her errors was, however, sound-based; her alphabetic skills had not yet emerged.

Frances' attempt to read simple nonwords supported this conclusion. She was able to read only one of the one-syllable words and was unwilling to attempt any two-syllable items. Her errors disclosed that she could decode most of the initial letters and some of the final letters but was unable to decode most vowels and blends. She made several reversal errors reading PAB as "bid" and SMADE as "seb". Finally, Frances made some odd errors reading MUF as "bife" and SKAG as "sculpt". The 'm' and 'b' confusion was one that frequently appeared in her spelling and stemmed from her inability to pronounce both of these sounds distinctly.

Tests of letter naming and letter-sound naming confirmed that Frances still had many gaps in her knowledge of letter–sound mappings. Although she knew the names of all the letters, she did not know the sound of the eight letters 'o', 'u', 'i', 'r', 'w', 's' and 'x', and was likely to have difficulty decoding words that contained these letters. When asked to write the 26 letter names, Frances was able to do so without error, but when requested to write the letter that represented a spoken phoneme, she could produce the correct letter only 42 per cent of the time. It appeared from these results that although Frances had competent letter-naming skills, she had not been able to use letter-name information to help her deduce the sounds of the letters, and had not yet formed reliable sound–letter mappings. Frances' poor performance when asked to write the letters that represented individual speech sounds suggests that her spelling would be weak.

Frances' spelling age of 6;2 years on the Graded Word Spelling Test (Vernon, 1998) confirmed this suspicion. She was able to spell only six words correctly and proved unable to produce plausible spellings for words that were not already stored in the lexicon. Her spelling attempts were almost always non-phonetic and could not be read by someone who did not already know the identity of the target. She spelled SICK ➤ <scak>, STORY ➤ <shroy>, GRASS ➤ <geasa>, BIT ➤ <peat>, DOWN ➤ <domen> and earth ➤ <ehar>.

One year later, Frances was asked to describe another cartoon story (Figure 6.3) in which a dog finds a baby bird that has fallen out of its nest and takes it to his master. Frances made 16 errors on the 40 words attempted, an error rate of almost 38 per cent. However, although a number of her errors were dysphonetic, for example <fied> (FOUND), <sedr> (SHOWED), <beg> (BEGAN) and <chiren> (CHILDREN), there were also some partially phonetic errors – <bieds> (BIRDS), <biad> (BIRD), <he's> (HIS) and <daid> (DID). Moreover, a number of words were correctly spelled (TREE, DOWN, NEST and SING), including PUT, an irregular word that needed word-specific knowledge. Several of Frances' spelling errors suggest that she was trying to remember what the words looked like rather than what they sounded like e.g. <somn>, <soma> (SOME) and <bog> (BOY).

In a tree soma (some) bieds (birds) wersing (were singing) one fall (fell) down a dog (boy) fiad (found) it and sedr (showed) a bog (boy) the boy saw the nest and put the biad (bird) wite (with) he's (his) Mum the Mum beg (began) to sing and some (so) daid (did) thee (the) chiren (children)

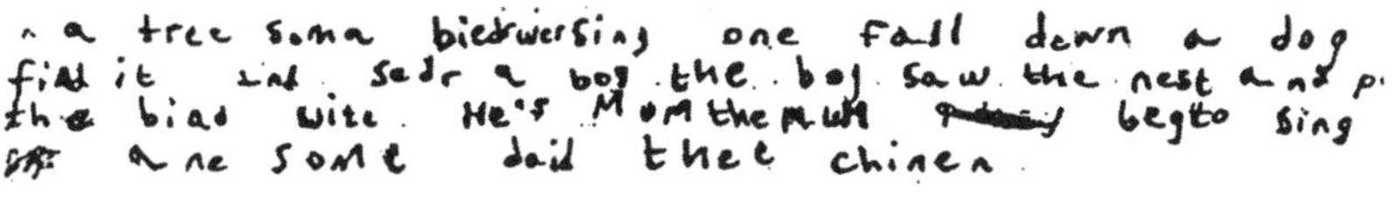

Figure 6.3 Frances' writing; aged 7 years.

Apart from the numerous spelling errors, Frances' writing shows that she totally disregarded punctuation and would require extensive instruction in its use. In addition, the occasional omission of syllables suggests that she would benefit from being taught to count syllables in words and to spell longer words syllable by syllable. She could also be asked to play word family games in which she had to identify the syllables, and could be helped to monitor each spelling when trying to generate new spellings.

Frances had a history of speech difficulties and, although no longer receiving speech therapy, had residual articulation difficulties that appeared to influence some of her spelling errors, especially the 'm', 'b' and 'p' confusion previously mentioned. The speech and language therapist's report noted that Frances had difficulty repeating words and non-words that contained clusters, she confused nasal sounds such as 'm' and 'n', and she made a number of other phonemic substitutions such as producing "f" for 'th', "the" for 'v' and "r" for 'w'. Such errors were also evident in her spelling.

On the *Neale Analysis of Reading Ability* (Neale et al., 1999), Frances scored an accuracy reading age of 7;3 years and a comprehension reading age of 7;0 years. From this result, it was evident that Frances was able to identify words much better if she had context to help her. Although she could not decode any unfamiliar words, she was able to guess a few words correctly.

Cognitive assessment showed that Frances had great difficulty with word and non-word repetition when compared with children of the same reading age. She also found it extremely difficult to think of words that rhymed with CAT, DOG or PIN. On the *Bradley Test of Auditory Organisation*, in which she had to identify the word that sounded different from the others (e.g. MAP, CAP, GAP, JAM or FISH, DISH, wish, MASH), she performed poorly compared with other children of the same 7 year reading level. Her difficulties with sound–letter mapping, decoding and reading unfamiliar words and nonwords were understandable given her basic phonological problems.

Conclusions

The assessment of reading and spelling and associated cognitive deficits is a crucial precursor of teaching. By adopting detailed assessment procedures and taking the time to undertake careful error analysis, it is possible to identify precisely the strategies used by each individual and to discern why he or she is not progressing normally. The next step is to devise a teaching programme that is tailor made to the child's or student's needs. The assessment procedure suggested above will take approximately 45 minutes to administer and another hour to score and interpret. Although this may seem a long time to spend on one child, the understanding gained from embarking upon such a diagnostic procedure should in the long run save time for practitioner and student alike.

Appendix 1: Standardized reading and spelling tests

Single-word reading tests

Raban B (1985) Macmillan Graded Word Reading Test: GWRT. London: NFER-Nelson.

Wilkinson GS (1993) Wide Range Achievement Test, 3rd edn: WRAT-3. Wilminton, DE: Jastak Associates, age range 5–75 years, normed in the USA.

Young D (1978) SPAR Spelling and Reading Tests. London: Hodder & Stoughton.

Decoding skills

Snowling MJ, Stothard SE, McLean J (1996) Graded Nonword Reading Test. Bury St Edmunds: Thames Valley Test Publishers; age range 5–11 years, normed in the UK.

Reading rate and accuracy

Torgesen J, Wagner R, Rashotte C (1999) Test of Word Reading Efficiency: TOWRE. Circle Pines, MN: AGS Publishing; age range 6–24;11 years, normed in the USA.

Prose reading

Neale M (1999) Neale Analysis of Reading Ability, 2nd edn revised: NARAII. Windsor: NFER-Nelson; age range 6–12 years.

Vincent D, De la Mare M (1989) New Macmillan Reading Analysis. London: NFER Nelson; age range 7;7–13;0 years.

Vincent D, De la Mare M (1990) Macmillan Individual Reading Analysis. Basingstoke, Hampshire: Macmillan Education; age range 5;6–12;11 years.

Spelling tests

Vernon PE (1977) Graded Word Spelling Test. London: Hodder & Stoughton.

Vernon PE (1998) Graded Word Spelling Test, 2nd Edition. London: Hodder & Stoughton.

Wide Range Achievement Test III (WRAT-III).

Young D (1978) SPAR Spelling and Reading Tests. London: Hodder & Stoughton.

Young D (1983) The Parallel Spelling Tests A and B. London: Hodder & Stoughton.

CHAPTER 7
Assessing children's reading comprehension

KATE NATION

The need to identify children who are experiencing difficulties learning to read should demand no justification. An accurate assessment of reading is crucial if children are to receive intervention that is specifically geared to improving their reading skills. Standardized reading tests are an important tool as they provide clear and objective estimates of a child's ability compared with that of other children of the same age. It is, however, important that appropriate tests are chosen, otherwise some children may continue through school with their difficulties unrecognized.

Broadly, it is possible to think of two sets of skills that a child needs to master to become a skilled reader of an alphabetic language. First and foremost, children need to learn to *decode*. Learning that letters map to speech sounds in a systematic way provides children with a rudimentary reading system that allows them to read words, even new words that they have never seen before. With practice and exposure to print, children's decoding skills soon become fast, flexible and efficient. However, the ultimate goal of reading is to understand what has been written, and although good decoding skills are an essential component of skilled reading, they are no guarantee that successful comprehension will follow. Thus, the other set of skills that children need if they are to read successfully are those concerned with *comprehension*.

Generally speaking, there is a strong association between decoding and comprehension: children who are good at decoding tend to have good comprehension, and children who are poor at decoding tend to have weak comprehension. For some children, however, the two sets of skills develop out of step. In dyslexia, a developmental disorder experienced by 3–10 per cent of children, decoding is slow, effortful and error prone (see Snowling, 2000, for a review). This type of difficulty is relatively easy to recognize in a classroom: the child with dyslexia who fails to develop the decoding skills necessary to 'sound out' new words is likely to be known to the teacher. In this case, a formal test of reading accuracy is likely to confirm that the child has a reading accuracy age lower than expected from his or her chronological age or general intellectual ability.

In contrast to children with dyslexia, some children decode well but have difficulty understanding what they have read. Approximately 10–15 per cent of children aged between 7 and 11 years have been identified as having specific reading comprehension difficulties (Nation and Snowling, 1997; Stothard and Hulme, 1992; Yuill and Oakhill, 1991). As these children have adequate decoding skills, many will not be recognized in the classroom as having any reading difficulties. Clearly, however, the fact that these children are failing to understand what they read suggests that they will begin to experience difficulties across the whole curriculum. In some senses, they will be more disadvantaged than the child with dyslexia whose difficulties are well documented.

This chapter begins by describing reading and reading-related skills in children who appear to show selective impairments of reading comprehension. As comprehension is a complex skill, it may be the case that different children fail to understand for different reasons. This heterogeneity is highlighted when we go on to consider the case studies of four children with poor reading comprehension. Finally, methods of assessing reading comprehension will be considered, and some commercially available tests will be reviewed.

Identifying children with poor reading comprehension

A number of studies have attempted to understand the nature and causes of reading comprehension failure. Unfortunately, most studies have included children who are poor at both reading comprehension *and* decoding. As a consequence, the results are difficult to interpret as poor reading comprehension is confounded by inadequate decoding skill. In a series of papers published over the past 20 years, Jane Oakhill and colleagues have shown how we can address questions concerning the cognitive and linguistic processes that contribute specifically to the comprehension component of reading by selecting children who have specific weaknesses in comprehension in the face of adequate decoding skill (Cain and Oakhill, 1999; Oakhill, 1982, 1984; Yuill and Oakhill, 1991).

Our approach to selecting poor comprehenders builds on the one developed by Oakhill and colleagues. The *Neale Analysis of Reading Ability* (NARA-II; Neale, 1997) provides a measure of reading comprehension that is relatively independent of reading accuracy. Children read a passage aloud, and any mistakes they make are corrected by the tester. It is possible to convert the number of words they read correctly to a reading accuracy standard score. They are then asked questions about the passage. Some of these can be answered by direct reference to information in the passage, whereas others require children to make inferences based on real-world knowledge. The number of questions answered correctly is used to derive an age-referenced reading comprehension standard score. Children whose reading comprehension scores fall substantially below their (normal range) score on tests tapping decoding skills can be classified as having specific reading comprehension difficulties.

Exploring the causes of children's reading comprehension difficulties

Arguably, the most important cause of reading comprehension failure in children stems from difficulties with decoding and word recognition: if children cannot read words with a reasonable degree of accuracy, their comprehension is likely to be compromised. Although there is good evidence to support this conclusion (e.g. Perfetti, 1985), the existence of poor comprehenders (children who read accurately but fail to understand what they have read) makes it clear that skills beyond those required for word recognition are needed if adequate comprehension is to follow.

An important question concerns the specificity of poor comprehenders' difficulties: are they specific to reading, or do poor comprehenders show a limited understanding of spoken language too? Typically, children selected on the basis of their poor reading comprehension show concomitant difficulties with listening comprehension. For example, Nation and Snowling (1997) asked children to listen to stories, and at the end of each story the children were asked a series of questions about the story. Poor comprehenders performed less well than control children on this test of listening comprehension. This finding suggests that poor comprehenders' difficulties with reading comprehension should be seen in the context of difficulties with language more generally (see Chapter 5 in this volume).

The importance of inferences

To understand language, it is often necessary to make inferences – to go beyond what is stated explicitly in the text or discourse to infer the intended message. Even very straightforward texts require inferences to be drawn. This point is nicely illustrated by Oakhill in her description of how the following story 'can only be understood against a background knowledge about birthday parties, the convention of taking presents to them, the need for money to buy presents, and so on' (1994, p. 822):

> Jane was invited to Jack's birthday.
> She wondered if he would like a kite.
> She went to her room and shook her piggy bank.
> It made no sound.

As this example makes clear, failure to draw inferences is likely to seriously impede comprehension. Oakhill (1984) presented data suggesting that poor comprehenders have specific difficulties drawing inferences. Building on earlier work by Paris and Upton (1976), she asked poor comprehenders and controls to read short stories and then answer questions about what they had read. The questions were split into two types: those which could be answered by literal reference to the text and those which required an inference. Poor comprehenders were worse than typically developing normal readers at answering both types of question. In a second condition in which the text remained in full view (allowing the children to look back at the story), performance on the literal questions improved, but the children still had marked difficulty making inferences. These findings demonstrate that poor comprehenders have difficulty drawing inferences when reading or listening, and it has been suggested that such difficulties are causally implicated in children's poor reading comprehension (Cain and Oakhill, 1999; Cain et al., 2001; Oakhill, 1982, 1984).

Oral language skills

Following on from the observation that poor comprehenders show difficulties with listening comprehension as well as reading comprehension, and that they are poor at drawing inferences when both reading and listening, a number of studies have examined components of poor comprehenders' oral language ability in some detail.

Nation and Snowling (1998b) investigated poor comprehenders' semantic skills – that is, their knowledge of and sensitivity to word meanings. When asked to decide whether two words mean similar things (e.g. *jacket* and *coat*, *small* and *little*), poor comprehenders were slower and less accurate than control children, and they produced fewer exemplars in a semantic fluency task. It is important to note, however, that the deficits observed in these experiments were not just symptoms of generally poor language; for example, deficits in semantic judgement and semantic fluency were accompanied by normal levels of performance on parallel tasks tapping rhyme judgement and rhyme fluency. Indeed, most of the available evidence suggests that poor comprehenders' phonological skills are similar to those seen in control children. This conclusion is based on a number of studies using a variety of different tasks including phoneme deletion, rhyme oddity, judgement and fluency, spoonerisms and non-word repetition (e.g. Cain, Oakhill and Bryant, 2000; Nation and Snowling, 1998b; Nation et al., 2004; Stothard and Hulme, 1995). Thus, poor comprehenders have difficulty processing aspects of language concerned with meaning. Such semantic impairments are consistent with mild-to-moderate deficits in receptive and expressive vocabulary that have emerged in some, but not all, studies (e.g. Nation et al., 2004; Stothard and Hulme, 1992).

Although Nation and Snowling characterized poor comprehenders as having poor lexical-semantic skills, subsequent research has revealed oral language weaknesses that are not necessarily restricted to the semantic or lexical domain. For example, Nation et al. (2004) found that poor comprehenders scored lower than control children on tests tapping morphosyntax and the understanding of non-literal aspects of language, as well as vocabulary. These findings are consistent with earlier work by Stothard and Hulme (1992) demonstrating group deficits on a test of syntactic comprehension, the *Test for the Reception of Grammar* (*TROG*; Bishop, 1983). For each TROG item, the child is shown four coloured pictures and has to select the picture that corresponds to a sentence read aloud by the tester. For example, the child might hear the sentence "The girl is pushing the horse" and be shown pictures of (a) a girl pushing a man, (b) a girl riding a horse, (c) a horse pushing a girl and (d) a girl pushing a horse. Grammatical complexity increases over the span of the test.

Not all studies have found deficits on the TROG test in children with poor text-level reading comprehension (e.g. Yuill and Oakhill, 1991). Inconsistent findings across studies are, however, difficult to interpret as performance levels on the TROG have typically been close to ceiling. A new edition of this test, *TROG-2* (Bishop, 2003), contains more items and is standardized through to adulthood. A recent study using this more sensitive test provides clear evidence pointing to syntactic comprehension impairments in poor comprehenders who on average gained a standard score of 80 (Cragg and Nation, in press).

There is thus considerable evidence supporting the view that poor comprehenders have oral language weaknesses. Nation et al. (2004) concluded that low language characterized poor comprehenders as a group, and their oral language skills were characterized by relative weaknesses in dealing with the non-phonological aspects of language, ranging from lexical-level weaknesses (vocabulary) through to difficulties with interpreting non-literal language.

From language to reading?

Given that oral language skills develop before children learn to read, it is tempting to suggest that poor comprehenders' reading skills are a product of their strengths and weaknesses in oral language. On this view, strengths in the phonological domain fuel the development of decoding and reading accuracy. In contrast, difficulties with wider aspects of language – impoverished vocabulary knowledge, difficulty inferring non-literal meaning, for example – lead to comprehension problems. These problems have their roots in oral language, but as written language is essentially parasitic upon spoken language, difficulties in reading and oral language comprehension are to be expected.

Although it is tempting to see difficulties with reading comprehension as a consequence of oral language weaknesses, an alternative perspective is that poor comprehenders' oral language weaknesses are the consequence of a lack of reading experience. Nagy and Anderson (1984) argued that, from the beginning of the third grade (around 9 years of age), the amount of free reading in which children engage is the major determinant of vocabulary growth. Preliminary data (Cain, 1994, cited in Oakhill and Yuill, 1996) suggest that poor comprehenders have substantially less reading and reading-related experience than control children. Although Cain's data need to be interpreted cautiously owing to the small sample size, they are consistent with a view that sees individual differences in reading comprehension failure becoming compounded over time. No longer-term follow-up studies of poor comprehenders have been published, but recent data we have collected confirm that poor comprehenders' difficulties with reading comprehension are not transient: 78 per cent of poor comprehenders originally tested at age 8–9 years still had significant comprehension impairments when tested later at age 13–14 years; a further 13 per cent continued to have milder weaknesses with reading comprehension.

Individual differences in poor comprehension

Reading comprehension is a complex process. To understand a written text, words need to be recognized and their meanings accessed; relevant background knowledge also needs to be activated, and inferences generated as information are integrated during the course of reading. In addition, control processes monitor both ongoing comprehension and the internal consistency of text, allowing the reader to initiate repair strategies (e.g. re-reading) if comprehension breakdown is detected (Hannon and Daneman, 2001; Palincsar and Brown, 1984). Given the complexity of comprehension, it seems likely that children may fail to understand what they have read for a variety of different reasons. Thus, any population of poor comprehenders selected via the screening method outlined above is likely to be heterogeneous. To illustrate the heterogeneity of poor comprehenders, four children will be described who all show substantial gaps between their at least average-for-age decoding and their impaired reading comprehension. All of them would be 'flagged' as poor comprehenders according to their pattern of reading performance. Yet, in other areas of development, the children are quite different and, arguably, the reasons why they find reading comprehension difficult may also be different.

David: a poor comprehender with relatively weak language skills

David is fairly typical of the poor comprehenders we recruit into our studies (see Nation, 2005, for a review). At age 9 years, his ability to read aloud single words presented one at a time out of context was average: he obtained a standard score of 100 on the *British Ability Scales* (*BAS-II*; Elliot, Smith and McCulloch, 1997) reading test. His reading comprehension was, however, poor: he achieved a standard score of only 70 on the NARA-II. His comprehension difficulties were still apparent 2 years later: on this occasion, his word reading score was 103 and his comprehension score 80.

Like many of the poor comprehenders described by Nation, Clarke and Snowling (2002), David's word recognition was in line with his overall IQ, but his reading comprehension was significantly lower than expected, given his cognitive ability. He also demonstrated a cognitive profile that is fairly typical of poor comprehenders: his visuospatial ability and non-verbal ability were average (100 and 101), but his verbal ability was below average (80). He also showed weakness on a range of tests tapping vocabulary knowledge and aspects of oral language comprehension, although his phonological skills were strong. For children like David, it is tempting to suggest that weaknesses in verbal ability constrain reading comprehension. Put simply, if a child has problems understanding spoken language, then difficulty understanding written language is not surprising.

Edward: a poor comprehender with weak cognitive ability

Edward presented with a reading profile similar to David's. At age 8;5 years, his single-word reading score was 103, but his reading comprehension score was 84. Like David, his poor comprehension persisted, and he achieved almost identical standard scores 2 years later; he also had poor verbal ability, achieving a standard score of 71 on the BAS-II verbal ability scale. Unlike David, however, Edward had general cognitive weaknesses that extended to the non-verbal (62) and visuospatial domains (80). In Edward's case, the gap between decoding and comprehension was not caused by surprisingly low reading comprehension: his poor reading comprehension was perfectly in line with IQ expectations. However, his reading accuracy was significantly *higher* than one would expect, given his IQ. Given that Edward has extremely well-developed word recognition skills (and phonological skills), relative to both his comprehension and general cognitive ability, his reading is characteristic of what one sees in children labelled as 'hyperlexic', a term used to describe exceptional word recognition skills in children who have otherwise limited cognitive abilities and behavioural abnormalities (see Nation, 1999, for a review).

Beth: a poor comprehender with non-verbal learning difficulties

Although she shared a reading profile similar to that of both David and Edward, the source of Beth's difficulties appears to be very different. At age nearly 10 years, Beth showed the classic profile of a poor comprehender, achieving standard scores of 78 on a test of reading comprehension and 106 on a test of word recognition. Unlike David and Edward, her vocabulary knowledge and other linguistic skills, including phonological skills, were average, and her verbal IQ was 97. However, her non-verbal abilities were less strong. On the BAS-II, she achieved a standard score of 86 on the non-verbal measures and 77 on the visuospatial measures. Thus, her cognitive profile is consistent with that typically seen in children described as having a non-verbal learning difficulty (NLD; Rourke, 1989). Although there have been no detailed studies of reading in children with NLD, the dissociation between normal word-level reading skills and impaired reading comprehension has been highlighted in clinical neuropsychological diagnostic schedules (e.g. Pelletier, Ahmad and Rourke, 2001; Rourke, 1989). Furthermore, researchers interested in hyperlexia have described a subgroup of such children who have NLDs (Richman and Wood, 2002).

It is interesting to note that we originally saw Beth when she was 7 years old. At that time, she appeared to have normal reading skills with standard scores of 105 and 103 on tests of word reading and comprehension, respectively. Indeed, she was a member of our control group of normal readers until further testing revealed that she did not meet our criterion of normal-range non-verbal ability. Why did her reading comprehension decline over time? One possibility is that her apparent decline is an artefact of test measurement error. This seems unlikely: not only do the tests have good psychometric properties, but her pattern of reading behaviour was also consistent across a number of different tests administered at each time point.

We suspect that declines in reading comprehension over time may be part of the developmental course of NLD. To have 'normal' reading comprehension at age 7 is not necessarily the same as having 'normal' reading comprehension at 10 years. In the early years, 'normal' reading comprehension may be achieved by capitalizing on adequate linguistic knowledge (e.g. vocabulary or sensitivity to grammatical word order). Children with NLD are not considered to have impairments with these aspects of language processing (e.g. Pelletier, Ahmad and Rourke, 2001). Arguably, however, as children get older, they are expected to be adept at the more complex aspects of comprehension, such as inference-making based on real-world knowledge and experience. Given the difficulties that children with NLD have with aspects of discourse, conversation and social perception (Worling, Humphries and Tannock, 1999), difficulty with 'higher-level' aspects of reading comprehension are not surprising. Similar pragmatic impairments have been reported in other groups of children who also have poor reading comprehension, such as high-functioning children with autism (Dennis, Lazenby and Lockyer, 2001) and children with early-onset hydrocephalus (Dennis and Barnes, 1993).

These ideas are speculative but could be tested empirically by assessing the reading comprehension skills of children with NLD longitudinally. In line with Beth's reading profile, we predict a decline in reading comprehension, relative to that of normally developing children, as the demands placed on reading comprehension increase as children get older. Additionally, it would be interesting to see whether the comprehension of children with NLD varies according to particular text properties. They may, for example, have a reasonable understanding of those aspects of the text that are fairly literal. On this view, comprehension only breaks down when understanding relies on the ability to make inferences.

Although David, Edward and Beth all have similar profiles of reading behaviour, the origins of their comprehension impairments may well be different. One feature that unites the children, however, is that none of them was recognized by their teachers as having a reading difficulty. David was thought to be a little fidgety and Edward considered unimaginative. Some concerns had been raised about Beth's clumsiness and her slightly insensitive social behaviour. But, in no case were these concerns serious enough to warrant referral to external specialist services, and in no case were difficulties with reading and language suspected. This was not the case for the next child though, whose difficulties were well recognized.

Duncan: a poor comprehender with autism spectrum disorder

We saw Duncan when he was almost 15 years old. His developmental difficulties were well documented, and he had been diagnosed with atypical autism during early childhood. His verbal and non-verbal skills were average, and his reading accuracy skills were well developed: he achieved standard scores of 115 on the two tests of reading accuracy we administered. Duncan's reading comprehension was, however, very poor. On the NARA-II test described above, his reading comprehension standard score was 70, barely at the level expected for a 6-year-old child. Unlike the children described above, our findings were entirely consistent with teacher and parent reports: in Duncan's case, his good reading accuracy had not been assumed to be an index of good reading comprehension.

There is a strong association between autism and hyperlexia. Many children who have a hyperlexic reading profile are autistic or show features of autism (Grigorenko et al., 2002). It is not clear why this is the case. Nation (1999) speculates that a number of factors may be important: a particular pattern of cognitive and linguistic strengths and weaknesses, a tendency to be interested in local features rather than global coherence, and a preoccupation with text and reading. As these features tend to cluster together in people with autism, patterns of hyperlexic reading are therefore more common in this group. An interesting question is whether these features also tend to characterize non-autistic children who have poor reading comprehension but good reading accuracy.

Although there is a large literature on hyperlexia, it is in the main limited to descriptions of the condition rather than attempts to understand the nature of reading behaviour in children considered to be hyperlexic (see Snowling and Frith, 1986). This is an important direction for future work. Similarly, it is important to keep in mind that although hyperlexia is more common in children with autism, most children with autism do not show hyperlexic reading. Very little is known about the characteristics of reading in non-hyperlexic autistic children.

Assessing reading comprehension

These case studies show very clearly that decoding skill is not always a good predictor of a child's reading comprehension ability: serious problems with reading comprehension are apparent in a substantial minority of children who otherwise appear to read accurately and fluently. Thus, a thorough assessment of a child's reading ability should include a test of reading comprehension. Together with assessments of the child's reading accuracy (see Chapter 6 in this volume), this will provide a comprehensive analysis of reading ability.

A number of reading comprehension tests are available commercially. They can be broadly split into two types: those which have a question–answer-type format, and those which use a multiple-choice or closed-type procedure. The NARA-II is an example of a question–answer-type test. As described earlier, children read short stories aloud. Mistakes are corrected by the tester, and the time taken to read the story is noted. After each story, comprehension questions are asked. Some of the questions may be answered using verbatim memory, whereas others require inferences to be made. Separate standard scores and reading-age equivalent scores are generated for text reading accuracy, reading comprehension and reading speed. It is suitable for children aged between 5 and 13 years.

The NARA-II provides a comprehensive assessment of component reading skills; importantly, it is a useful tool in that it highlights those children whose component skills may be developing out of step (e.g. poor comprehenders). In addition, it is normed against an IQ battery, the BAS-II (Elliot, Smith and McCulloch, 1997). It is thus possible to ask whether a child's reading skills are commensurate with his or her general cognitive ability (Nation, Clarke and Snowling, 2002). However, it takes approximately 20–30 minutes to administer, and as it is administered individually, it is rather time-consuming for routine use in the classroom. In addition, Stothard and Hulme (1991) raised some concerns over the reliability of the two parallel forms, and they also found that Form 2 was biased against boys.

The *Wechsler Objective Reading Dimensions* (*WORD*; Rust, Golombok and Trickey, 1993), which may be administered only by psychologists or other suitably qualified professionals, measures three components of literacy, each measured by an independent test: Basic Reading (single-word reading), Spelling and Reading Comprehension. As with the NARA-II, reading comprehension is assessed via a question–answer-type format: children read short passages and are then asked a single question per passage to assess their comprehension. Raw scores are converted to standard scores and reading-age equivalents. The test is graded in difficulty, covering the age range 6–16 years, and the reading comprehension subtest takes about 10–15 minutes to administer. As the WORD is normed against the *Wechsler Intelligence Scale for Children*, it is a useful tool allowing psychologists to explore whether children's reading ability is significantly different from the level expected from their IQ.

Although the NARA-II and the WORD Reading Comprehension subtest both assess comprehension by asking children to answer questions about text that they have read, there are important differences between the two tests that need to be kept in mind when interpreting children's performance. In the WORD test, reading errors are not corrected, and indeed the children are allowed to read silently should they desire. Thus, if the child makes many reading errors, reading comprehension may be severely compromised. For example, a child with dyslexia may perform poorly not because she does not understand the passages, but because of the heavy demands placed on her decoding skills. In such a case, it would be wrong to interpret poor performance as evidence of comprehension weaknesses. In contrast, in the NARA-II, the tester is instructed to correct any words a child fails to read correctly. Arguably, this provides a more accurate estimate of comprehension, one less contaminated by decoding ability.

Another important difference between the two tests of reading comprehension concerns the type of comprehension question they contain. Bowyer-Crane and Snowling (2005) analysed the nature of the comprehension questions in each test. Only 14 per cent of the questions in the NARA-II could be answered on the basis of literal information provided in the text, whereas 32 per cent of the WORD questions could be answered this way. Bowyer-Crane and Snowling (2005) also found that the NARA-II contained more knowledge-based inference questions. Such inferences are essential to the text comprehension process, and they can only be answered correctly by reference to the reader's real-world knowledge. In contrast, the WORD test was characterized by questions tapping elaborative inferences. Unlike knowledge-based inferences, elaborative inferences are not necessary for text comprehension but instead serve to enrich a reader's representation of the text. Interestingly, children selected as poor comprehenders on the basis of their poor performance on the NARA-II did not necessarily perform poorly on the WORD comprehension test. This finding is consistent with research discussed earlier highlighting the difficulties that poor comprehenders have with drawing necessary inferences (e.g. Oakhill, 1984). It also serves to highlight that different tests measure different aspects of reading comprehension, and, as Bowyer-Crane and Snowling (2005) caution, 'practitioners need to be aware that the use of a single test of comprehension may not be adequate to assess a child's specific educational needs' (p. 199).

In contrast to the question–answer format of both the NARA-II and the WORD, many group-administered reading tests have a multiple-choice sentence-completion format. Each item typically contains a sentence with a blank space, and the child has to choose the appropriate word from a list of four or five distracter items (e.g. 'He ran home _____ to show his mother the letter' quick, quickly, quite, slow, quiet). The *Suffolk Reading Scale* (Hagley, 1987), a popular reading test used in British schools, is an example of such a test. It has three different levels to cover the range from 7 years to 14 years of age, and within each level, there are two parallel forms. The time allowed for the test is 20 minutes, and children are encouraged to continue with the test until the time limit is reached.

Despite the popularity of this type of test, important questions need to be asked concerning their validity. As they are group-administered, it is impossible to ascertain (on the basis of the test result alone) why a particular child performs poorly. It is important to consider what underlying skills each reading test is measuring and to question fully why a child may succeed or fail at a particular test. As sentence context needs to be understood in order to complete the Suffolk Reading Scale, it is tempting to assume that the test is measuring reading comprehension skill and to interpret satisfactory performance on this test as indicative of satisfactory comprehension. However, Nation and Snowling (1997) reported that performance on the Suffolk Reading Scale was predicted by reading accuracy (as measured by non-word reading or the recognition of single words) but not by listening comprehension, suggesting that it is more sensitive to individual differences in reading accuracy rather than reading comprehension. More worrying, children with reading and listening comprehension impairments generally performed at an age-appropriate level on the Suffolk Reading Scale. Thus, children with severe comprehension difficulties can score well on a sentence-completion test. Conversely, children with dyslexia may perform poorly on sentence completion tasks because of the demands they place on decoding skills, rather than because they do not understand the sentences.

In summary, although group-administered tasks are useful for screening a large number of children to identify those with reading difficulties, such tests do not detail the nature of a child's difficulty. Moreover, Nation and Snowling's (1997) findings offer a cautionary note as they show that reading comprehension difficulties are not always revealed by group-administered tests. It thus seems that individually administered tests of comprehension are required if the difficulties of poor comprehenders are to be identified and their needs met. Finally, regardless of how a reading comprehension impairment is identified, it is important to remember that the underlying causes of the impairment also need to be identified. As is clear from the four case studies described earlier, comprehension may fail for various reasons. If appropriately targeted interventions are to be put into place, it may be necessary to investigate oral language skills, cognitive skills such as attention, memory and executive function, and general behaviour, in addition to a thorough assessment of literacy (see Chapters 5 and 8 in this volume).

Conclusions

Identifying children who read well but fail to understand what they have read raises many theoretical questions and, of course, practical concerns. First and foremost, poor comprehenders exist. Our screening methods suggest that approximately 10–15 per cent of the population of 7–11-year-old children have specific reading comprehension weaknesses. These children demonstrate that the possession of fluent reading accuracy is no guarantee that successful comprehension will follow. In our experience, many of these children are not identified as having a reading comprehension difficulty. Why might this be? Arguably, the most obvious index of a child's reading ability is how accurate he or she is at reading words and texts. Children with these obvious difficulties are likely to be very noticeable in the classroom. In contrast, poor comprehenders read accurately and fluently. Their difficulties are seldom recognized in the classroom, and it is only when they are tested that their underlying difficulties with reading comprehension are revealed. Thus, one practical application of our work is to suggest that classroom assessments of children's reading make every effort to assess the comprehension of extended text or discourse, rather than word recognition or sentence comprehension (Bowyer-Crane and Snowling, 2005; Nation and Snowling, 1997).

A related point concerns the developmental course of poor reading comprehension. With the exception of some of the studies investigating extreme cases of hyperlexia in clinically referred children, most studies of poor comprehenders have been concerned with children in the middle-to-late primary years. An interesting and important question concerns what happens to these children as they get older. Their difficulties are unlikely to be transient: both David and Edward above showed consistent patterns of poor reading comprehension over time, and preliminary data from our longitudinal sample suggest that David and Edward are not atypical. This is worrying given that, as children get older, so much of the curriculum comes to depend heavily on reading comprehension. Although it is an empirical question, it seems likely that poor comprehenders will face educational difficulties across the whole curriculum as they get older.

It is clear that reading comprehension is a complex process, a corollary of which is that children may fail to comprehend for a number of different reasons. The four children considered in this chapter all showed reading comprehension skills that lagged well behind their ability to decode and recognize print. However, the four children are very different, and potentially the reasons why they failed to comprehend may also be different. Many poor comprehenders show oral language weaknesses and, for a substantial minority, their level of language impairment is fairly severe (Nation et al., 2004). For other children, however, their difficulties may be a consequence of more general or non-linguistic factors. For some children, their reading profile may need to be considered alongside other developmental difficulties such as NLD or autism. Another possibility is that some poor comprehenders lack appropriate environmental input or support. An important task for future research is to begin to tease apart these different routes to poor comprehension. This will help to identify early risk factors associated with poor reading comprehension; in turn, these should point the way to methods of effective assessment and intervention for children with poor reading comprehension.

CHAPTER 8

Short-term memory: assessment and intervention

MAGGIE VANCE AND JANE E. MITCHELL

Children and adults with language and literacy difficulties often show considerable difficulty with short-term memory (STM), as described by the individuals themselves and by their teachers and clinicians. Assessment findings often show weaknesses in performance on STM tasks, such as recalling digits in serial order (digit span). In this chapter, we will describe some of the theoretical perspectives on STM and the nature of the difficulties experienced by some children, before proceeding to discuss suggestions for assessment and intervention. In order to assess and remediate STM problems, it is vital to have a good theoretical understanding as there is no simple prescription that suits every person. An understanding of which problems in the classroom are caused by STM as opposed to long-term memory difficulties is also necessary for planning appropriate intervention.

Deficits in STM will have an impact on any task that involves listening and comprehension, including understanding instructions, videos and stories. In reading, STM is needed during decoding, in particular for remembering which sounds (phonemes) have been identified while analysing the subsequent letter strings before synthesizing the word's pronunciation. In spelling, the child will have a visual record of which letters (graphemes) he or she has reached in the word. For reading comprehension, children need to remember previous information and context, and in writing, to remember their ideas about what they are going to say. STM is essential for the completion of mental arithmetic and for copying from the board. It can also affect other aspects of learning, for example the acquisition of new vocabulary and concepts. In contrast, difficulty in remembering what was done in the last lesson, or even earlier that day, and recall of vocabulary, spellings or facts that have been learned previously can be considered to be failures of long-term memory, as can some word-finding difficulties and problems with revision or the recall of information during exams. Bringing the right books to the lesson, remembering to take home letters and turning up to appointments also reflect long-term memory problems. However, short-term and long-term memory interact, and therefore STM difficulties will affect consolidation in long-term memory, and long-term memory difficulties will affect STM performance (Hulme, Maughan and Brown, 1991).

Models of short-term memory

Much of the current research into STM is based on the working memory model, first described by Baddeley and Hitch (1974). This is designed to account for the limited capacity of STM in the temporary storage of material. The model proposes three components (Figure 8.1): a core system, the central executive; and two slave systems, the visuospatial sketch pad (retaining visual and spatial information) and the phonological loop, which maintains speech-based material in STM. More recent modifications to the basic model, such as the episodic buffer will not be discussed here.

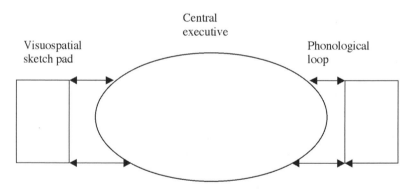

Figure 8.1 Working memory model (adapted from Gathercole and Baddeley, 1993).

The central executive is a complex system that controls the slave systems and is therefore involved in the processing of information that is being retained in STM. It is thought to select, control and monitor attention; it is, for example, involved in switching from one task to another, and in selectively attending to incoming information while rejecting other information, as well as in manipulating information in long-term memory systems (Baddeley, 1996).

The phonological loop (Figure 8.2) consists of a store in which material to be remembered is held in a phonological form for between 1.5 and 2 seconds (Baddeley, 1990). A sub-vocal rehearsal process involves 'repeating'

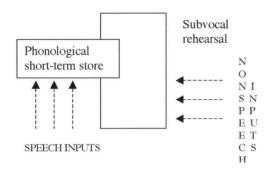

Figure 8.2 Phonological loop (diagram from Gathercole and Baddeley, 1993).

the material to be remembered, usually subconsciously or with an 'inner voice'. This rehearsal process refreshes material held in the store, allowing it to be maintained for longer. Visual material that can be encoded verbally, such as written words or pictures, may also be retained by the phonological loop (Gathercole and Baddeley, 1993). The model suggests that such visual input is first coded in a speech-based form by 'naming' the pictures or words through the sub-vocal rehearsal process. From about 7 years of age, this may be the primary means of recalling nameable visual information (Palmer, 2000a), whereas the visuospatial sketchpad receives visual material either directly from perception or from generated visual images (Baddeley, 1990; Baddeley, Wilson and Watts, 1996).

The working memory model provides a useful framework for a discussion of how STM functions. First, it is helpful to distinguish between the terms 'short-term memory' and 'working memory'. To an extent, these concepts overlap, but it is important to distinguish them. Swanson (1993, p. 87) defines STM as a 'small amount of material held passively and then reproduced in untransformed fashion', for example, when a telephone number is remembered for the time taken to dial the number. In contrast, working memory is defined as holding 'a small amount of material in mind for a short time, while simultaneously carrying out further operations' (Swanson, 1993, p. 87). A good example of the use of working memory comes from considering performance during a mental arithmetic task. Following presentation of the numbers, each has to be held in temporary storage prior to its use in the calculation. The products of each calculation similarly have to be held in store during further processing stages. The arithmetic process thus requires not only STM, but also the allocation of attention during processing operations; it therefore poses complex working memory demands. Within the working memory model, the operation of the phonological loop accounts for performance on simple STM tasks, and is related to memory span, whereas complex working memory tasks also involve the central executive.

Second, it is important to consider how the storage of material relates to its processing. Here it is useful to think of a limited-capacity mental resource that is used for both the storage and processing of material, with some trade-off between the two. Thus, if the processing of material is relatively 'easy', more resource is available for storage than if processing is more 'difficult'. Brady (1991) illustrates this idea by representing the working memory system as a 'pie'; if perception and/or encoding of the material to be remembered requires one quarter of the 'pie', three-quarters are left over for recall. If encoding is easier, and takes up a smaller proportion of the 'pie', more of the resource becomes available for working memory operations (processing).

It follows that, in contexts where encoding is difficult, perhaps because of within-child factors such as processing deficits, or because of external factors such as background noise, the ability to remember the material will be reduced. Thus, poor working memory resources may result either because of processing inefficiency within a standard capacity, or from a reduced overall storage capacity (de Jong, 1998). To take an example from the reading process, a poor reader will expend much of the available resource on decoding, leaving little capacity available for remembering the words, with knock-on effects for comprehension (see Chapter 7 in this volume). The solution to this problem is to achieve a higher level of automaticity of decoding skills, such that decoding utilizes less capacity and frees up more resources for text comprehension and memory. Memory can also benefit from a 'reviewing' process, in which material to be learnt is re-examined at optimum intervals for learning. Further descriptions of this process are available in Buzan (2003), and Mitchell (2000) shows a practical method by which this process can be facilitated for children with dyslexia and other learning difficulties.

Short-term memory versus long-term memory

The STM system store is limited in capacity and therefore in the amount of information that can be stored at any time. STM is also fleeting, possibly lasting only 1.5–2 seconds, as suggested above. This temporary nature of STM means that unless information is transferred to long-term memory, it will be lost. Baddeley (1990) describes different kinds of long-term memory, such as semantic and episodic memory. Remembering what was done in a lesson the previous day taps into long-term memory, as does holding on to a verbal message for the 5–10 minutes it may take to deliver it. In reading a sentence, paragraph or story, earlier-occurring words and information may require retention in long-term memory. Where the transfer of information from STM does not occur automatically, active intervention may be required.

It is generally accepted that STM skills and deficits have an impact on learning and on long-term remembering (Bristow, Cowley and Daines, 1999; Levine, 1990). Material to be learnt or remembered in the long term must be retained in the short-term while long-term memory representations are established. To illustrate this relationship, one can view STM as a postbox, with the size of the posting slot reflecting the individual's STM capacity. Information destined for long-term memory is 'posted' into the STM. If it is too big to fit through the 'slot' (over-size for current capacity), it cannot get through to long-term memory. If the material is broken down into small enough chunks to fit through the 'slot', it may be able to move through the system into longer-term store.

Repeated presentation of the same material, or rehearsal, may not be enough for a transfer from STM to long-term memory for children with language or literacy difficulties. A child may have repeated exposure to a word or concept and still not learn it, or may copy a spelling hundreds of times but still not remember it. A different approach is needed rather than yet more practice. It has been known for many years that transfer to long-term memory is facilitated by how deeply material is processed. Craik and Tulving (1975) presented people with experimental word lists and asked them either to fit each word into a sentence (semantic processing), to identify whether it was written in upper or lower case (visual judgement), or to decide whether the word rhymed with another word (phonological coding). The people who had processed the words semantically showed a better incidental learning of the words, suggesting that processing at the level of meaning has a more beneficial effect on longer-term remembering than does visual or phonological processing of the same material. This finding has important implications for teaching children who have specific learning difficulties.

Development of short-term memory

Children can remember more pieces of information as they get older. Gathercole (1999) reports that 4-year-old children can recall two to three items, 12-year-olds can recall about six items, and by 15 years of age, STM is at adult levels. Miller (1956) was the first to suggest that adults can recall seven, plus or minus two, items and this has not been refuted. It is important to have realistic expectations for what it might be possible for children of different ages to remember and to acknowledge that, within the range of normal variation, even some adults who function well in the real world may have a span of only five items.

An examination of why STM improves with age may give pointers for intervention. One clear change appears to be in the use of sub-vocal rehearsal. Evidence from a number of studies suggests that sub-vocal rehearsal becomes established at about 7 years of age (Gathercole and Hitch, 1993) and appears to have a positive effect on STM capacity. At this stage, visual material is coded verbally by naming the items and is retained within the phonological loop. There is individual variation in this development, with such use of phonological coding occurring in some children from the age of 5 years (Palmer, 2000a).

Other factors such as focus of attention, strategies, knowledge, processing speed and efficiency also result in increased memory span with age. Cowan (1997) highlighted the role of attention in remembering. He described an early study by Macoby and Hagan demonstrating that older children are more able to focus attention on relevant aspects of the material to be remembered, and to ignore distractions, than younger children. Older children also develop more strategies such as linking, grouping and chunking that can reduce memory load. For example, chunking of items may occur when familiar units are recognized: '118118', a six-digit string for a 5-year-old, may be recognized by an adult as one item in STM – for example, as a telephone directory enquiry number in the UK – leaving space for several more.

The use of visual memory strategies also increases with age. Palmer (2000a) reported that children as young as 3 years of age made some use of strategies of 'seeing the pictures in their heads' for recalling pictures, and the use of this kind of strategy increased up to 6 years of age. Pickering (2001) also noted a developmental increase in memory for non-nameable visual material and discussed possible mechanisms to account for this, including increased knowledge and a greater facility for shape and pattern recognition, the use of visuospatial rehearsal strategies and increased processing speed allowing children to respond more quickly during recall.

In a similar vein, Schneider and Sodian (1997) discuss four phases of strategy use in children taught memory strategies. In a first phase of 'median deficiency', even children instructed in a memory strategy may fail to improve memory performance. In a second phase of 'production deficiency', children may use a memory strategy when prompted, but not spontaneously. In the third 'utilization deficiency' phase, strategic activity occurs but does not benefit recall; and finally there is a final stage of 'mature strategy use'. As we shall see, intervention in children with STM difficulties involves making explicit some of the strategies that develop more automatically in others.

Short-term memory and literacy

A number of studies have shown significant relationships between STM skills and reading and spelling in children (e.g. Leather and Henry, 1994;

Passenger, Stuart and Terrell, 2000). This relationship appears to be predictive. Thus, Grogan (1995) found that early verbal and visual STM skills (at age 4;6) were related to reading scores at age 7, and Singleton, Thomas and Horne (2000) found that visual and verbal STM skills at age 5 years were more predictive of later reading test results (at age 8) than were rhyming skills (note, however, that they did not measure phoneme skills, which may mediate this relationship; McDougall et al., 1994).

Significant relationships have also been found between STM and measures of phonological awareness (Oakhill and Kyle, 1999; Singleton, Thomas and Horne, 2000). STM, reading and phonological awareness may rely on the same underlying 'skills'; in particular, given the importance of the sub-vocal rehearsal process, speech input- and output-processing skills can be expected to play a key role in STM (Watson and Miller, 1993). Furthermore, Snowling and Hulme (1994, p. 23) suggest that: 'We might consider STM mechanisms to be no more than a by-product of the mechanisms ... that exist primarily for the perception and production of speech.'

Regardless of the precise causal relationships between speech processing, phonological awareness, STM and reading, what is, however, clear is that good STM skills are likely to aid the development of phonological awareness skills as well as reading, spelling and wider literacy skills. The corollary of this is that children with dyslexia perform less well on STM tasks than children who have literacy skills within the normal range (Brady, 1991; Wagner and Torgesen, 1987, see Cain, Oakhill and Bryant, 2004). Studies show poorer performance on word and digit span tasks (generally regarded as phonological loop tasks) for children with dyslexia compared with those with more average literacy skills (e.g. de Jong, 1998). Moreover, STM deficits in dyslexia appear to persist into adulthood (Pennington et al., 1990; Ramus et al., 2003). However, other aspects of working memory may also be important, and children with reading difficulties have been reported to show central executive deficits (de Jong, 1998; Palmer, 2000b, 2000c; Pickering and Gathercole, 2001). Arguably, such deficits may prevent such children from switching between visual and verbal strategies, and thereby the inhibition of less useful visual coding strategies.

In contrast to the verbal memory deficits that characterize dyslexia, there is a general consensus that visuospatial skills are as good as those of children of the same age who are average readers (Pickering and Gathercole, 2001). In fact, some studies suggest that children with dyslexia appear to have superior visuospatial memory skills (Palmer, 2000b; Witruk, Ho and Schuster, 2002) and that they do make less use of the phonological coding of visual stimuli (Holligan and Johnston, 1988; Rack, 1985). In line with this, there seems to be a preference for the visual coding of words by poor readers (Johnston and Anderson, 1998, Palmer, 2000c). Where visuospatial memory skills are relatively intact, it can be useful to harness them to boost STM performance. It is, however, important to bear in mind that some people with reading difficulties have poorer visual than verbal memory (Fawcett, Singleton and Peer, 1998; Goulandris and Snowling, 1991), emphasizing the need for individual assessment and intervention that takes account of individual cognitive profiles.

Principles for assessment and intervention

Materials

A number of research findings in STM have implications for the selection of tasks and materials for STM work. Children may be able to remember more or fewer items, depending on the characteristics of the items themselves. There is, for example, an effect of word length on remembering. More items will be remembered from lists of short, single-syllable words than from lists of longer two- or three-syllable words (Baddeley, 1990). This effect may extend to the number of phonemes within the words. Vance (2001) found that young children could remember more words from lists of single-syllable words with three phonemes (e.g. CUP) than from lists of words with four phonemes (e.g. DRUM).

Another way in which the phonological structure of words can affect recall is the phonological similarity effect. Lists in which the words are phonologically similar to each other (e.g. HEAD, RED, BED) are remembered less well than lists in which the words are not phonologically similar (e.g. BED, TREE, CAR) (Baddeley, 1990). Similarly, in remembering pictorial or visual material, there are visual similarity effects (Hitch et al., 1988) such that sets of items that look similar (e.g. RULER, PENCIL, COMB) are recalled less well than sets of items that look dissimilar (e.g. BALL, RULER, HOUSE). Where the recall of sequences of letters is required, both the visual similarity effect (e.g. 'p', 'q' versus 'p', 's') and the phonological similarity effect (e.g. 'p', 'b' versus 'p', 's') could affect remembering.

It is clear that familiarity will have an effect on how many words will be remembered, more familiar words being recalled more easily than less familiar words (Roodenrys et al., 1994). There is also an effect of lexicality, with lists of words recalled more easily than lists of non-words (Hulme, Maughan and Brown, 1991). In using sets of words, pictures or objects for assessment or intervention, variable performance may occur if, for example, the lists used are mostly of longer words on one day and shorter words on another. A hierarchy of difficulty can be employed for teaching and therapy whereby lists that are likely to be easier to recall are followed by lists containing material likely to be harder to recall.

Modality of presentation

Both presentation and response mode may also affect recall. Items can be presented visually as pictures or objects, spoken words, or objects presented for touching. The child's response could be to identify visual material that matches what she remembers (multiple-choice answer), to say what she has remembered, or to touch, make or do something to show what she has remembered. Any combination of input and output can be presented (Figure 8.3), and this combination will affect how many items the child can remember. Vance (2001) found that a group of children aged 4–5 years, who were developing normally, recalled significantly more items when word lists were spoken with a picture-pointing response; the next best recall was for spoken word lists (auditory input) with a spoken response (verbal output); and the poorest recall was for a visual (picture) input and spoken response.

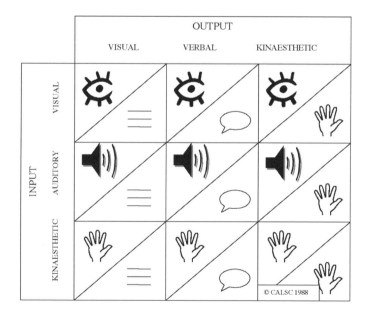

Figure 8.3 Combinations of different input and output modalities in short-term memory tasks.

To summarize, in terms of presentation the child may 'see', 'hear' or 'feel' the items to be remembered, and in response may be asked to 'pick out', 'say' or 'make' the answer. In individuals with STM difficulties, there may be different, individual patterns of which is easier and which is harder. Patterns are likely to reflect learning style, existing strategies and compensations, and individual strengths. A child may, for example, be able to follow "Go and get a test-tube and Bunsen burner" (spoken input and kinaesthetic output) but not be able to repeat a sentence of a similar length (spoken input and spoken output). It is important to note under which conditions a child performs most successfully. These strengths can then be used by parents and teachers, particularly for tasks where recall is important. Allowances should be made for weaker combinations. If, for example, visual output is more difficult, the child may benefit from covering up the answers when completing multiple-choice questions, deciding the answer and then looking for it among the given alternatives, rather than completing it in a conventional way.

Processing

Material may not be processed in the expected way with different presentation and response modes. As has been described above, visual stimuli can be retained in a spoken form (i.e. within the phonological loop), and this is in fact the usual pattern in individuals who do not have language and literacy difficulties, after the age of about 7 years. Spoken stimuli can be

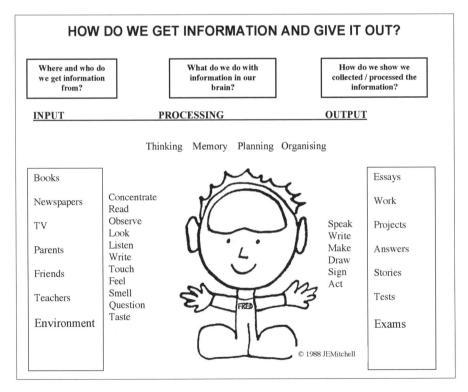

Figure 8.4 An information-processing model of short-term memory.

retained by a visual strategy, probably within the visuospatial sketchpad, and this may happen in individuals with strong visual learning style preferences. Where a visual presentation is used and the pictures or items are left on display while the instruction is given, the child will have visual support for recall. For example, asking the child to "Give me the red pencil and the blue pencil" when the pencils are in view is a different task, requiring different strategies for recall, from one in which the pencils are hidden in a pencil box. That processing is not the same because input or output can be discussed and explained to children with the help of a diagram such as 'Fred' (Figure 8.4).

A holistic view of short-term memory

Many factors can impact on a child's ability to remember and/or to learn, including the child's visual, verbal and cognitive skills, the child's state of health, motivation and confidence. In addition, the distractions within the environment, or the child's ability to filter these out, the child's comfort with the situation and the child's relationship with the therapist or teacher can affect performance. Searleman and Herrman (1994) and Baddeley (1990) discuss the effects of stress and emotion on memory ability. For example, people with depression show reduced recall and fail to use appropriate strategies, such as grouping, to aid recall. In carrying out memory intervention, it will be important to generate a positive attitude in the child, to build confidence and to make intervention contexts safe and enjoyable (see Chapter 13 in this volume).

Assessment of memory skills

A range of materials can be used to assess verbal STM in children. The most traditional measure of the phonological loop is digit span, in which the child hears a list of digits and then repeats them. Such measures are incorporated into the majority of IQ tests and memory batteries, such as the *Wechsler Intelligence Scale for Children III* (*WISC-III*; Wechsler, 1992), the *British Ability Scales II* (*BAS-II*; Elliott, Murray and Pearson, 1983) and the *Working Memory Test Battery for Children* (*WMTB-C*; Pickering and Gathercole, 2001). These tests usually start by presenting two digits and, if the child repeats these successfully, moves on to three digits and so on until the child is unable to repeat the list correctly. Word span, in which lists of words are spoken for serial recall, is an alternative to digit span and can be a more sensitive measure of STM capacity. Examples of such tests can be found in the *Ann Arbor Learning Inventory* (*LI*; Vitale and Bullock, 1996) or the WMTB-C.

Tests of verbal STM can be usefully supplemented by non-word repetition tasks that assess phonological memory, such as the *Children's Test of Nonword Repetition* (*CNRep*; Gathercole and Baddeley, 1996), in which the child hears a nonsense word and repeats it verbatim. Typically, nonwords of increasing length are presented (Gathercole et al., 1994). There is a large body of evidence showing that children with language learning difficulties (e.g. dyslexia and specific language impairment) have difficulty on such tasks (Bishop and Snowling, 2004), but there is some debate over the proper interpretation of these findings. Specifically, it is not clear how far non-word repetition performance reflects memory and how much it is influenced by speech-processing skills (Edwards and Lahey, 1999; Vance, 2001). If children are poor at non-word repetition, this may reflect a speech-processing deficit rather than poor STM. Similarly, some people might consider repeating sentences to be an assessment of STM (as in the Clinical Evaluation of Language Fundamentals subtest Repeating Sentences; Semel, Wiig and Secord, 1995). Performance on this task is, however, likely to reflect the child's language skills as much as STM skills (for example, the child's syntactic knowledge; Sturner et al., 1993).

Some assessments, for example the WMTB-C and the *Cognitive Profiling System* (*CoPS*; Singleton, Thomas and Leedale, 1996), also target visuospatial STM memory skills. In addition, the central executive component of the working memory system can be assessed using more complex memory tasks. For example, the digit span backwards task from the tests found in IQ batteries requires the child to retain a string of digits while reversing their order for the response, and this processing may involve the central executive. A test of backward recall is included in the WMTB-C (see above), as is another working memory task (Sentence Span), in which the child hears a series of sentences and is asked to say whether each is true or false and then to recall the last word of each sentence at the end. For example, "Ducks swim on <u>water</u>" (true/false), "Cars have <u>ears</u>" (true/false), and a final recall of '<u>water</u>', '<u>ears</u>'. A satisfactory performance on this task relies on good language skills as well as STM for understanding the task instructions, understanding the sentences and making true/false judgements.

A list of published assessments of STM in children is given at the end of this chapter. Although published assessments can establish whether or not a child has a STM deficit, and something about the nature of the difficulty, the score itself may not be as useful as noting the child's strategies, pattern of performance and behaviour during testing. For example, does he whisper the words to himself while doing the task? It may be useful to ask the child, "How did you remember that?" to see what strategies he or she is aware of using. Informal assessment can also help to establish a child's individual profile of STM function. Hypotheses about the child's preferred processing styles can be evaluated by noting the child's ability with different modes of presentation and response, as outlined above, to identify particular strengths and weaknesses. This will enable the teacher or therapist to identify which strategies can best be introduced to the child in intervention. As discussed above, a child may use a visual strategy to remember in an auditory sequential STM test. This should not be viewed as 'cheating' or 'incorrect' as the child is using a strategy that is successful for them.

Intervention for children with memory difficulties

Research evidence suggests that, although it may not be possible to increase actual memory capacity, developing the use of memory strategies can improve STM performance. Turley-Ames and Whitfield (2003) found increases in memory span in undergraduate students as a result of instruction in the use of rehearsal strategies, with more effect for participants who had lower spans before the instruction. A linking strategy, in which the students were encouraged to make up a sentence or a story using the material to be remembered, also had a significant effect on span. McNamara and Scott (2001) also found an improvement in span following training in the use of linking for undergraduates, whereas there was no effect of straightforward STM practice when strategy instruction was not given. Brady and Richman (1994) evaluated intervention with children with reading difficulties. The use of visual imagery had a greater effect on improving STM than did developing verbal rehearsal for those children who had more generalized language difficulties. For children whose spoken language was not impaired, but who had STM difficulties, the reverse was true, with development of use of a verbal rehearsal strategy having the greatest effect. It seems that intervention that focuses on developing the use of strategies can have a beneficial effect on STM. This approach is used in programmes such as *Memory Bricks* (Mitchell, 1994) and *Mastering Memory* (Mitchell, 2001).

Whether or not improved STM has a beneficial effect on reading and language is open to debate. Nevertheless, it is valid to target STM improvement in its own right in children with language-difficulties because of its role in a wide range of activities. Anecdotal evidence suggests that it can have a positive effect on children's self-esteem and their ability to function within the school environment and in everyday life. It may also enable better learning (e.g. in 'posting' information into long-term memory) and reduce frustration caused by poor memory for instructions and other material.

Facilitation

One approach to the management of STM difficulties is to facilitate remembering by differentiating the teaching and structuring the environment. This is appropriate when the main aim is to improve a child's functioning in the classroom. Helping the child to attend more effectively, and guiding the child to focus on important information in the classroom, may improve memory. Children often do not need to remember all the detail of information they hear, only key items. The teacher can use phrases that signal this, such as "Pay attention to . . ." or "This is the important bit of the lesson, remember this if nothing else . . .". Children may also be encouraged to focus on what they are likely to be asked about and to concentrate on just these bits of information, thus reducing overall memory load.

Differentiation should teach to students' strengths, use their preferred modality, chunk information to an appropriate size and present it at the preferred speed. This might include using visual or kinaesthetic presentation styles, removing distractions, using simple vocabulary, simple grammar and short sentences, and speaking more slowly or more quickly. It will be helpful to familiarize the child with new materials/situations and to use familiar contexts to teach new information. For example, use familiar structures to teach new vocabulary or written words, familiar words to teach new grammatical structures, and familiar learning activities and contexts to teach new concepts or information. It will also be helpful to aim ultimately for automaticity of what is taught, so that material is over-familiar and will therefore be processed more efficiently. Children's output processing can be facilitated by using their best output modality, as determined in assessment.

Other support can be given in the teaching of content so that it is more deeply processed and more easily remembered. Examples of this type of support are the use of mnemonics such as 'big elephants can always understand small elephants' for the spelling of 'because', or the use of a story or characters, as in the *Letterland* or *Jolly Phonics* schemes, to remember letter shapes and sounds. This may aid children's recall of specific content later, but they may not be able to generate similar reminders for themselves without more intervention. The use of memory aids, such as diaries, lists or the *Student Organiser Pack* (Mitchell, 1988), will also aid the recall of timetables, homework and 'things to be done'. Adults tend to use this kind of support automatically, but many children do not.

Facilitation offered to younger children without explanation is, although useful to aid the recall of specific material in specific contexts, unlikely to improve underlying memory difficulties and the ability to generalize. As children get older, the facilitation can be made more explicit so that they develop some understanding of what can help them to remember, and skills are then more likely to be generalized.

Metacognitive memory training

The aim of metamemory work is to provide children with strategies that they can utilize for themselves to support memory. A metacognitive approach can be used with children from about 5 years of age. Intervention teaches the strategies for STM that people who do not have STM deficits use automatically. Initially, the normal developmental sequence of strategies can be followed, just as one might use a normal developmental sequence to teach language and phonological awareness explicitly. By the time a child is 10–12 years old, all the strategies of memory can be included, and work can continue into adulthood if needed. It should include developing an understanding of how memory works (Joyner and Kurtz-Costes, 1997). A key principle in this work is that intervention is mediated and not taught, so that the child 'owns' the skills and strategies for him- or herself. Children individually find and prove to themselves which strategies are most effective, allowing confidence in the use of these skills to develop and the children to take control and recognize that they can remember things when they want to. It is not usually possible to carry out this kind of intervention in class as a more individual approach to the development of strategies is needed. It is important to make strategies explicit and then to practise strategies in activities within the classroom for generalization. The focus is on the process of recall rather than the content to be remembered.

Metamemory work will encompass a number of areas. Flavell and Wellman (1977) suggest three components of metamemory. First, children should be encouraged to consider how, when and why they might remember or forget, and recognize, for example, what they remember more easily. Second, discussion with the child might explore task variables, for example the fact that more familiar items are easier to remember and that it is easier to recall the gist of a story than remember it word for word. Last, Flavell and Wellman (1977) suggest the importance of strategy knowledge.

The development of metamemory can be supported by an explicit explanation of different kinds of memory, such as the difference between short-term and long-term memory, and of different models of memory. A diagram of an information-processing model of memory (such as that in Figure 8.4 above), encompassing input, processing and output, has been found to be useful in this context. It can be used to explain how memory works to children, parents and others. For younger children, the model can be built up in stages, using appropriate vocabulary. Older children may be able to understand the whole of the three-part process, and for some it helps them to recognize what they are experiencing. For example, Paul, aged 9 years, responded to an explanation of this model by saying, "Now I see all my memory isn't rubbish, I can input stuff, but the hard bit is finding it again to output when I need to."

Sarah, aged 11 years, described herself as being in a greenhouse: in class she could see the teacher talking but realized that she was not taking in information via the auditory route and so was not processing or remembering what the teacher said. The difference between not inputting (i.e. acquiring) information and having difficulty in outputting information (i.e. recall) is an important distinction. To intervene effectively, assessment should distinguish between these. Bristow, Cowley and Daines (1999) provide a description of ways to differentiate between input and output. Joyner and Kurtz-Costes (1997) give a fuller description of the development of metamemory. The website www.understandingdyslexia.co.uk gives some useful analogies that may also help children and their parents to understand how memory works.

Memory strategies

Individuals are likely to prefer different strategies according to their learning style and processing strengths and weaknesses. Careful assessment and observation, as described earlier, will aid the choice of strategies to be introduced. Observation of the child's response to activities in which these strategies are used will allow the intervention programme to be adapted to suit the child.

Strategies should be developed initially in practice task situations, for example remembering a sequence of very familiar pictures or words. Assessment findings will determine the number of items first presented, and this can be gradually increased as strategies become established. Tasks should allow the child to work through a hierarchy of difficulty, using simple lists as described above to develop the strategies. As the use of a strategy develops, there should be an interaction between difficulty and list length, so that initially a simple list increases in number and then, as more complex material is presented, a shorter list length is used and gradually increased again.

Other ways in which recall can be expanded is with the use of lists of words, symbols or letters that are likely to be more difficult for the child, or by manipulating characteristics of the material, such as increasing word length and using less familiar items. The linguistic and perceptual difficulty can also increase. For example, a set of pictures of a BLUE BALL, BLACK BALL, BLUE BOOT and BLACK BOOT will be more difficult than a set of pictures that do not require both adjective and noun to be recalled, such as SHEEP, HEN, DUCK, CAT (Figure 8.5).

Although it is important to teach memory strategies explicitly without focusing on content, the transfer of strategies, once learned, out of practice tasks to 'real life' should be introduced as soon as appropriate. The benefits of STM work may not be maintained unless work is also done to

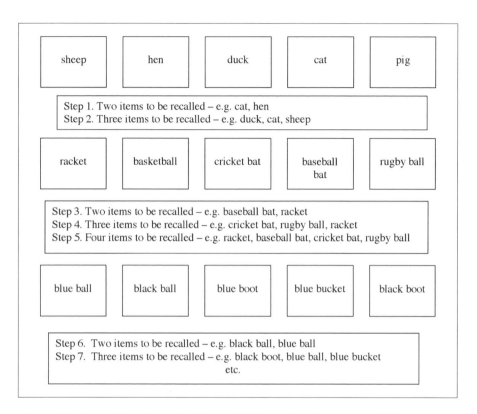

Figure 8.5 Illustration of manipulations of list length and increasing difficulty of item lists presented for recall. The child is asked to remember two or more pictures, as indicated, from the array presented.

transfer the strategies taught to automatic long-term memory, i.e. the child will need to 'remember how to remember'. This can be done by the process of reviewing, as described by Mitchell (2000). Transfer of memory strategies to long-term memory will also facilitate transfer and generalization to everyday situations. That is, it is important to ensure that the child can explicitly recall and describe the 'rehearsal' strategy he or she is using.

Tricks and techniques such as the *Number Rhyme System* and *Roman Room System* (Buzan, 2003) appear to be useful for some individuals. Here, the child is required to associate items to be remembered with those in a familiar sequence (e.g. 'one's a bun ➤ two's a shoe ➤ three's a tree'). However, such techniques may not be so helpful for children with severe memory difficulties because of problems in 'remembering' the linking item and manipulating it together with the information to be remembered in working memory. Some older children find these techniques fun to learn and confidence-boosting in a relatively short amount of time. A few like using them for school work, but for the majority there is too much work involved for these methods to be used independently and automatically as part of their everyday repertoire.

As with any intervention, it is important for both the teacher/therapist and child to ensure that the aims of activities are explicit. Games such as 'I went to Market', in which participants attempt to recall a shopping list of increasing length, or 'Pairs', in which participants take turns to select two face-down cards to try to find matching pairs of pictures, can be used. If, however, the child does not realize that the activity is one in which memory strategies are being practised, there is unlikely to be any beneficial effect or possibility of transfer. For the therapist or teacher, it must be clear what aspects of memory are being targeted. For example, is the input visual or verbal? Is the strategy being practised rehearsal or linking? If work is done on visual memory, it is unlikely to improve auditory memory. A child may become more adept at playing 'Pairs', as a visuospatial exercise in which the positions of face-down cards need to be remembered, but not generalize this to visuosequential memory in tasks such as spelling.

There are several strategies commonly used for STM recall that can be explicitly taught to children.

Naming or labelling

This is usually the first strategy to develop and may be observed in children as young as 2 years of age. The child is accessing semantic knowledge by naming the item(s), and this supports recall. Intervention at this level may not be needed. If it is, the child can be encouraged to label by asking, "What's that picture?", "And that one?". The effectiveness of such a simple strategy can be demonstrated to children by asking them to remember a set of pictures when they are named and asking them to recall a similar set that were not named. Discussion with them can enable them to identify which was easier or harder.

Rehearsal

Rehearsal is an extension of the naming strategy and, as noted above, seems to occur at around 7 years of age in children who are developing normally. There is a wide range of individual variation, and many children seem to be aware of using this strategy themselves. For example, Palmer (2000a) found that many 6–7-year-olds reported that they were "trying to hear the name of the picture in my head". It is, however, a strategy that can be encouraged in children younger than 7 years (Bristow, Cowley and Daines, 1999). With visual material, the child names the items, and with verbal material, he or she repeats back what needs to be recalled. People working with children with language and literacy difficulties often suggest that they have not developed the use of this strategy. Mitchell (2001) describes two kinds of rehearsal: of each item immediately after it is presented, and of the list cumulatively. Sub-vocalization of the rehearsal may need to be explicitly taught, moving from saying the material out loud, to saying it in a whisper, then saying it in your head and finally using a whisper in your head. The rehearsal strategy may be useful in class, for example for remembering some instructions while turning to the right page in the book, or for remembering the numbers in a sum while doing the sum. For some people, however, this strategy may not be useful for long-term memory and learning, and a deeper processing of the material while it is being held in STM is needed, such as processing it for meaning and structure.

Visualization

Visualization is found in some children as young as 3 years who reported that they were trying to see "the pictures in my head" (Palmer, 2000a) and is a common strategy by the age of 6 years. It may be a more automatic strategy than rehearsal for children with dyslexia, so that intervention may involve the validation and expansion of a strategy that the child is already using. The strategy can be used with visual material, by noticing visual characteristics, or with verbal material by creating a picture in ones head. Children can be encouraged to use a visual strategy by asking them to describe the picture and talking about size, colour, what looks the same, what looks different, and so on (see Mitchell, 1994). The *NeuroLinguistic Programming Spelling Strategy* (outlined in the *Magical Spelling Pack*; www.arkellcentre.org.uk) uses visualization techniques to help children to recall spelling patterns and irregular spellings, and is advocated by many practitioners.

Bristow, Cowley and Daines (1999) describe the use of icons and self-generated visual material to aid recall, and this is potentially very useful for children with poor written language skills. For example, children are given a grid into which they can draw their own icons as they listen to a story, and they then answer questions to see how much is recalled. With practice, children may become able to create the icons, or pictures, in their heads. This strategy is an important one as, in school contexts, much material is presented verbally, whereas a child's individual strengths may lie in visual or kinaesthetic processing.

Linking

Linking material to be remembered is useful for short-term recall. It has been used successfully with children with spoken language difficulties (Rinaldi, 1992) and with children with dyslexia (Wilson and Moffat, 1984). Connections or associations are made between the items to be recalled. The strategy can be used to link items on a 'things to do' or shopping list, or to remember factual information. For example, when remembering a sequence of items, a link can be made between the first two items and then between the second and the third, the third and the fourth, and so on. An alternative form of linking is to make a story that links the items to be remembered. For example the items, CAT, TREE, FOOTBALL are more easily remembered through the sentence "My <u>cat</u> Miffy looks behind a <u>tree</u> to find my <u>football</u>", than as three separate items.

The linking strategy may be usefully applied to spellings and may help to facilitate transfer to long-term memory. For example, to learn the spelling of 'stationery', one could use 'the kind of station<u>e</u>ry that means envelopes has an e, as in envelopes'. New vocabulary may be linked with known vocabulary, such as the SOURCE of a river linked to 'sauce' (presuming the child knows and suggests this word him- or herself) and visualized as a sauce bottle spilling blue liquid for the start of the river. (This example was generated by a child to help himself remember how to say the word and remember its meaning; he was not at a stage where he could be expected to spell it as well.)

Chunking

Chunking is the dividing up of information into sections so that a smaller number of 'units' are being stored for recall. It allows the recall of material in sequential order. For example, in remembering the telephone number 01748526135, the numbers can be chunked as 01 74 85 26 13 5. For individual children, the size of chunk that they can recall should be established. Intonation can also be used to aid chunking. It is a useful strategy for copying from the board, as the child can retain the spelling or the word in the correct order. Alternatively, if the child organizes the figures into an 'area code' and 'two lots of three numbers', 01748 526 135, this chunks the 11 digits into three groups that resemble a UK telephone number. Adding a semantic structure can aid the transfer to long-term memory.

Grouping

Grouping involves the organization, reordering or categorizing of material and cannot usually be completed quickly enough for STM tasks. Material may not be retained in sequential order. Grouping is, however, an essential skill, useful for study and for the learning and transfer of information into long-term memory. A range of criteria or characteristics can be used for grouping, such as visual, auditory (e.g. the sound of the first grapheme), semantic, word family or emotional response (like/dislike). Careful questioning, such as "Are there any that could go together?" or, more specifically, "Are there any with the same first sound?", will enable children to construct groups. Children should then be encouraged to develop their own ideas about how any set of items can be grouped.

Transfer and generalization

Moely et al. (1992) found that children who were taught strategies, but not overtly encouraged to use them, seldom generalized their use. When, however, children were encouraged to do so, they were more likely to use strategies effectively in different situations. Transfer and generalization are discussed by Mitchell (1994, 2001) and by Lake and Steele (2000), the latter using the Feuerstein term 'bridging' to describe transfer.

If STM activities are presented as 'games' with no explanation of their purpose, children may not see the relevance of the activities for improving their STM. Transfer of the skills developed may not occur unless the value of what is being taught is made explicit to the child. Children's memory skills may not improve in class after time spent on popular memory games such as 'Kim's Game', 'Pairs', and 'I Went to Market' in small group or individual lessons. For transfer and generalization to occur, it is important to introduce STM work as being useful and relevant to the child, explaining that this work will help him or her to remember in a range of different situations. Various questions can promote discussion that enables children to see how strategies can be useful, such as "When your teacher tells you to do things in class and you are not sure what to do because you have forgotten what she said, how do you feel?", "Would you like to remember what people tell you to do better?" or "What's hard in the classroom?" Memory work can then be introduced with an explanation of why you are doing the activities, what they are for, how they will help in real life, and how this is something that the children can use for themselves. It may be helpful to refer back with individual children to the list of things they have noted as being difficult as STM strategies are practised, and to discuss contexts in which the strategies could be used. This may counteract the children's belief that they have a poor memory and that there is little they can do about it. Conscious knowledge about short-term and long-term memory strategies will allow the child to help him- or herself to remember.

An essential element of STM intervention is to help the child to 'remember when to remember' so that strategies are used in classroom and everyday contexts. Parents and other staff working with the child can often help with this process, if instructed appropriately. Discussion on "How are you going to remember this?" before starting a task or giving an important instruction in individual work, in the classroom or at home will prime the child to consider what strategies he or she can use. The revision of memory strategies to ensure transfer to long-term memory has been mentioned above (Mitchell, 2000). If attention is not paid to this phase of the learning cycle, the work done assessing and teaching the strategies of STM will be wasted as the strategies will not be transferred to automatic long-term memory and generalized to everyday use.

Conclusions

Children with language and literacy difficulties may experience significant difficulties with STM. Careful assessment can indicate the nature of these difficulties and the child's existing profile of strengths and weaknesses. It is important to consider the range of ways in which information is processed. Metacognitive memory training encompasses developing the children's understanding of how memory works and their ability to use a range of strategies that they have not accessed automatically. It can provide children with STM difficulties with skills that support not only their ability to remember material in the short term, but also the transfer of material to long-term memory. This can have beneficial effects on recall and learning, and on a child's self-esteem. Metamemory work carried out by a therapist or teacher can achieve results because strategies are taught explicitly to individual children for them to take control of for their own use. The ideal situation for the maximum transfer and generalization of skills is when teachers, parents and others understand how STM functions and understand the individual child's pattern of strengths and weaknesses. This allows strengths to be utilized and strategies provided to support weaker skills in everyday situations. Facilitation within the classroom can also aid the child's ability to recall material. Other techniques, such as the use of memory aids, can further support memory.

Appendix 1: Resources and publications

Intervention in memory difficulties

Bristow J, Cowley P, Daines B (1999) Memory and Learning A Practical Guide for Teachers. London: David Fulton Publishers; provides explanations of different aspects of memory and very practical suggestions for strategies to use in the classroom.

Buzan T (2003) Master Your Memory. London: BBC Books; describes some of techniques for remembering.

Buzan T (2003) Use Your Head. London: BBC Books; describes the transfer of material to long-term memory by reviewing.

Johnson M (1997) Lost in a moving stream – auditory sequential memory deficits. Speech and Language Therapy in Practice Winter: 18–21; discusses issues in assessment and intervention in STM for children with language impairments.

Lake M, Steele A (2000) Improving Memory Skills. Birmingham: Question Publishing; presents the philosophy of adapting and bridging, with some useful activities to develop strategies. (The order of presentation within the text may not the most helpful one. We recommend choosing activities according to the hierarchy presented in this chapter.)

Levine M (1990) Keeping a Head in School. Cambridge MA: Educators Publishing Service; provides practical suggestions for maintaining attention, explanations of different aspects of memory and ideas developing memory.

Levine M (1993) All Kinds of Minds. Cambridge MA: Educators Publishing Service; a book of stories for children about a range of learning difficulties, including those with poor memory skills.

Malone G, Smith D (1996) Learning To Learn: Developing Study Skills With Children who Have Special Educational Needs. Tamworth, Staffordshire: Nasen; describes the process of learning and how to develop learning skills, using case studies.

Mitchell JE (1994) Enhancing the Teaching of Memory Using Memory Bricks. London: Communication and Learning Skills Centre; describes an intervention to develop strategies to support short-term memory.

Pearce H (1998) Developing a 'Learning Culture' in Your Classroom. Wyton, Cambridgeshire: School Support Agency; outlines practical ideas on using mind maps, memory techniques, etc.

Saunders K, White A (2002) How Dyslexics Learn. Evesham, Worcester: Patoss; illustrates the importance of motivation, with hints on learning and memorizing spellings and maths, and revision for examinations.

Squires G, McKeown S (2003) Supporting Children with Dyslexia. Birmingham: Questions Publishing; provides ideas for facilitating learning together with useful strategies for mainstream classrooms.

Intervention resources

Jolly Phonics. Jolly Learning Ltd, Tailors House, High Road, Chigwell, Essex, IG7 6DL,UK; www.jollylearning.co.uk

Letterland, Collins Educational, HarperCollins Publishers, Westerhill Road, Bishopbriggs, Glasgow, G64 1BR, UK; www.letterland.com

Magical Spelling Pack, Helen Arkell Dyslexia Centre, Frensham, Farnham, Surrey, GU10 3BW, UK; www.arkellcentre.org.uk

Mastering Memory v4 (2002) A computer-based therapy tool for children and adults that presents material visually, auditorally and both together, in sequential form. The manual describes how to develop memory and memory strategies, and to transfer skills to the classroom and everyday life. Communication and Learning Skills Centre, PO Box 621, Sutton, Surrey, SM1 2DY, UK; www.calsc.co.uk

Memory Booster (2004) Computer-based games for children, with some mention of memory strategies. Material is presented visually but not sequentially so differs from Mastering Memory (see above). Beverley, East Yorkshire: Lucid Creative Limited; www.memory-booster.com

Time2Revise (2000) CALSC: Communication and Learning Skills Centre, PO Box 621, Sutton, Surrey, SM1 2DY, UK; www.time2revise.co.uk

www.understandingdyslexia.co.uk – a downloadable leaflet, part of which gives useful analogies for explaining memory.

Materials to support kinaesthetic and visual learning

Active Designs, produce tactile curriculum materials for vocabulary and concepts. Unit 6, Home Farm Business Park, Church Way, Whittlebury, Northants, NN12 8XS, UK; www.activedesigns.co.uk

Cued Articulation and Cued Vowels by Jane Passy, a series of hand postures that can support sound–letter learning and phonics. STASS Publications, North Road, Ponteland, Northumberland, NE20 9UR, UK; www.stasspublications.co.uk

Edith Norris Letter-case, Helen Arkell Dyslexia Centre, Frensham, Farnham, Surrey, GU10 3BW, UK; www.arkellcentre.org.uk

Lakeland Educational, produce dry-wipe jigsaws and other useful materials. Casterton Grange Cottage, Casterton, Kirkby Lonsdale, Cumbria, LA6 2LD, UK; www.lakelandeducational.co.uk

Upwords, uses letter tiles to build up word families/patterns. Secret Games Shop, 20 Osborne Road, Crowborough, East Sussex TN6 2HN, UK; www.secret-games-shop.co.uk, Winslow Press and in toy shops.

Wikki Stix (RNIB), enable a kinesthetic approach to learning letter shapes. The Green Board Game Company, Unit 112A, Cressex Business Park, Coronation Road, High Wycombe, Bucks, HP12 3RP, UK; www.greenboardgames.com

Books including references to memory

Carter R (1998) Mapping the Mind. London: Phoenix; provides a layman's guide to the neuroanatomy of memory.

Grauberg E (1998) Elementary Mathematics and Language Difficulties. London: Whurr; contains a chapter on memory and how it relates to mathematical learning.

Greenfield S (1997) The Human Brain: A Guided Tour. London: Phoenix; discusses different types of memory, such as STM and long-term memory, and how they interact.

Henderson A (1998) Maths for the Dyslexic. London: David Fulton Publishers; includes a description of different learning styles and how anxiety can affect memory.

Rose S (1992) The Making of Memory: From Molecules to Mind. London: Bantam Books; retraces, from a neuroscientist's perspective, the roads leading to our current understanding of memory.

Searleman A, Herrman D. (1994) Memory from a Broader Perspective. Singapore: McGraw-Hill; explores a wide range of issues from theoretical models, through descriptions of different kinds of memory and ideas about intervention, to the effects of emotion on memory.

CHAPTER 9

Phonological awareness and reading intervention

PETER J. HATCHER

It is now widely accepted that training in phonological skills is more effective when combined with the teaching of reading (Ball and Blachman, 1991; Bradley and Bryant, 1983, 1985; Byrne and Fielding Barnsley, 1989; Cunningham, 1990; Hatcher, Hulme and Ellis, 1994; Iversen and Tunmer, 1993). Indeed, this view is supported by the findings of a meta-analysis (National Reading Panel, 2000) that evaluated the effects of phonemic awareness instruction on learning to read and spell. Using 52 published intervention studies, the outcomes from 96 treatment and control groups were compared using a standardized effect size unit called Cohen's d (in which 0.20 is small, 0.5 is medium and 0.8 is large). According to this analysis, the mean effect size on reading for phonological awareness training that makes explicit links with letters ($d = 0.67$) was found to exceed that for phonological awareness training alone ($d = 0.38$).

This chapter focuses on one such approach that we have found to be effective in a number of evaluation studies. I begin by describing the Reading Intervention programme in detail, outlining procedures for assessing children entering the programme, teaching reading strategies and ways of monitoring progress. I go on to describe empirical evidence for the efficacy of the programme before discussing a case study of a severely delayed reader who received it.

The Reading Intervention programme

Assessment

Reading Intervention begins with an assessment of a child's reading, writing and spelling attainments and of his or her strengths and weaknesses in tackling words that are difficult to read or write. The assessment provides normative data for evaluating progress during an intervention. It also provides criterion-referenced data that can be cross-referenced (between tests) for reliability and integrated within a profile of strengths and weaknesses in using text, word and letter strategies. These data are used to derive the first lesson plan. Thereafter, the content of lessons is determined in response to children's reading behaviour. The purpose and a brief description of each assessment measure is presented.

Concepts about print

The purpose of the concepts about print test is to determine whether children have mastered basic book concepts such as directional rules and the function of punctuation marks. An awareness of concepts about print is predictive of future reading development (Tunmer, Herriman and Nesdale, 1988) and is considered to be one of the foundations upon which visual and sound skills, in learning to read and write, are built (Adams, 1990). The test used is based upon Clay's (1985) measure but employs Brown's (1996) book *Look What I've Got!* as the text. Children are asked a series of questions, such as 'Where should I begin?' as the teacher reads the book to them. The test yields information about directional rules, the one-to-one matching of spoken and printed words, the use of meaning to predict unknown words, concepts such as 'first' and 'last', punctuation marks and letter and word awareness.

Early word recognition

The *Early Word Recognition Test* (Hatcher, 1992) comprises 42 words that are commonly encountered in children's early reading books. The test provides an indication of progress in acquiring a bank of recognizable words. It is highly correlated with the *British Abilities Scale* (*BAS*) Word Reading Test (Elliot, Murray and Pearson, 1983) but is more sensitive to differences in attainments at an early stage of learning to read. The test card contains 14 rows of three words and is presented with either one line of print at a time, using a card with a cut-out window, or on seven cards each containing two lines of print. Children are asked to name any words that they know, and their score is the total number of words correctly identified. As with any measure of single-word reading, a profile of strengths and weaknesses in word-reading strategy can be identified from children's responses.

Running record

The running record is a key component of the initial assessment, and of subsequent lessons, as it measures the level of difficulty of a text for a child and provides information about his or her strengths and weaknesses in reading it. The record provides a framework for identifying whether children notice that they are making errors, whether they attempt to correct them, clues that are being used to read difficult words and whether they use the cues in conjunction with each other.

Children are required to read a book, although there may be as few as 20 or so words in children's first books, or a passage of up to 100–200 words from a book. They are asked to do this without any help from the teacher, who records their 'error' (e.g. omissions and insertions of words) and 'self-help' (e.g. sounding-out and self-correction) behaviour using a code. The record yields a percentage reading accuracy score that determines whether the text is at an easy, instructional or difficult level for the child, as well as data that can be analysed to determine whether the child is using appropriate directional movement in reading, the type of clues being used to read difficult words and whether the child is using self-correction and cross-checking strategies. An example of a completed running record is presented in Figure 9.1.

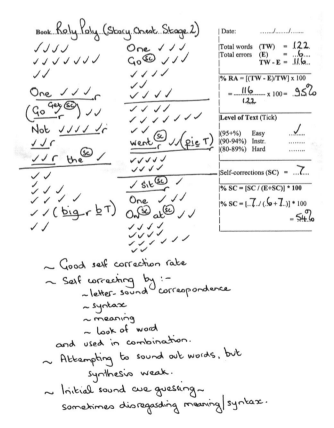

Figure 9.1 A running record.

Letter identification

The purpose of the letter-identification test is to ascertain the number and identity of printed letters that can be articulated by name and/or sound. Letter identification is a strong predictor of progress in learning to read (Gallagher, Frith and Snowling, 2000; Muter et al., 1998; Share et al., 1984). In fact, based upon her review of the literature, Adams (1990) asserts that it is an absolute prerequisite. Children are presented with a printed card containing the 26 lower- and upper-case letters, in the order used by Clay (1985), and are asked to identify as many of them as they can. Having established their preferred mode of identification (that in England following the implementation of the National Literacy Strategy (Department for Education and Employment, 1998), is commonly 'by sound'), any remaining letters that can be identified by that mode are recorded. Children are then asked to look at each letter and to identify as many as they can using the other mode. The test provides a score out of 104 and a helpful insight into which letters might be taught at the start of the intervention.

Written language

The test of written language requires children to write a short story. This test provides information about their level of written language (which may range from writing a few letters to a paragraphed story), as well as their handwriting, spelling, punctuation and ability to read what they have written. When children cannot think of a story, they are read a story about a monster-man with green spiky hair and are encouraged to draw a picture about the story and to write as much as they can about it. They are encouraged to write as much of a difficult word as they can and to put a dash for the rest of it. Afterwards, they are asked to read the story out loud. Their handwriting, language level, punctuation, spelling and reading behaviour are related to attainment criteria. For example, for spelling, a record would be kept of whether children used the initial, final or medial sounds to spell difficult words.

Early writing vocabulary

The measure of early writing vocabulary provides an indication of children's early progress in acquiring a bank of words that they can write, and of whether they exhibit difficulty in forming letters and writing from left to right. Children are required to write their name and any other names or common words that they might be expected to know, and they receive a score for the number of words spelled correctly. The most important information gathered from this test is probably, however, the identity of the words a child can write and evidence of the way in which they form letters when writing.

Phonological awareness

The *Sound Linkage Test* (Hatcher, 2000a) is a normative and criterion-referenced test that measures children's development in acquiring phonological skills. It is another key test because phonological awareness is an integral component of learning to read (Blachman, 1997; Goswami and Bryant, 1990; Rack, Hulme and Snowling, 1993; Wagner and Torgesen, 1987). The Sound Linkage Test has seven subscales, each comprising six items, that measure syllable blending, phoneme blending, rhyme, phoneme segmentation, deletion, transposition and spoonerisms. The 42 item test can be used to determine the point at which training in phonological skills might begin and to measure progress in acquiring phonological skills during the intervention.

Sounds in writing

The Sounds in Writing test provides an indication of the degree to which children are able to use their awareness of sounds to write unknown words. As already noted, it is now accepted that sound linkage (Bradley and Bryant, 1983; Hatcher, Hulme and Ellis, 1994; National Reading Panel, 2000) is an integral component of learning to read. In the test, children are encouraged to write a difficult passage (e.g. A FOX CUB JUMPED OVER THE FENCE. IT RAN ALONG THE PATH.). Their spelling is used to determine whether they can segment spoken words, or parts of words, into sounds and record them as printed words or parts of words.

At the end of the testing period, which often takes place over two or three 35 minute sessions, children are also asked to complete normative measures of word reading and spelling so that progress during the period of intervention can be related to national norms (see Torgesen et al., 2001). The assessment therefore yields a considerable amount of information, some of which may be common to two or more tests.

The next phase is to summarize the 'useful' and 'problem' strategies employed by children under the headings, and subheadings, for Text, Word and Letter strategies. The subheadings for text strategies are Concepts about Print, Directional Movement, Spatial Layout, Error Substitutions, Self-corrections and Cross-checking. The subheadings for word strategies are Word Recognition, Spelling, Writing Direction, Sounds in Words and Writing. For Directional Movement, for example, a teacher might find pertinent information on the record sheets used for the Concepts about Print and running record assessments. For the heading Letter Strategies, information might be found on the record sheets for the running record, letter identification, written language and early writing vocabulary measures. An example of a page from a completed summary sheet is shown in Figure 9.2.

Word strategies

Word recognition (see Early word recognition, Running record, Written language)

Useful strategies
~ beginning to build a stock of words known by sight.
~ initial letter-cue reading.
~ beginning to build a stock of writing vocabulary words – both regular & irregular. Aware of importance of letter order.

Problem strategies
~ will accept a word read by initial letter-cue guessing that does not fit the text in meaning or syntax.

Spelling, and writing direction (see Written language, Early writing vocabulary)

Useful strategies
~ attempting to write unknown words using sounds.
~ aware of doubling of letters, position of each letter in a word.
~ beginning to write familiar 'letter strings'.

Problem strategies
~ able to identify syllables in words, but not all phonemes.
~ not able to link letters with sounds beyond cvc level.
~ reversal of p/q.

Sounds in words and writing (see Sound Linkage test of Phonological Awareness,

Sounds in writing)

Useful strategies
~ able to write up to a 4 phoneme word
~ able to identify & blend syllables.
~ developing ability to reflect upon and manipulate sound structure of words.

Problem strategies
~ some grasp of phoneme blending & segmentation; extension required.
~ extension of use of letter strings, letter/sound linkage.
~ phonemes omitted in words >4 phoneme – no use of syllable division to aid retrieval of sounds.

Figure 9.2 A summary of a child's word-reading strategies.

Finally, the teacher's task is to complete a first lesson plan based upon the assessment information. An example can be seen in Figure 9.3. The profile of strengths and weaknesses revealed by the assessment is helpful

Suggestions for a first 35-minute lesson plan for .... *Amy* ....

	Book level (**13**) and suggested titles	Reading items or strategies, one or two only, to be taught if an opportunity arises
Reading easy books (books than can be read with greater than 94% accuracy), or shared reading	1 *The Big Toe* 2 *Bubble Bath* 3 *The Wobbly Tooth.*	~ use initial sound cue & meaning strategies (already used) to predict an unknown word.
Where applicable, **book to be read at the instructional level** (90-94% accuracy) with the teacher taking a running record. The book should have been introduced and read by the child before the first session. Book level (**14**) and suggested title *Little Red Hen.*		~ praise letter/sound & meaning cross-checking strategy to show that this is a good strategy to use & try again.
Letter knowledge	Identification (letter to be practised)	Formation (letter to be practised)
	p — consolidation of *p* before introducing *q*.	
Phonology	Activities to be undertaken from Sections 1 to 9 of <u>Sound Linkage</u> Section 2 Activity 3 — Syllable blending.	
Writing a story (letter or word to be practised)	*pat* (*hat, fat, mat* etc.)	
Phonological linkage (see Section 10 of <u>Sound Linkage</u>) where applicable	use known word 'sat' (reading/writing) to produce words with similar letter string 'at'.	
Cut-up story (State the objective.)	—	
Introduction to a new book at the instructional level (90-94% accuracy) **Attempt at reading and shared reading**	Book level (**14**) and suggested title	
Comments	Aim = ~ to build on existing skills ~ develop awareness of word structure (sound linkage) ~ to encourage extension of existing text strategies, by showing that they can be used in different ways.	

Figure 9.3 Suggestions for a first 35 minute lesson plan.

for completing the first lesson plan, as is a table that links areas of reading difficulty to strategies that can be used to facilitate progress. These are listed in areas such as letter identification, learning new words, hearing sounds in words, word analysis and text reading.

In a programme that comprises 48 sessions each lasting 35 minutes, the first four are taken up with the assessment of children's reading and writing and the derivation of the first lesson plan. Thereafter, sessions 5–48 follow a similar format and consist of three main sections. The middle section involves work on letters, sounds and writing, and the first and last are spent reading text. The sequence of activities is:

- the reading of a familiar book;
- the teacher taking a running record of the child reading the previous session's new book;
- letter identification;
- phonological awareness training activities;
- writing a story;
- cutting up the story;
- being introduced to a new book;
- attempting to read the new book;
- the shared reading of the new book.

Section 1: Reading text at the easy level, and recording children's reading behaviour

Section 1 comprises two activities: re-reading a familiar book and re-reading a book at the instructional level while the teacher takes a running record. The two activities are expected to be complete in about 9 minutes.

Re-reading an 'easy' book

Each session begins with children reading a book (or books) that can be read with at least 95 per cent accuracy (one or fewer errors in 20 words). The purpose of this is to provide an opportunity to rehearse known words in as many different contexts as possible and to read with fluency, phrasing and comprehension. Teachers are expected to praise children for aspects of their reading that are being consolidated. For example, if a child corrects an error for the first time, the teacher would make a positive comment about that. Where children do not have sufficient reading skills to read a book, the teacher might share a book with them and ask them to point to letters or words, or to guess the identity of a word based on the meaning and syntax of a sentence.

Reading the book introduced at the end of the previous session

Having read one or more easy books, children read the book that was introduced during the third part of the previous session. While they are reading, teachers use a coding system to record the children's responses to between 100 and 200 words of text. Clay (1985) refers to this as taking a 'running record'.

If a book is read with 90–94 per cent accuracy (commonly referred to as the instructional level of reading), teachers introduce another book from the same level at the end of the session. When children have read books fluently and with greater than 94 per cent accuracy on two or more consecutive sessions, a book at a higher level may be introduced at the end of the session. To facilitate finding books at an appropriate level, teachers are provided with a list of about 1800 books categorized according to a formula (Hatcher, 2000b) that is predictive of the New Zealand Ready to Read books (New Zealand Department of Education, 1987). The formula yields 30 finely graded book levels up to a reading age of 9 years and may be used beyond that level. The list of books currently graded is available on the Internet at two addresses:

- www.dyslexia-inst.org.uk/graded.htm
- www.cleo.ucsm.ac.uk/content/sen/cpsbooklist

In addition to helping to determine a book's 'reading level', the running record provides data about children's reading behaviour. It should, for example, enable teachers to determine the degree to which children have mastered concepts about print, letter identification, phonic decoding and the use of visual, syntactical and text meaning cues to decode difficult words. At a later stage of reading acquisition, teachers would look for evidence that children are using these strategies in combination. Having completed the running record, teachers praise children for implementing skills that they are acquiring or consolidating and select one or two teaching points that will be maximally effective.

At a very early stage of learning to read, children might spend time on a letter, a word, print directionality or one-to-one finger-pointing to words in the text. Children who are more advanced in their reading might be encouraged to acquire phonic skills. Normally, they might be expected to identify the sounds (initial, final or medial) associated with single letters within printed consonant-vowel-consonant words, and then either vowel digraphs, such as "ee" in <keep>, or initial and final blends, such as "fr" in <frog> and "nd" in <hand>. They would then move on to initial triple blends, the final <e> rule, silent letters, prefixes and suffixes. For further reading on phonic skills, the reader might like to consult the materials by Davies and Ritchie (1998), Hornsby and Shear (1980), Lloyd and

Wernham (1994) and McGuinness (1998) (see also Chapter 10 in this volume).

In addition to paying attention to letter–sound relationships, children might be encouraged to search for visual, semantic or syntactic clues, or to cross-check pairs of these clues when reading unknown words in text. The essence of this level of work is to encourage children to question whether what they are reading makes sense, whether it sounds right and, of particular importance, whether their attempts at unknown words correspond to the letter–sound sequence of printed words. For example, if a child reads the sentence <He jumped over the wall> as "He jumps over the wall", the teacher might praise the child for correctly articulating the first part of the word JUMPED and ask her to look at the word again to check whether it ended with a 's' sound as in JUMPS. A teaching point might then be made out of changing the suffix <ed> of words such as JUMPED, BUMPED and PUMPED to an <s>.

Section 2: Letters, sounds and writing

Section 2 comprises four activities: letter identification, phonological awareness and linkage, writing a story and the cut-up story. The four activities are expected to be completed in about 17 minutes.

Letter identification

Where necessary, the middle part of every session begins with children learning the names and sounds of letters and how to form them. Although letter–sound identification is very important for reading and spelling, letter names are less confusing than letter sounds when writing irregular words such as THE, ONE and SAID. Letter identification is accomplished through a multisensory approach (feeling, writing and naming) and through the construction of individual alphabet books containing pictures and words associated with each letter. Materials that have been successful in helping with letter identification include the *Active Literacy Kit* (Bramley, 1998) and *Jolly Phonics* (Lloyd and Wernham, 1994). The letter chosen might have been derived from the running record or from a previous session, and examples of the letter might be searched for in text in the third part of the session.

Phonological awareness training

The training in phonological awareness involves a graded sequence of purely phonological activities (Hatcher, 2000a), derived from the work of researchers such as Lundberg, Frost and Peterson (1988) and Yopp (1988), and letter–sound linkage activities. The activities are divided into nine sections:

- the identification of words as units within sentences;
- the identification and manipulation of syllables;
- phoneme blending and linkage with letters;
- the identification and supply of rhyming words;
- the identification and discrimination of phonemes;
- phoneme segmentation and linkage with letters;
- phoneme deletion and linkage with letters;
- phoneme substitution and linkage with letters;
- phoneme transposition and linkage with letters.

The grading of the activities is important. One of the requirements for children to be able to manipulate letter–sound relationships in literacy is for them to be able to isolate phonemes within words (phoneme segmentation). On entry to school, some children are not aware that the sentence CAN I HAVE A BISCUIT PLEASE? contains a number of separate words, let alone that the word CAN contains three sounds: 'c-a-n'. For such children, it may be more important to develop lower-order phonological skills, for example an awareness of words and syllables, than to attempt to associate letter shapes with sounds that they cannot discriminate within words.

One of the early sound linkage activities requires children to push plastic counters into a line of squares marked on a card (Figure 9.4a) while simultaneously saying each word of a sentence. For example, given four counters and the sentence THAT IS MY BIKE, children are expected to push the counters into the squares while simultaneously saying each of the four words. Once children are able to complete such activities with 75 per cent accuracy, they are encouraged to listen for, and to manipulate, syllables in words. Tasks within this section include children clapping in time with rhythmic rhymes (e.g. "One, two, three, four, five; Once I caught a fish alive"), blending syllables to form common words (e.g. "tel-e-vi-sion" to "television"), syllable segmentation using plastic counters, and syllable deletion (e.g. deleting the word FARM from FARMHOUSE to leave the word HOUSE).

After becoming proficient at manipulating syllables, the children progress to blending sounds into words. Phoneme blending is generally easier for children than phoneme segmentation and may be carried out without an awareness of phoneme units. At first, children are simply shown two pictures and asked to identify which of the two they think teachers are trying to say. In Figure 9.4b, for example, they would be expected to choose the picture of a BOY rather than the picture of the SEA when teachers articulate the sounds "b-oy". The blending activities progress to manipulating five sounds to produce words such as CARPET and WHISKER. The section concludes with activities in which the sounds associated with two- and three-letters words are blended to yield word pronunciations, for example <rug> ➤ "r-u-g" ➤ "rug".

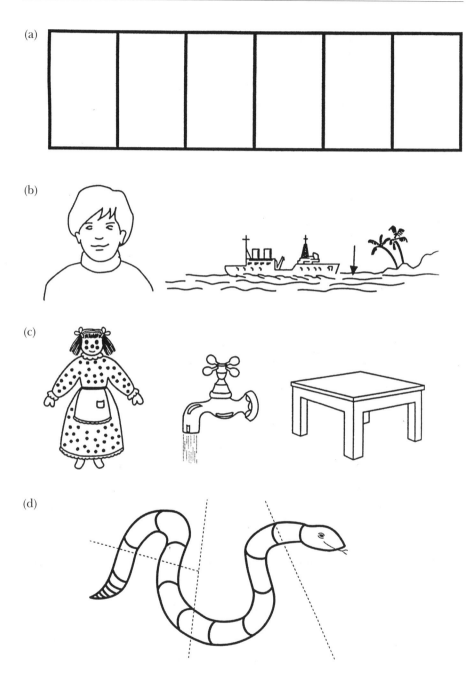

Figure 9.4 (a) Diagram of boxes for pushing counters while segmenting sentences or words. (b) Pictures for blending the words 'b-oy' and 's-ea'. (c) Pictures for discriminating two of three words (doll, tap, table) with the same initial sound. (d) Pictures used, prior to work on phoneme segmentation, to introduce the concept of 'breaking things up' (from Hatcher, 2000a).

Children find it easier to segment words into onset-rime units (e.g. C-AN, M-AN and P-AN) than they do to segment them at any other point. The ability to segment final (CA-N) and medial sounds (C-A-N) emerges later. For this reason, after the phoneme-blending activities, children progress to the identification and supply of rhyming words. One of the rhyming tasks requires them to complete rhymes such as MRS BROWN WENT TO TOWN WITH HER FACE PAINTED – . Another requires them to identify which of three words rhymes with a stimulus word. For example, given the stimulus word HOUSE, the word MOUSE would be the correct response from MONKEY, DOG, MOUSE.

The introduction to individual speech sounds (phonemes) is undertaken by varying the speed with children say words such as FISH, SNEEZING and SUPERMAN. With the aid of pictures, they are then encouraged to listen for specific sounds at the beginning (e.g. 'ssss' in SNAKE, and 'ffff' in FAN) at the end and in the middle of words. Following success with this type of activity, children are asked to discriminate between words on the basis of their initial, end and medial sounds. For example, when presented with a set of three pictures for DOLL, TAP and TABLE (Figure 9.4c), they are asked to touch the two pictures with the same sound at the beginning (TAP and TABLE). A related but more difficult task requires them to indicate which of four words ends with a different sound. For example, SHOOT would be the correct response given the words KNIFE, SHOOT, SCARF, LEAF.

By this time, children should be ready to complete phoneme segmentation exercises, such as indicating the beginning, end or medial sound of a target word. They might, for example, be asked to indicate what sound the word WINDOW begins with. After being introduced to the concept of breaking up words through 'cut-up pictures', of for example a SNAKE (Figure 9.4d), children progress to segmenting words while simultaneously pushing counters into a phoneme frame. For the word LOCK, for example, children would be given three counters and expected to say "l-o-k" slowly, while simultaneously pushing the counters into the squares. Letter–sound linkage activities begin with children being encouraged to identify two of three printed consonant-vowel-consonant words that begin with the same sound (e.g. FIB and fun in the printed words <den, fib, fun>).

The ability to delete or substitute phonemes within words and to transpose phonemes between words normally develops after children have begun to read. Exercises in these sections of the programme include deleting sounds from words, for example 'g' from GOLD, to produce another word, OLD; changing sounds within words, such as the 'a' to an 'ee' sound in BATTLE to form the word BEETLE; reversing the sounds of words, as required to change SAIL to LACE; and transposing the initial sounds of words, for example 'd' and 't' in DOWN TRAIN to produce TOWN DRAIN. Letter–sound linkage activities extend to forming two words using plastic letters (e.g. RED JAM) and transposing the initial letters to form new words (as in JED RAM).

Writing a story

Children are required to write a short story of one or two sentences on the bottom page of an unlined exercise book that has been turned through 90 degrees. The top page is used as a practice pad. One of the aims of the activity is to help children add to the list of words that they can write fluently. When using the practice pad, teachers generally use the multisensory approaches described by Clay (1985) and by Bryant and Bradley (1985) to help children to acquire an initial sight vocabulary. Clay's procedure of 'trace and say, imagine and say, look and say, and write and say' draws children's attention to the overall appearance of words. Bryant and Bradley's approach of 'look and say, write and say the letter names, and look and say' draws their attention to words being formed of sequences of distinct letters.

In either case, children are encouraged to write the words in as many other settings as possible (e.g. using sand, chalk, paint, windows with condensation, plastic letters, large crayons and felt pens, etc.), as well as in their story, and the word would be added to a list of words that is accessible to teacher and child. The first words selected might include those from early reading books or from the list of high-frequency words advocated in the National Literacy Framework (Department for Education and Employment, 1998).

Once children are able to identify letters by sound and are proficient at phoneme segmentation, they are introduced to the notion of using sounds to write words. Using simple, phonemically regular words that children wish to write in their stories, teachers draw a phoneme frame on the practice pad that includes a box for each sound segment of a word. They articulate the word slowly and encourage children either to push counters into the boxes or to listen for a sound, think (and possibly practise) how it would be written and consider in which box the corresponding letter should be written. Children might initially be able to write only the first or last sound. The correct sequencing of letters is attended to after they are able to write each of the letters in the right box without too much trouble.

During the writing-a-story activity, children may also be introduced to 'phonological linkage' activities such as Bradley's plastic letter technique (Bryant and Bradley, 1985). Bradley's technique involves choosing a word from one of a set of words known to a child (e.g. HEN from HEN, MEN, PEN) and encouraging them to form the word with plastic letters. The child is encouraged to make further words from the same set until such time they realize that the task requires only a change to the first letter of the word. This type of work runs in parallel with the phonological awareness exercises in which, for example, a child might be segmenting words using the phoneme frame and counters.

Once children have completed their story, they are encouraged to read it aloud. If necessary, they are asked to point to each word while doing so. If one-to-one reading and finger-pointing is difficult, teachers write the story on card and cut the card into language units (e.g. phrases or words) for children to reassemble. The children then either check their responses by placing the segments on top of, or below, the teacher's model, or simply read the words aloud. The cut-up-story activity remains part of each session until one-to-one finger-pointing has been established, or it may be continued until teachers are assured that children are able to recognize their story words out of context.

Section 3: Introduction to a new book

Section 3 comprises three activities for the children: being introduced to a new book at the instructional level, reading the book on their own and reading it with the teacher. The three activities are expected to be completed in about 9 minutes.

Being introduced to a new book

When introducing a new book, teachers assist children in discussing the plot and draw their attention to any unusual language within the book. This helps children to be aware of words and ideas that will enable them to respond to clues in the text.

Attempting to read the new book

After the book has been introduced, and with support being given when difficulties are met, children are encouraged to read the story on their own. Teachers will almost certainly derive a teaching point from this. Children's attention to letter–sound relationships may, for example, be encouraged. Finally, teachers and children read the books together to encourage fluency of reading.

Reading progression within the programme therefore follows Clay's (1985) cycle of consolidating children's reading strengths with material that can be read with more than 94 per cent accuracy, working to overcome confusions and learning new skills with text that can be read with 90–94 per cent accuracy, and identifying the set of skills to be taught at the next level through a running record of children's responses to text at that level. Most importantly, it also includes additional phonological and phonological linkage activities that are linked to children's writing and reading.

Who benefits from reading intervention? Evidence-based practice

An important question concerns the extent to which phonological awareness training linked to letters, given by class teachers, helps to facilitate reading in young children who are less than 5 years of age on school entry. There is evidence that such training has an effect on the development of phonological awareness (Byrne and Fielding-Barnsley, 1995; Foorman et al., 1997; Whitehurst et al., 1999), but it is not clear that the training generalizes to performance on standardized measures of regular and irregular word reading. One study in which generalization did occur was that of Blachman et al. (1999). In this study, however, the children were aged 5;6 years on school entry. It therefore remains an open question whether phonological skills training and linkage work is of help to children who enter school before this age. From a practical point of view, it is also of interest to know whether such training might help to prevent reading delay in children at risk of experiencing difficulty in acquiring literacy when they enter school.

In England, much of the good practice in intervention studies has been embodied in the National Literacy Strategy (Department for Education and Employment, 1998), which now comprises three types of provision, described as 'waves' (Department for Education and Skills, 2003a). The first wave is a daily hour of literacy teaching for all children. The second is a selection of small-group intervention programmes that are, by revising earlier learning objectives, designed to enable children to 'catch up' to an average level of reading ability. One example of this is the Early Literacy Support (ELS) scheme for children in their second year of school (Department for Education and Skills, 2001a). Children who require a Wave-2 programme are likely to have reading skills below the 25th percentile but with additional help are expected to attain skills closer to the 50th percentile. The third wave comprises programmes such as the Reading Intervention programme that was used in Hatcher, Hulme and Ellis (1994), described above, and we have data to support the effectiveness of this intervention programme below.

It is equally important to gather data on the effectiveness of programmes such as the ELS scheme. In an attempt to compare the effects of the ELS scheme with an alternative sound-linkage strategy, we recently compared the effects of the ELS scheme with a programme of Reading Intervention that was modified for group teaching so that it was more similar to that of a Wave-2 programme. Given the similar content of the two programmes, it is not surprising that we found that both programmes were associated with significant improvements in literacy of an order in keeping with our 1994 study (Hatcher et al., in press). In the next sections, we describe the findings of these studies.

The First Cumbria:York Study

The purpose of our first Cumbrian study was to compare the effects of three forms of structured reading intervention on children experiencing difficulty in learning to read. A total of 128 7-year-old children with reading quotients of less than 86 (the poorest 18 per cent of readers) on the *Carver Word Recognition Test* (Carver, 1970) were divided into four groups of 32. The four groups were matched on IQ, reading ability, age and gender, and were randomly assigned to one of three experimental teaching conditions – 'reading with phonology', 'reading alone' and 'phonology alone' – or to a control condition at time 1 (t1). Following a 20-week period of intervention, the children were reassessed (t2) on the same measures of reading, spelling, maths and phonological awareness that had been administered at t1. In order to determine whether the effects of the intervention were long-lasting, measures of reading and spelling were taken again 9 months after the period of intervention (t3).

The measures of reading included a test of early word recognition (words commonly found in children's early reading books) (Hatcher, 1992), the BAS Word Reading Test, a test of single-word reading (Elliot, Murray and Pearson, 1983), the Neale Analysis of Reading Ability, a test of text-reading accuracy and comprehension (Neale, 1989) and a test of non-word reading that included items such as <um>, <bac>, <blod> and <unplint>. We used the *Schonell Graded Word Spelling Test* (List B; Schonell and Schonell, 1956) to measure spelling and the *BAS Basic Number Skills Test* (Elliot, Murray and Pearson, 1983) to measure arithmetic.

We used four measures of phonological processing to monitor the children's development of phonological skills. These included a modified version of Bradley's (1984) *Sound Categorisation Test* and tests of phoneme blending, segmentation and deletion. The sound categorization test was used to measure children's ability to recognize rhyme and alliteration in spoken words. The phoneme blending test measured children's ability to blend a sequence of sounds into non-words, and the non-word segmentation test required children to segment non-words into separate sounds while pushing a coin forward as they spoke each sound. Finally, a modified version of Bruce's (1964) *Word Analysis Test* was used to measure children's ability to delete sounds from spoken words.

During the period of intervention, the experimental groups received 40 teaching sessions of 30 minutes each over 20 weeks. Children in the control group received the support they would normally have received in school. The 93 children in the three experimental groups were taught by 23 teachers who had been released from their normal duties for training and to implement the teaching. Each of the teachers worked with 2–9 children and generally taught the same number of children (1–3) from each of the experimental groups. The children in the 'reading with phonology' group were taught to use visual reading strategies (after Clay, 1985), phonological awareness, and how to make the link between sounds and the written forms of words (Hatcher, 2000a). Details about the 'reading with phonology' programme are provided in a preceding section. The 'reading alone' group received 'the same' reading training as the 'reading with phonology' group, apart from the omission of any reference to let- ter– sound association activities and phonological awareness. These children received no phonological awareness training or phonological linkage activities. The 'phonology only' group undertook the phonologi- cal awareness training without any reference to reading.

The aim of the study was to assess the differential effectiveness of the three training programmes in enhancing progress in acquiring literacy. The results for text reading, spelling and maths are presented in Figure 9.5. The results for the other measures of reading were similar to those for text-reading.

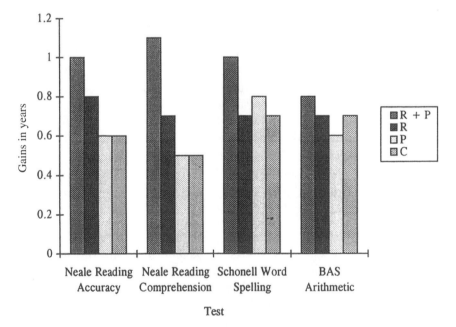

Figure 9.5 Average gains in reading, spelling and arithmetic for the four groups, reading and phonology (R + P), reading alone (R), phonology alone (P) and control (C), following the period of intervention.

It was found that, on each of the five literacy measures, early word recog- nition, word reading, text reading, non-word reading and spelling, the 'reading with phonology' group made greater progress than the control group. It was also the case that, for word and text reading and spelling, the 'reading with phonology' group made greater progress than each of the other groups (Hatcher, 2000c). The success of the 'reading with phonology' group in learning to read and spell clearly could not be attributed to the reading element of its training alone. Neither could it be attributed to the phonological element. The 'phonology alone' group did not make significantly greater progress than the control group on any of the measures of literacy. It did, however, make significantly greater progress than the control group in developing phonological awareness. At t2, the 'phonology alone' group performed better than the other groups on a composite score derived from the measures of sound deletion, sound blending, nonword segmentation and sound categorization (Figure 9.6).

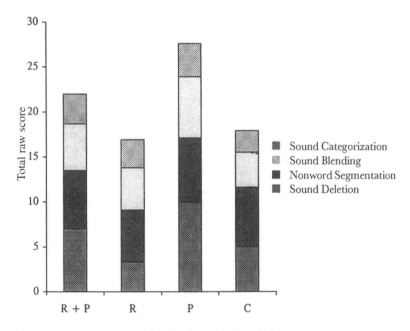

Figure 9.6 Average raw-score gains in phonological ability for the four groups, reading and phonology (R + P), reading alone (R), phonology alone (P) and control (C), following the period of intervention.

The results support the view that phonological awareness training is most effective in enhancing progress in literacy when it is combined with the teaching of reading and writing. Two other important points must be considered. The training effect was specific to literacy and not attributable to factors such as teacher expectations. None of the treated groups performed better than the control group on the maths tests at t2. Also, with reading, but not spelling, the effect was long-lasting. The 'reading with phonology' group continued to outperform all other groups on text-reading accuracy and comprehension at t3 (Hatcher, 2000c). These findings are in keeping with a study by Iversen and Tunmer (1993) and with research that has found phonic methods to be more effective than methods that omit phonic teaching (Adams, 1990).

The results of our study are educationally, as well as statistically, significant. An inspection of Figure 9.5 shows that the 'reading with phonology' group made over a year's progress in text-reading accuracy and comprehension between t1 and t2 (7.43 months), although the teaching lasted for just 20 weeks. This amounts to gains of approximately 1.7 months for each month of elapsed time. In contrast, the control group made gains of just 0.9 months per month.

The second Cumbria:York study

The purpose of our second intervention study was to determine whether phonological awareness training linked to a structured approach to teaching reading (inclusive of phonics) would lead to reading gains in 4–6-year-old children in mainstream classrooms. We also wished to determine whether such training would be beneficial for children at risk of reading failure, and the optimal phonological unit (rhyme or phoneme) for linking sounds to print.

In this study, 20 classes of children (each from a different school) were allocated to four groups, based upon measures such as general IQ, letter identification and phonological awareness. The groups were randomly allocated to one of three intervention conditions – reading with rhyme and phoneme, reading with rhyme, and reading with phoneme – or to a taught control condition 'reading'. The period of intervention lasted for five terms (terms 2–6), with the children being assessed prior to the intervention at the end of their first term (t1, mean age 4;65 years), at the end of their third term (t2, mean age 5;25 years) and at the end of their sixth term (t3, mean age 6;22 years). To assess any durability of effects on reading, the children were also reassessed mid-way through their eighth term (t4, mean age 6;93 years).

The measures of reading included our test of early word recognition (Hatcher, 1992), the BAS Word Reading Test (Elliot, Murray and Pearson, 1983) and the *Graded Nonword Reading Test* (Snowling, Stothard and McLean, 1996). Phonological skills were assessed using two measures of rhyme awareness (detection and production) and two measures of phoneme awareness (initial and final phoneme deletion) that were based on the *Phonological Abilities Test* (Muter, Hulme and Snowling, 1997). Each of the measures was supplemented by the addition of more difficult items (e.g. after Snowling et al., 1994). The *BAS Basic Number Skills Test: Test C* (Elliot, Murray and Pearson, 1983), supplemented by easier items to avoid floor effects, was used to measure arithmetical skills, and the *English Picture Vocabulary Test* (Brimer and Dunn, 1973) was used to provide a measure of receptive vocabulary. We also measured letter identification using 12 letters at t1, and 26 letters at subsequent times of testing.

During the period of intervention, which lasted for 14.5 months, the reading programme involved children being taught as a class, in groups and as individuals while the phonological awareness programmes were taught to groups of 10–15 children for three 10-minute sessions per week. The same amount of teaching time was dedicated to the teaching of reading in all four conditions. During the time that the experimental groups received work on phonological awareness, the control groups spent additional time on reading. The reading programme, adapted from the approach used in our first study, included work on concepts about print, letter identification, words, writing and spelling (including phonics), and text reading. The 'reading with rhyme', the 'reading with phoneme' and 'reading with rhyme and phoneme' programmes included identical work on reading but were supplemented by structured packages of either rhyme and rime-linkage training, phoneme and phoneme-linkage training, or both.

The first aim of the study was to assess whether the addition of phonological awareness training benefited young children at an early stage of learning to read. We also wished to determine whether children who were at risk of reading delay would show particular benefits. We therefore conducted two sets of analysis, one for the children judged to be developing normally (N = 273) and one for children considered to be at risk of reading failure (the poorest third of children based upon scores for receptive vocabulary, letter identification, rhyme and phoneme skills; N = 137). In each analysis, we compared the effects of the intervention for the experimental groups, across the times of assessment, with the progress of the control group.

After controlling for any significant school effects (Rasbash et al., 2000), and differences between the groups on receptive vocabulary at t1, it was found that, within the sample of normally developing children, the groups that had received training in rhyme manipulation developed enhanced rhyme skills, and the groups that had received training in phoneme skills developed enhanced phoneme skills, relative to the control group. However, the effectiveness of the phonological awareness training had no significant effect on the chilren's reading. There was no significant difference between the progress of the three experimental groups of normally developing children relative to the control group. It would seem that if structured phonic work is included in a reading programme, the majority of children do not need training in phonological awareness in order to master the alphabetic principle.

Similar analyses were conducted for the at-risk children. On this occasion, the group that had received 'reading with rhyme and phoneme' training exhibited greater progress in acquiring rhyme skills than the control group, and all three experimental groups exhibited significant growth in phoneme skills compared with the control group. The fact that all three experimental groups, including the rhyme group, made significant progress in acquiring phoneme skills may be due to the fact that, in rhyming tasks, onsets are frequently single phonemes (e.g. 'k' and 'p' in CAT and PAT). Our analyses of progress in word reading were carried out on a composite reading score, derived from the full sample of 410 children, with a mean of 100 (standard deviation = 15). The mean standardized scores for the at-risk sample are shown in Figure 9.7.

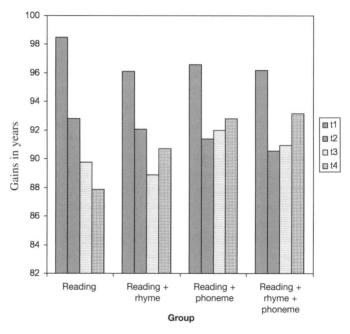

Figure 9.7 Progress in the word reading of at-risk children (N = 137) relative to the total sample of 410 children (data from Hatcher, Hulme and Snowling, 2004).

From Figure 9.7, it is clear that although the children were making progress over time, their reading scores were falling behind relative to those of their normally developing peers. After controlling for any significant school effects, it was found that the groups that had received training in phoneme manipulation developed enhanced reading skills relative to the control group. This suggests that, for the at-risk children, the additional training in phoneme manipulation, and phoneme–grapheme linkage skills, was effective in reducing the extent to which children of average and above-average potential accelerate ahead of them. The effect of the intervention was also specific to literacy. Relative to the control group, none of the experimental groups made significantly greater gains in arithmetic skills between t1 and t4. The effects on reading cannot therefore be attributed to general differences in teaching received during or after the period of intervention.

The absence of any generally beneficial effects of phonological awareness training on reading for normally developing children is in keeping with other reports that training in phonological awareness may yield only small or possibly no immediate gains in reading (Byrne and Fielding-Barnsley, 1995; Olson et al., 1997). Providing additional phonological awareness training may therefore be redundant for most children. In contrast, there is support for providing at-risk children with such training, and particularly for training in phoneme manipulation and phoneme-linkage skills.

The gains of the at-risk children in the second Cumbria:York study were quite substantial. At t4, the average BAS Word Reading Test standardized scores for the four groups were 94.93 (reading with rhyme and phoneme), 94.63 (reading with phoneme), 93.25 (reading with rhyme) and 91 (reading alone). The average difference in standardarized score between the two successful groups of at-risk children and the 'reading alone' group was 3.8 points. On average, the children were achieving at a level that was equal to or better than that of about 36 per cent of children of their age. Had they not received the additional phonological skills training, they would have been doing as well as or better than about 27 per cent of children of their age.

The educational implications of our study are that it is possible to identify children who are at risk of reading delay and to halt the decline in performance in (at least some of these) young children, relative to their peers, if they are presented with a structured programme of phoneme and reading training at school entry. Arguably, if the same amount of phoneme training were to be presented over a shorter period of time and to smaller groups of children (National Reading Panel, 2000) or to individuals, the effects would be larger. Another possibility is that, for very young children, programmes of phonological awareness training should be confined to the teaching of phoneme blending and segmentation in preference to metacognitive skills across a wide range of activities (National Reading Panel, 2000).

The North Yorkshire study

The purpose of this study (Hatcher et al., in press) was to compare the effectiveness of the *Early Literacy Support* (*ELS*) programme (Department for Education and Skills, 2001a) and a modified programme of Reading Intervention in enabling 6-year-old children to catch up to an average level of reading. Based upon the ELS screening criteria for children who are exhibiting below-average levels of literacy, the study began with 16 schools nominating 6-year-old children to take part. We had no control over the assignment of children to groups in that five schools opted to provide Reading Intervention, five to provide the ELS programme and six to provide both forms of intervention. Based upon the percentage of children receiving free school meals, there were, however, no significant socioeconomic differences between groups, and the groups did not differ in terms of the age and level of education of the teaching assistants. Neither did the two groups of children differ significantly on age and measures of receptive vocabulary, phoneme manipulation, letter identification, reading and spelling at t1. Following a 12-week period of intervention, the children were reassessed (t2) on the measures of phoneme manipulation, letter identification and reading. In order to determine whether the effects of the intervention were long-lasting, measures of letter identification and reading were taken again 3 months after the end of the intervention.

Letter identification was assessed using lower-case letters in the order used by Clay (1985), and our measures of reading included the Early Word Recognition Test (Hatcher, 1992) and the BAS-II Word Reading Test (Elliot, Smith and McCulloch, 1997). Phoneme-manipulation skills were measured using the blending, segmentation and deletion subscales from the Sound Linkage Test of Phonological Awareness (Hatcher, 2000a), and receptive vocabulary was measured using the *British Picture Vocabulary Test* (*BPVS-II*; Dunn et al., 1997). Finally, phonetic spelling was assessed using a measure in which children were encouraged to write words such as SKATEBOARD and were awarded points based on the phonetic plausibility of their spelling (after Snowling, Gallagher and Frith, 2003).

Each teaching programme was implemented over the same 12-week period between t1 and t2, in the second term of year 1. The ELS programme involved children working in groups of six for 60 daily 20 minute teaching sessions. The modified Reading Intervention programme required children to work on alternate days in groups of six, for a total of 30 sessions each lasting 20 minutes, and on the intervening days individually with the teaching assistant for a total of 30 sessions each of 20 minutes.

Both programmes include many of the ideas from Reading Recovery (Clay, 1985). Both, for example, include training in phonological and grapheme-linkage skills, recognition of the names and sounds of letters, reading and writing common words, the use of phonic and other strategies to check and self-correct words, the reconstruction of written sentences that have been segmented into words and guided reading. However, whereas the content of the ELS is scripted, the content of the Reading Intervention programme is determined by the teaching assistant after an assessment of each child's strengths and weaknesses in the use of text, word and letter strategies in reading and writing, and in response to progress during the intervention. The Reading Intervention programme also requires more attention to the development of phoneme manipulation and linkage skills (after Hatcher, 2000a).

The aim of the study was to assess the differential effectiveness of the two training programmes in enhancing progress in acquiring literacy. The results for phoneme manipulation, letter–sound identification, reading and spelling are shown in Figure 9.8. Statistical analyses that took account of the equivalent scores at t1, and also spelling scores at t1, confirmed that there was an association (in favour of the Reading Intervention group) between the group and the learning of letter sounds. Otherwise the two groups did not differ on any measure at t2. Further analyses confirmed that both groups made significant progress on all measures between t1 and t2. For reading, the children progressed from a BAS standardized word reading score of 94.2 at t1 to 100.2 at t2, and with a score of 101.4 at t3, they maintained that level of reading for at least 3 months. The rate of gain of 0.3 SS points per hour of intervention accords with that for our first Cumbrian study (0.31) and is in keeping with the rate of gain reported by Torgesen et al. (2001) for successful programmes of intervention. The gains were also maintained for at least 3 months after the period of intervention.

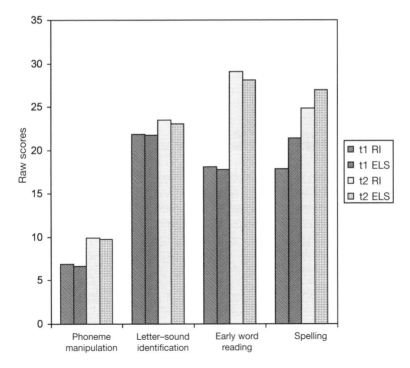

Figure 9.8 Mean scores for phoneme manipulation, letter–sound identification, early word reading and spelling for the two groups (data from Hatcher et al., in press). ELS, Early Literacy Support; RI, Reading Intervention.

From a practical point of view, it is important to remember that the programmes of intervention were implemented by teaching assistants and to note that their success testifies to the important pedagogical role that they are able to play in schools. Whether the children caught up to the point where they were literally reading at the mean level for their age is not clear, however, as we found that in a sample of 303 children, of the same age and from the same schools as the intervention groups, the mean standardized score on the BAS was 107.36. Relative to these children, it might be argued that our sample progressed from a reading score of 86.8 at t1 to 92.9 at t2 and may have required the interventions to be effected over a longer period of time.

The fact that both programmes were associated with acceptable gains in phonological skills, reading and spelling should not be surprising. They exhibit much the same content, having been derived from Reading Recovery (Clay, 1985) and from recent research (e.g. Hatcher, Hulme and Ellis, 1994). Subject to the limitation of our design not including an unseen control group, schools might have confidence in the ELS programme and may feel that, on the grounds of cost, it is the preferred option for children in their second year of school, whose reading is marginally below average. An advantage of Reading Intervention is, however, that learned skills may be generalized to individuals at any stage of learning to read, and, in keeping with the results of our first Cumbrian study, Reading Intervention might be expected to be particularly helpful to those who exhibit greater difficulty in learning to read.

'Sound linkage' – a case study

While group results are crucial for evaluating the effectiveness of a teaching programme, a case study can provide an understanding of what is happening to an individual as he or she proceeds through the programme. David, a child with severe reading difficulties, provides a good example of how reading and phonological awareness training can bring about change during the course of a sequence of teaching sessions.

David's slow progress in acquiring literacy was apparent before he was 6 years old. At 5;9 years, he was not only delayed in his literacy attainments, relative to his friends, but also exhibited poor articulation of some words (e.g. "taktor" for TRACTOR) and spoonerisms in his speech (e.g. "par cark" for CAR PARK), and was slow in his verbal responses to questions. He was also tearful about going to school. On the positive side, he was noted to enjoy modelling, drawing, book illustrations and being read to by his mum.

Some 6 months later, according to his performance on the BAS (Elliot, Murray and Pearson, 1983), David was found to exhibit average general reasoning skills. However, he performed at a below-average level on the visual IQ scale and on subtests that measured the ability to remember a series of spoken numbers, to copy a series of shapes and to read single words. Aged 6;3 years at the time of testing, David was credited with reading at less than the 5 year level. He was also noted to be poor at phonological awareness tasks. Although able to blend syllables, he did not appear to be able to blend phonemes into words, to detect the odd word out in a three-word rhyme-oddity task or to segment words into phonemes.

At the time of the pre-intervention assessment, when he was 6;7 years, David knew most of the concepts about print, but he was not able to point to words as they were read or to make a return-sweep at the end of lines of print. Neither was he able to name or give the function of punctuation marks. He was able to articulate the sounds commonly associated with 19 lower- and 16 upper-case letters, to write a few words, such as <in>, <it>, <Tom> and <me>, and to use initial and final sounds when writing unknown words (e.g. <rn> for RAN). He tended to write upper- and lower-case letters indiscriminately, to mirror-write some letters, to muddle the order of letters in words and to omit spaces between words. He wrote <tehD the-ost> (see Figure 9.9a) for the sentence THE BEAR FRIGHTENED THE GHOST. David was able to read about six words from the Early Word Reading Test. He articulated two of the words, WENT and STOP, after naming the letters according to their sound ('wuh' 'eh' 'nuh' 'tuh' → "went"). He was not able to blend three phonemes into words. Not surprisingly, perhaps, David tended to rely on pictures as clues to text reading.

After the pre-intervention assessment, David received 36 teaching sessions of 35 minutes each. During the first few sessions, his teacher followed a multisensory approach to building a basic sight vocabulary, encouraged David to finger-point while reading, to finger-space when writing or reassembling cut-up stories and to segment spoken sentences into words using counters. He also learned to name and to form letters. After 12 sessions, David was able to point to words as he read but still needed prompting to leave spaces between words when writing. He had progressed from writing simple sentence structures, such as I SEE THE CAT, to more complex forms, such as IF ITS A BADGER YOU CAN SEE, PLEASE TELL ME (Figure 9.9b and 9.9c). He was also using initial sounds as clues in his reading and being prompted to use end sounds. He was also learning how to use capital letters and full stops.

David continued to exhibit difficulty in attending to sounds in spoken words. By session 24, he had only just mastered the ability to identify the medial words in sentences of four words, to tap the syllabic rhythm of poems and to blend three phonemes into words. Nevertheless, his concentration and confidence with phonological awareness tasks had improved. He was also becoming more confident with text, looking carefully at the ends of

(a)

teho.- - - - - - - -

frightened teh-ost

the bear   the ghost

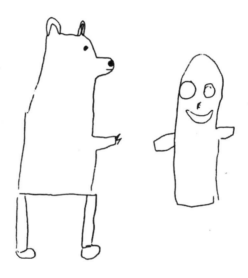

(b)

I see the cat

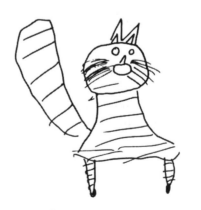

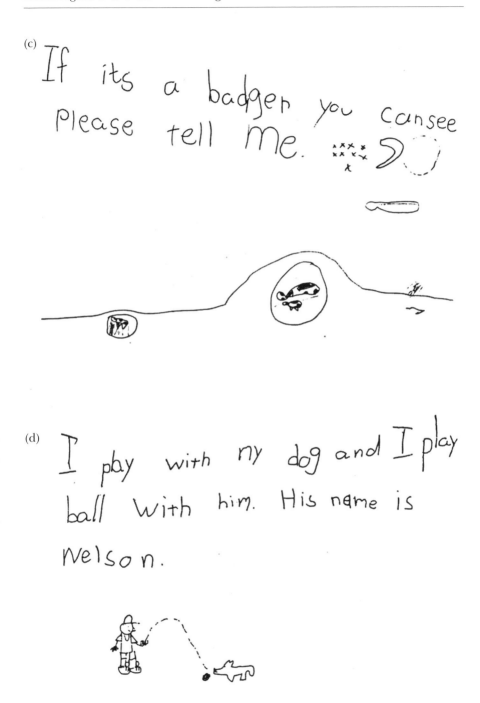

Figure 9.9 (a) Example of David's writing prior to the intervention. (b) Example of David's writing with support in the first week of intervention. (c) Example of David's writing after 12 sessions. (d) Example of David's writing after 36 sessions of intervention.

words as well as their beginnings and correcting some of his errors, although picture and meaning clues continued to be his preferred option. By session 36, David's writing had also shown further improvement (Figure 9.9d).

After the 12 week period of intervention, David was reassessed on the attainment measures employed at t1. On the Sound Linkage Test of Phonological Awareness, he was credited with being able to segment words into phonemes (score 6/6) and with some ability to delete phonemes from words to make new words (3/6). He did not exhibit these skills at t1. His spelling had improved dramatically. He was able to write 'unknown' words using sequences of four sounds and, aged 6;10 years, was credited with an average performance (6;8) on the Schonell spelling test. He was also able to write sentences and to leave spaces between words.

David's word reading was also found to have improved significantly. His reading age of 6;5 on the *Burt Test* (Scottish Council for Research in Education, 1974) was again within normal limits. He continued, however, to exhibit weaknesses. He exhibited difficulty in naming letters, in giving the sounds associated with certain letters ('P', 'B', 'D', 'T', 'G', 'J', 'p', 'b', 'd', 'q') and in reading text. Consequently, his teacher felt that David would need to follow the programme of reading intervention until he had reached a higher level of text reading and was no longer dependent upon her for encouragement and support. There is no doubt, however, that the reading with phonological awareness training programme had had a significant impact upon his progress in acquiring literacy during the 12 weeks of intervention.

Conclusions

It is clear that, over the past 10 years, the importance of phonological awareness and letter–sound linkage for reading acquisition has been accepted. Both components have been included in the UK's National Literacy Strategy (Department for Education and Employment, 1998) and in Wave-2 programmes such as the ELS scheme (DfES, 2001a). In our own studies (Hatcher, Hulme and Ellis, 1994; Hatcher, Hulme and Snowling, 2004), we are now able to differentiate between the phonological needs of young children who are developing normally and of those who are delayed or are at risk of developing reading delay. Explicit and extended training in phonological awareness and sound linkage may be unnecessary for normally developing children who follow a literacy programme that includes phonics, but it is beneficial for children who are experiencing, or are likely to experience, difficulty in learning to read. We also provide evidence in support of phoneme- rather than rime-linkage for these children at school entry.

The active implementation of these findings in schools is encouraging, but, from personal observation, there needs to be a cautionary note. English is not an orthographically transparent language. If the sounds in a word such as SAID are articulated as "suh-a-i-duh", they can rarely, if ever, be blended to yield the correct articulation for that word. Two points follow from this. When articulating the sound of a consonant, the sound should be pronounced, so far as possible, without adding a vowel. Thus, the letter 's' should be articulated as "sss" not "suh". The second point is that letter names should play a role, particularly in the identification of letters and in the spelling of irregular words. Children need to use both letter names and sounds in an informed and flexible manner.

Finally, there is no reason why the Reading Intervention approach should be confined to school-aged children who have a specific difficulty in acquiring literacy skills. We have evidence (Hatcher, 2000d) that, for children diagnosed as having low IQ (mean IQ = 66, range 55–75), a programme of Reading Intervention can be a powerful way of enhancing progress in learning to read and to spell.

Appendix 1: Resources and materials for teaching reading

Bramley W (1998) Active Literacy Kit: Essential Foundations for Literacy. Cambridge: Learning Development Aids.

Clay M (1985) The Early Detection of Reading Difficulties, 3rd edn. Tadworth, Surrey: Heinemann.

Davies A, Ritchie D (1998) Thrass Wordchart. Chester: THRASS.

Department for Education and Skills (2001) The National Literacy Strategy Early Literacy Support Programme. London: DfES.

Hatcher PJ (2000) Sound Linkage: An Integrated Programme For Overcoming Reading Difficulties, 2nd edn. London: Whurr.

Hornsby B, Shear F (1980) Alpha to Omega, 3rd edn. London: Heinemann.

Lloyd S (1994) The Phonics Handbook. Chigwell, Essex: Jolly Learning.

McGuinness D (1998) Why Children Cannot Read. London: Penguin.

CHAPTER 10

Spelling: challenges and strategies for the dyslexic learner and the teacher

CLAIRE JAMIESON AND SARAH SIMPSON

Spelling in English is by no means straightforward. An awareness of the complexities of the English writing system will guide discussion in this chapter. There will be an emphasis on the role of different aspects of language in the acquisition of the skills and the knowledge required for proficient spelling. The particular difficulties that the dyslexic learner can be expected to encounter will be identified, and principles to guide teaching and promote learning will be illustrated. The respective roles of the speech and language therapist (SLT) and the teacher will also be considered. As a basis for intervention, some practical teaching strategies, set within a graded summary of English spelling patterns and conventions, will be offered.

It is difficult to isolate a discussion of spelling and its development from one of reading because of the constant but changing interaction between these skills (Frith, 1985). From a developmental perspective, Bryant and Bradley (1985) have suggested that students having difficulty in the acquisition of literacy skills may be failing to use 'the right skill at the right time' and that it is the merging of skills required for reading with those required for spelling that is problematic for some children. Therefore, although the complexities of the English spelling system can be discussed in isolation, the teaching of reading and spelling must go hand in hand and should not be separated.

Complexities and challenges

The English spelling system: a challenge for all

Spelling in English involves representing words with sequences of symbols according to a number of conventions. It is complex because it is in part systematic and in part a result of historical accident. The conventionally correct spelling of a word may simply reflect its pronunciation but can also reflect its grammar, its meaning, the language from which the word was derived or any combination of these. To complicate matters further, some of these influences may be in conflict with one another. In fact, spelling so frequently fails to reflect current pronunciation that basic sound–symbol correspondence is a relatively unreliable cue to accurate spelling.

There is, for example, a straightforward relationship between the individual sounds of the word BAT and the letters used to represent them. The same is not true, however, for the word PLOUGH – although the spelling <plow> is used in American English. Similarly, it is by understanding the way in which spelling reflects grammar and meaning, through the use of suffixes and prefixes to represent morphemes, that the competent speller comes to appreciate that although the word WALKED may sound as if it ends with the sound /t/, it must be spelled with the letter sequence '-ed' to reflect the past tense.

Thus, spelling is more than a transcription of speech. The way in which words are spelled in English (i.e. their orthography) reflects phonology (sound structure), morphology (grammatical markers) and semantics (meaning), and also provides clues to etymology (the origin of words).

Sounds to symbols: two-way mapping

At a basic level of spelling, learning to represent sounds with letters requires a two-way mapping between phonology and written symbols, and it is here that difficulties will first be encountered by the child with any sort of limitation in phonological skills.

Before a child is in a position to attempt to represent spoken words in writing, some knowledge of the relationship between sounds and letters is needed. This knowledge may be limited to a relatively small set of letter names and sounds, and the child may know the names of some letters but not their sounds, or alternatively their sounds but not their names. Acquiring such knowledge requires phonological learning. For all learners, some letter–sound associations are more evident and easier to learn than others. For example, the initial sound in the names of letters such as 'b', 'd', 'p' and 't' is the same as the sounds these letters represent; the letters 'f', 'l', 'm' and 'n' end with the sounds they represent, whereas, on the other hand, the names of letters such as 'w' and 'y' are positively misleading. Hence, the spelling by Hamish, a normally developing boy of 5;6 years, of WAS as <yoz> – the word has been successfully segmented into its three component sounds: the initial sound has been represented by a letter whose name starts with the target /w/ sound, whereas the medial and final letters accurately reflect the word's pronunciation.

Once some letter–sound associations have been learned, the novice speller is in a position to make some first attempts at writing words to convey a meaning or message. It is at this point that demands on phonological skills increase, as the child must now segment the target word into, at the very least, its salient sounds and then represent these sequentially with symbols. Initial spelling attempts reflect a knowledge of both letter names and sounds, and an approximation of a word such as CAR as <cr> would not be unusual.

The task of segmenting the speech stream into words, and words into sounds, is a challenging one for the pre-literate child with a limited knowledge of the way in which abstract sounds can be visually represented by concrete symbols. Sounds within words overlap, with features of one affecting features of not only the following sound, but also the preceding sound. It is for this reason that segmenting clusters of consonant sounds such as the initial /sp/ in SPOT or the final /nt/ in WENT is so often unsuccessful in the early stages of literacy development, resulting in SPOT → <sbot> and WENT → <wet>. In the first case, the aspiration (a little puff of air) on the /p/ is not realized and the sound produced is closer to /b/ than /p/, whereas in the second example, the nasal /n/ sound influences the quality of the preceding vowel sound and is barely perceptible as a sound in its own right, therefore being difficult for the early speller to appreciate.

As the knowledge of letter–sound associations grows and, for most children, phonological segmentation skills develop, more of the sound structure of a word can be represented. At this point, ELEPHANT as <lft> could be considered a reasonable approximation. The word appears to have been segmented successfully into three syllables, and each of these has been represented with a letter. Indeed, it is possible for the word to be understood by a reader familiar with the emergent spelling of an early writer. At this stage, it is the consonant sounds that are most likely to be represented as these are more salient in terms of both their sound and their articulation, although in the case of <lft> for ELEPHANT, the first two letter names start with vowel sounds, which may have misled the child into believing that the vowels have actually been represented.

For a child who has struggled to learn letter names and letter–sound associations, the task of segmenting a word into syllables and sounds will present the next challenge. Not only is it likely that syllables will be omitted or sequenced incorrectly, but there is also the very real possibility that the phonological representation that the child has stored for a target word is actually incorrect or imprecise. For Craig (aged 7;9 years), with an early history of delayed and disordered speech development and a number of residual, imprecise pronunciations, his representation of SUDDENLY as <sudlee> matches the way he actually pronounces this word. Similarly, his representation of CAME as <game> indicates that he continues to confuse the voiced /g/ with its voiceless counterpart /k/.

Two-way mapping between sounds and symbols allows children to express their ideas in a written form that others can decipher, but it is only an initial springboard to spelling. What children are doing at this stage amounts to a rather simple form of transcription from speech to writing.

Phonology, morphology and orthography: three-way mapping

This simple form of transcription does not involve a need for any awareness of word meanings or word structure. Very quickly, however, it becomes important for children to recognize that, for example, the /s/ sound at the end of CATS is represented by the letter 's', and that this symbol actually represents 'more-than-one-ness', or plurality. Its use can therefore be generalized to other words: HAT/HATS, MUG/MUGS, PIG/PIGS. Children who might initially have written PIGS as <pigz>, accurately reflecting the sounds in the word, no longer do so once the concept of the letter 's' as a plural symbol has been understood. This is the beginning of morphological awareness, which gradually increases to include a knowledge of a range of prefixes and suffixes including '-ing', '-ly' and '-ed'.

Because the addition of suffixes or prefixes to root words sometimes involves relatively complex spelling rules, such as dropping, doubling or changing letters, a focus on morphology may seem more suitable for older children than for those in their first years at school. There is, however, no reason why very young children should not develop simple mappings between sounds, symbols and morphemes, and begin to use these in their writing. For example, '-ed', '-ly' and '-ing' can be added to words ending in a digraph or cluster without the need to apply any spelling rule.

Early theories of spelling development (Gentry, 1982) suggested that spelling skills developed in a series of stages, with children acquiring and applying a different set of strategies at each stage. Alphabetic strategies were thought to emerge before orthographic strategies, and these included the representation of morphemic units in writing (Frith, 1985). It is now more generally agreed that, from a very early age, children draw on a number of strategies and a range of knowledge in order to represent spoken words in written form and that this knowledge includes morphological awareness (Varnhagen, McCallum and Burstow, 1997). The rationale for relating spelling to morphology at a very simple level as soon as children start to learn to write is therefore justified in developmental terms.

The relevance of a word's linguistic structure to its spelling, and the importance of introducing grammatically related concepts at an early age, is recognized in the way in which reading and spelling are now taught in England, Wales and Northern Ireland, within the framework of the National Literacy Strategy (Department for Education and Employment, 1998). The National Literacy Strategy specifies termly attainment targets for the 7 years of primary school. For example, a target for 'word recognition, graphic knowledge and spelling' in year 1, term three (when children are aged between 5 and 6 years) specifies that pupils should be taught 'to investigate and learn the spellings of words with "s" for plurals'. This involves teaching children to look beyond the phonological structure of words and to consider how graphemes can also convey grammar and meaning. The teaching of spelling is thus integrated with the teaching of grammatical concepts from a very early stage.

A knowledge of the morphemic structure of words, although not absolutely essential for competent spelling at a more advanced level, is a useful tool for generating or deducing the spelling of words not previously learned. For example, when first encountering the word DISCRETION in speech, the writer with an awareness of the use of the spelling pattern '-tion' at the end of a noun is less likely to spell the word as ending in <shun>. Morphological awareness and the three-way links between phonology, morphology and orthography should therefore be fostered at all stages in the teaching of spelling.

For learners with dyslexia, the first and most evident difficulties will arise with sound–symbol mapping and phonemic segmentation. Although these can be directly attributed to a weakness in phonological awareness, the subsequent failure to integrate a developing awareness of sounds with a knowledge about morphemes (such as plural '-s' and past tense '-ed'), is another barrier to acquiring competence in spelling. Spelling errors such as <my sisted code jane> (MY SISTER'S CALLED JANE) made by Lucy (aged 8;4 years) indicate that she has not grasped the rationale for adding the past tense '-ed' to the word CALL. There is no doubt that, by this stage, she will have been taught how to use '-ed', and indeed she may well be attempting to do so in writing <sisted>. Lucy is now at risk of misapplying the spelling rules she has been taught because of her 'fuzzy' grasp of both the phonological and the morphological principles underlying them.

An early misunderstanding of morphological structure combined with poorly specified phonological representations can lead at a later stage to errors such as <I haven't the foggious idea>. Here, Ashley (aged 15 years) demonstrates her implicit knowledge of a common adjective ending in '-ous', as in OBVIOUS, but it is the wrong one. Ashley has well-specified orthographic knowledge, in that she is able to write the '-ous' suffix correctly. She also has morphemic knowledge, in that she is implicitly aware that '-ous' is an adjective ending. However, Ashley's mappings between phonology, morphology and orthography are not well enough specified for her to realize that her target is FOGGIEST.

It is thus evident that the teaching of spelling to learners with dyslexia must simultaneously promote the mappings of graphemes to sounds, develop an explicit awareness of the way in which parts of words are used to convey different aspects of grammar and meaning, and relate phonological and morphological information to the conventions and rules of English spelling.

Meeting the challenges

In this section, the assessment of spelling and the qualitative analysis of errors are addressed in detail as this will inform subsequent teaching. General principles to guide teaching style and focus are then given, and the role of the SLT is discussed.

Assessment

In order to be well structured, a programme of intervention should be based on a detailed assessment of the individual's performance in all aspects of literacy attainment and cognitive style, including phonological awareness.

The starting point for teaching spelling will depend on the results of a qualitative assessment of current spelling knowledge, through which the learner's areas of difficulty and attainment can be ascertained. Although one purpose of assessment is to identify what the learner does not appear to know, it is equally important to establish which spelling patterns have been learned so that teaching can focus on gaps in knowledge. A standardized spelling test may be useful for relating a learner's knowledge to that of his or her peers, but it will be unlikely to provide sufficient information to guide teaching intervention. Ideally, spelling should be assessed both at single-word level and in the context of a piece of writing. Correct spelling in free writing is a better indication that learning has been consolidated than is performance at single-word level, because of the need to focus on composition at the same time as on spelling. Inconsistent spelling in free writing is a clear indication that knowledge is insecure. Discussion with the learner about any rationale for spelling errors can also yield very useful information.

The testing of single words is important because it enables the assessor to control the grading and range of the words presented. The *Manual for Testing and Teaching English Spelling* (Jamieson and Jamieson, 2003) provides finely graded sets of test words for initial assessment, with a parallel test for monitoring learning.

The analysis of errors made in assessment allows inferences to be made about the strategies that a learner is probably using, throwing light on the development of phonological, morphological, semantic and orthographic linkage processes.

Below, the errors of four dyslexic learners are discussed with view to planning intervention:

Darren (aged 7 years)

Data from the *Graded Spelling Test* (Vernon, 1998):

SICK	\<sikl>
STORY	\<stort>
COLD	\<clode>

The word before SICK was MILK, which Darren spelled correctly, so there is a strong possibility that his spelling \<sikl> simply involved a repetition of the letters in the previous word. While trying to write STORY, he said he could not remember what the last letter was. He tried the letter 'e' but thought it did not look right. He settled on the letter 't' and seemed happy with this. Darren's spelling of COLD indicates that he is aware of the letters in this word, but not of their order; he may also have been taught about silent 'e'. The most important observation about Darren's spelling is that he is not able to follow a sequence of sounds and reflect this in his writing. He relies on remembering how the words look – a strategy that is extremely unreliable when not combined with other cues. Darren will certainly need training in phonological awareness.

John (aged 9 years)

Data from free-writing:

HORSES	\<horsiz>
COLLECTED	\<cletid>

Both these errors reflect sound structure (even though COLLECTED would be considered to have three syllables, it is often pronounced with only two). John's errors are related to a lack of morphological awareness (suffixes of '-es' for plural and '-ed' for the past tense), which will need to be addressed as a core part of intervention.

Mikey (aged 16 years)

Data from coursework (free writing):

SHRAPNEL	\<shracknel>

This error is indicative of a 'fuzzy' phonological representation that has not been modified through an exposure to this word in print. This is unlikely to be because the word has not been encountered, but Mikey is probably unaware of the detail within letter sequences as he reads. There would appear to be less interaction between Mikey's reading and spelling skills than would be expected at his stage of development.

MESSIAH   <messier>

This is an invented spelling reflecting sound structure. Mikey's explanation indicated that that his spelling was based on both semantic and morphological cues (a MESSIAH brings a message; -er is a suffix for someone who does something, e.g. BAKER, RIDER).

NEANDERTHAL   <meanderthal>

This error is another example of a 'fuzzy' phonological representation (/m/ for /n/) promoted by an 'invented' semantic representation: these people 'meandered around' – but Mikey's orthographic knowledge is otherwise perfect.

PINKING (shears)   <clinking> (shears)

Once again, Mikey's error indicates a fuzzy phonological representation, also attributable to semantic interference (the scissors making a clinking noise).

Mikey's spelling errors are not random – indeed, they are highly systematic – but it is only through his explanations that the full rationale can be elicited. Phonological, morphological, semantic and orthographic cues are being used, but one sometimes overrides the other, leading to errors. The information gained from discussing Mikey's spellings with him is invaluable. Intervention for Mikey will need to focus on teasing apart conflicting representations.

Peter (aged 18 years, undergraduate student)

Data from the graded spelling subtest of the *Wide Range Achievement Test* (*WRAT III*; Wilkinson, 1993):

QUANTITY   <quanty>

Here Peter demonstrates some orthographic knowledge ('qu' + 'a', final 'y'), but he does not reflect syllable structure.

CHARACTER   <carhater>

In this attempt, syllable structure is reflected, but the sequence of sounds in the target word is not represented; Peter has remembered that the letter 'h' occurs somewhere but is relying on visual memory, which is not sufficiently explicit. He does not extend his knowledge of 'ch' being pronounced as /k/ (e.g. as in CHRISTMAS or CHRIS) to include this word.

DECISION   <dicssion>

Again, syllable structure is not reflected. Peter may know of the '-ssion' spelling pattern (as in MISSION and SESSION), but this is misapplied.

ENTHUSIASM   <emphuism>

This is another example of Peter's failure to reflect the syllable structure of words in his writing. He may be confusing 'emphasis' with 'enthusiasm', hence the letters <ph> substituted for the letters 'th'. Alternatively, he may pronounce 'th' as "f", selecting the letters <ph> to represent this sound.

Peter's errors indicate either that his phonological representations are fuzzy and that he has difficulty mapping sound sequences to letter sequences, or that his difficulties arise at the mapping stage because of his tendency to rely on visual memory for spelling. He has some knowledge of spelling conventions, but this is often misapplied. For Peter, intervention needs to focus on strengthening the links between phonological units (syllable and phoneme) and orthographic units, many of which will relate to morphology.

These examples illustrate different cognitive profiles at different stages of development, highlighting the changing manifestation of dyslexia in spelling and the range of difficulties experienced by individuals, and demonstrating the importance of tailoring intervention to suit individual needs.

Principles underlying intervention

Differentiation

As most teaching is likely to take place in the classroom, consideration needs to be given to providing a suitable framework for learning for children with dyslexia. Broadly speaking, there are three different focus points to consider in differentiation, all of which are also relevant in small-group work or one-to-one teaching. These are the profile of the learner, the learning objectives and teaching style, that is to say, the learner, the content and the teacher.

To take account of individual need, it is important to have an understanding of the learner's language development, cognitive strengths and weaknesses, any additional barriers to learning such as dyspraxia or attention deficit hyperactivity disorder (ADHD), educational attainment, personality, motivation and social skills. This information may have been elicited through formal psychological assessment, but it may also be gathered on a more informal basis.

Learners with strong visual skills and artistic talent will respond to the use of colour and pictorial aids; children who lack motivation may become more inspired if teaching is related to their hobbies or interests; others may respond well to the use of information and communication technology in teaching. Pupils with ADHD may need regular breaks, and activities within lessons will need to be paced to take account of their short attention span.

Suitable learning challenges should be set so that teaching will take place at the instructional level. If tasks are too easy, motivation will be lost; if they are too difficult, frustration will ensue. Learners who have received ongoing intervention to promote the development of literacy skills will often have covered the same ground over and over again. It is important to establish, before embarking on teaching a particular rule, that learning targets have not already been reached. If learning has not taken place despite previous attempts, new teaching methods should be considered.

Having considered the profile of the individual and the importance of setting appropriate targets, the rest of this section will be devoted to teaching style. Learning takes place through all sensory modalities but primarily through auditory, visual and kinaesthetic channels. Ideally, all should be stimulated to reinforce the learning of new information. Even young children should be encouraged to take responsibility for their learning, and to do this they need to understand what they are being asked to do and why. Teaching needs to be structured so that each piece of new information builds logically upon previous knowledge. Spelling cannot be taught in a vacuum but needs to be integrated with spoken language, with reading and with the wider curriculum. These fundamental teaching principles are expanded below.

Multisensory teaching

The rationale for multisensory teaching is now familiar to teachers and therapists, and the success of this approach to teaching learners with specific learning difficulties is well documented (Rack and Hatcher, 2002). There is no doubt that learning is facilitated when more than one, preferably three, sensory channels are activated. When teaching at the word level, the well known 'look, cover, say, write, check' spelling method uses simultaneous visual, auditory and kinaesthetic feedback, in an endeavour to support memory and lead to automaticity in producing particular letter sequences. A number of methods such as this have been found to be effective.

Teaching methods for learners with dyslexia must balance the need for training in areas of weakness with making maximum use of compensatory strengths; a multisensory approach offers the opportunity to do this. This approach encourages the learner to integrate information from auditory, visual and kinaesthetic channels and thus make that all-important connection between reading and writing.

Metacognitive teaching and active learning

Many learning programmes for spelling, including commercially produced work sheets, rely on learning through practice. Spelling patterns and rules are gradually absorbed through a 'drill' approach, and although spelling proficiency may increase, learning takes place in the absence of any real mental engagement on the part of the learner. There is, especially in the early stages, a tendency to underestimate the importance of adopting a metacognitive approach to teaching.

A metacognitive approach encourages the development of problem-solving strategies, rather than focusing on the training of specific skills. Borkowski (1992) outlines such an approach in general terms and explains how it teaches children to monitor and regulate their own performance, to take more responsibility for their own learning, and to devise ways of organizing a framework of knowledge on to which new knowledge can be mapped.

In order to maximize generalization of learning, the development of explicit awareness and knowledge is important at all stages of the learning process. Learners should, from the outset, be encouraged to be reflective, observant and exploratory in their learning. They need to know and understand why certain knowledge must be acquired; they should be aware of the teaching methods being used, and they should be able to explain what they have learned.

Luke (aged 6;9 years) had a very clear grasp of the range of skills he would need to become good at reading and spelling, so he was happy to practise these in his individual lessons. This was because he had made, with the help of his teacher, a mind map of the many and varied skills required to become good at football, a subject about which he was both passionate and knowledgeable. The analogy worked well. He realized that, contrary to his first suggestion that to become a good reader and speller you just had to 'grow older', he would become better at reading and spelling through recognizing words, knowing his letter sounds, breaking words into syllables, building words up from syllables and so on. He was thus able to see the rationale for the various activities in his lessons, and his cooperation and enthusiasm were harnessed.

Learners with dyslexia need to be aware of the nature of their difficulties; they need to be encouraged to talk about why spelling is important, and they need to be helped, through teaching, to gain an insight into why spelling in English is so difficult. The priorities for learning and individual perspectives, particularly of older learners, ought to be taken into account when planning teaching. To ensure that learning has taken place, pupils can be encouraged to play the role of teacher and to explain how particular spelling patterns work. They should also be asked for feedback about their learning so that teaching can be modified to reflect individual needs.

A metacognitive approach to teaching spelling involves developing an explicit awareness of letter sequences and spelling patterns, and making observations about the contexts in which these patterns occur. This applies at all levels of attainment and development, but it is even more important for dyslexic children or for those who, in the first 2 years of primary school, are perceived to be at risk of literacy difficulties, as such children will not acquire the ability to spell simply through exposure to print. Metacognitive techniques should therefore be used in conjunction with multisensory teaching methods. Explicit understanding is particularly relevant when teaching grammatically related spelling rules, such as adding suffixes for plurals and tenses.

Structured, sequential and cumulative teaching to promote consolidated learning

For new spelling knowledge to become properly assimilated, especially in the case of learners with dyslexia, much overlearning and practice is required. Teaching needs to be *structured*, with a clear rationale for the content of lessons and the order in which material is taught. Teaching should also be *sequential*, with a logical progression from one target to the next, and it must be *cumulative*, ensuring that new information is introduced only when previously taught material has been fully absorbed.

To ensure that knowledge is secure, much overlearning and formative assessment will need to take place. It is not sufficient simply to check that the words covered in the previous week have been learned, but reference needs to be made, on an ongoing basis, to all work covered until it is clear that this has been fully accommodated. Learners may be successful in their spelling when tested, but they may not be able to spell the same words correctly in a less structured format such as free writing. It is important to verify that learning has taken place first at the word level, through short tests, then at sentence level, perhaps through dictation, and then at text level, through observing spelling in free writing. Spelling patterns can be considered properly learned when they are consistently applied in writing outside spelling lessons.

It is important to limit the introduction of new information to a pace that will not cause confusion. It is not generally a good idea to teach more than one spelling pattern or rule in a lesson. It is also important not to teach easily confusable spelling patterns together, for example double 'e' (-ee-) as in KEEP, and the letter sequence '-ea-' as in REACH. This may be a useful technique when teaching pupils whose literacy skills are developing normally, but it can lead to confusion for those pupils experiencing difficulty. Some of the more complex suffixing rules are likely to take three or four lessons to complete.

An integrated approach to teaching

Integrating spoken and written language

No matter where the learner's strengths and weaknesses lie, it will be necessary to make links with his or her underlying spoken language skills so that both the content of lessons and the exercises used for practice are as meaningful as possible. In particular, it is important for teachers of spelling to be aware of learners' vocabulary levels. Many consonant-vowel-consonant (CVC) words that regularly appear in spelling worksheets (e.g. BAN, WED, RIG, LOP, PUN) are of such low frequency that children working at a basic level are likely to perceive them as non-words. Although extending vocabulary is a valuable teaching target, the random inclusion of such words in exercises to practise spelling patterns results in a drill-like approach, in which reflective engagement on the part of the learner is not fostered.

Integrating word-, sentence- and text-level learning

Spellings may be introduced at the level of the single word but quickly need to be used in the context of phrases and sentences. Working at single-word level is initially important as it draws attention to spelling patterns and leads to learning through analogy. However, unless the crossover to text level is made quickly, learning is likely to be confined to the bottom-up, 'drill' context, in which relevance and wider application are not apparent.

Integrating reading and spelling

The skills involved in learning to read and spell are related but different, in that reading primarily involves the recognition of whole words and of letter sequences, whereas spelling demands specific, explicit knowledge. There is, however, constant interaction and much overlap between the two sets of skills, which can be used to good effect in teaching.

As children in the very early stages of learning to read tend to rely on recognizing whole words (in the absence of effective decoding strategies), their spelling is unlikely to improve through noticing, for example, consonant clusters ('st', 'pl') or vowel digraphs ('ai', 'oy') while reading. They are more likely to gain an explicit awareness of these basic phonic principles through the act of writing, so in the early stages of literacy development (and reflecting Frith's, 1985, model), spelling should be the starting point. An implicit awareness of more complex spelling patterns appears to develop as a result of reading experience. Through this implicit awareness, learners may know that they have spelled a word incorrectly simply because it does not 'look right'.

This awareness does not develop in the same way for learners with dyslexia, who continue to rely on recognizing words by their general 'shape', supported by context. Adults with dyslexia often claim that they do not have any difficulty with reading, and that their only persisting problem is spelling. Although it may be true that reading does not pose a problem for them, an assessment of adults' reading generally reveals high levels of inaccuracy, a tendency to substitute words that are visually similar to the target, and a lack of effective strategies for decoding unfamiliar words. It is therefore important, when teaching spelling to people with dyslexia, to draw attention to letter sequences and spelling patterns in text to foster an awareness of the detail within letter sequences.

Integrating cognitive strengths and weaknesses
It is difficult to know whether intervention is best aimed at training in areas of weakness (e.g. phonological awareness) or promoting cognitive strengths (e.g. visuospatial skills) to support learning. To some extent, this depends on the stage of development of the learner, as well as on the severity of the difficulties. Although it is important to incorporate and integrate both remediation and compensation in teaching, the balance between the two is likely to change over time.

When working with young children who have been identified as dyslexic, or at risk of literacy difficulties, a focus on areas of weakness is likely to be beneficial. Training in phonological awareness, especially when linked to alphabetic knowledge, is known to promote the development of literacy skills (Hatcher, Hulme and Ellis, 1994; see also Chapter 9 in this volume). Teachers should, however, also try to harness the cognitive strengths of young children to support their learning.

When working with older learners or adults, the balance is likely to shift gradually from training in areas of weakness to the development of compensatory strategies based on cognitive strengths. Success in training adults in phonological awareness is likely to be limited, and there may come a point when continuing on this path becomes frustrating, tedious and generally counterproductive. At this stage, there is often more to be gained by focusing on strategies for spelling such as words in words, mnemonics or visual imagery to reinforce learning.

Integrating the teaching of spelling with the curriculum
When the teaching of spelling takes place outside the classroom, it is important to relate the content of lessons to the wider curriculum to ensure that vocabulary is relevant and to maximize the opportunity for the generalization of skills. Spelling patterns or rules can be based on subject or topic words; sentences for dictation can relate to material being covered in, for example, history or geography, and curricular texts can be used for identifying particular spelling patterns.

Roles and responsibilities

For many years, it was assumed that if children were taught to read, they would automatically learn to spell, that spelling was simply the inverse of reading. Currently, however, it is acknowledged that the processes of reading and spelling are as different as they are similar, and that spelling is better taught than caught. Teaching children how to spell is therefore now a core part of the literacy curriculum, and as such spelling instruction is the responsibility of the teacher. It is, however, also now generally accepted that reading and spelling are dependent on the integration of a range of linguistic skills, and that children whose speech and language development are compromised in any way may be at risk of literacy learning difficulties. For this reason, it is becoming increasingly recognized that there is a role for the SLT in facilitating the literacy learning of some children (Simpson, 2000).

The role that the SLT takes in a child's literacy learning will vary according to the child's age and stage of learning, and the nature of his or her underlying language difficulty. It may focus on prevention, assessment or intervention; it may involve taking a direct or an indirect approach. In addition, it may focus on the child, the parent or carer, or the teacher. It will also vary according to the SLT's own particular areas of expertise and local service delivery policies.

SLTs are in a position to identify, and train others to identify, preschool children with speech and language difficulties who are at risk of dyslexia. It may be appropriate for them to offer early intervention or to train others to intervene. Research has shown that where phonological processing deficits are identified early, and programmes in which phonological awareness training is integrated with the early teaching of literacy are carried out, the knock-on effects on children's long-term literacy learning are positive (see Ehri et al., 2001, for a review). Research has also shown that such programmes do not need to be delivered by an SLT in order to be effective (Gillon, 2002). There is therefore a clear place for the SLT, with his or her specialist knowledge about both spoken and written language, in the training of parents, carers, teachers, learning support assistants and specialist teachers.

Once the child is at school, the primary responsibility for literacy teaching will rest with the school, supported by the parents or carers. The way in which the school meets this responsibility will depend on the individual child's particular needs, together with school policies and staffing. In some cases, a specialist teacher may be involved; in others, a learning support assistant may be available. The SLT can still, however, play a role in both identification and intervention. The extent and nature of the SLT's involvement with individual children with literacy learning difficulties will depend upon whether the child is currently on the SLT's caseload, has a history of SLT or has not previously been known to the SLT services. At this stage, the SLT's role is most likely to be consultative and may involve both collaboration and training.

It is sometimes the case that parents or carers prefer to take responsibility for meeting a child's language and learning needs by making arrangements for teaching and or speech and language therapy to take place out of school. When this arises, it is important that they ensure the teacher has appropriate skills and qualifications, is able to devise plans for skill generalization, does not teach the child without reference to his or her wider curricular demands, and is willing to collaborate and liaise with the other professionals involved in the child's learning.

Practical strategies for addressing the challenges

Principles to guide differentiation and good teaching practice have been discussed; these principles will need to be applied when implementing some of the practical suggestions for intervention offered in the following section.

Early teaching and phonological linkage

In the early stages, a child at risk of dyslexia can be expected to have difficulty in learning letter names, making letter–sound associations, segmenting words into sounds and blending sounds into words. Confusions over letter names and sounds, phoneme segmentation and identification, and the orientation of letters will interfere with spelling attempts and may make them appear bizarre. Where letters represent more than one sound, or a sound can be represented by more than one letter, the difficulty will be compounded.

Teaching the alphabet and letter names

The classic longitudinal study conducted by Bradley and Bryant (1983) was one of the first to emphasize the importance of combining the training of phonological skills with the teaching of reading and spelling. Similarly, Hatcher, Hulme and Ellis (1994) have found that training poor readers in phonological skills in isolation from reading and spelling skills is less effective than training that makes explicit the links between these skills. The value of using plastic letters in such training is now well attested. These can be physically manipulated both to demonstrate the importance of letter orientation and to draw attention to the relationship between a particular sequence of symbols and the sounds that they represent.

A commonly adopted technique for teaching in the early stages involves asking the child to work with you to set out part of the alphabet, naming the letters as you do so (Jamieson and Jamieson, 2003). Initially, a group of four or five letters may be sufficient to work with at a time. Taking a metacognitive approach, as already described, the teacher can explain to the child how the 26 letters of the alphabet can be combined in hundreds of ways to represent the 44 sounds of the English language, and in thousands of ways to spell all the words in English – that letters are the building blocks of learning to read and spell.

As the sequence of one group of letters is learned, another group can be introduced. In this way, a knowledge of the sequence of the alphabet can gradually be built up. As the child becomes more familiar with the sequence, games can be played to consolidate the child's learning. The teacher can, for example, ask the child to look away while a letter is removed, moved or repositioned, and the child is then asked to recite the alphabet while pointing to the letters and so 'spot the change'. Alternatively, as the child becomes more confident, the teacher can use a stopwatch to record the time taken to set out a section; charting the times on a graph, or in some other visual way, will provide a record of progress, which is motivating for the child. At the same time, there can be a discussion and demonstration of the need to know the sequence of the alphabet in order to use a dictionary, telephone directory or reference book.

Sound–symbol correspondence

Once the child has made a start on learning the names of the letters, the plastic letters can be used to start teaching some sound–symbol correspondences, taking care to make consonant sounds without an accompanying neutral vowel sound. At this point, it may help the child to develop phoneme awareness if obvious articulatory gestures relating to the place and manner of articulation and voicing quality are pointed out, and comparisons are drawn between sounds (Lindamood and Lindamood, 1998). It may also be helpful if actions or pictures are linked with the sounds, or semantic associations are forged; this can be done through the use of schemes such as *Jolly Phonics* (Lloyd and Wernham, 1994), *Cued Articulation* (Passy, 1993a) or the *Nuffield Dyspraxia Programme* (Williams, 2004). The distinction between vowels and consonants can also be made and discussed at this point.

There is currently some debate about whether it is more appropriate to focus on small phonological units (phonemes) or larger units (rimes) when teaching reading and spelling (Deavers and Solity, 1998). It is generally accepted that, with the dyslexic learner, sound–symbol correspondence and early spelling strategies should be taught in a way that is known to be developmentally appropriate. Goswami and Bryant (1990) describe three separate levels at which words can be segmented: into syllables ('ca-ter-pill-ar'), intra-syllabically into onsets and rimes ('c-at') or into phonemes ('c-a-t'). As there is a substantial amount of evidence to suggest that phoneme awareness develops later than the awareness of larger phonological units (awareness of syllables and rhyme), it follows that if onset/rime segmentation places fewer demands on the learner than phonemic segmentation, it is appropriate, when working with pupils with dyslexia, to use these units as a springboard to teaching phoneme awareness and sound– symbol correspondence.

A further rationale for teaching the dyslexic child at the onset/rime level is offered by Tunmer (1994). He notes that short vowels are more stable when produced as part of a rime. Also, such an approach facilitates the learning of consonant blends and is a useful way of encouraging the child to appreciate letter sequences as it raises an awareness of orthographic units that are greater than single sounds mapped to single letters.

There is no set order in which sound–symbol correspondences should be taught, but it will be important to avoid teaching those which look or sound alike in too close proximity. It is also helpful to ensure that the combination taught allows some common, high-frequency words to be represented. Broomfield and Combley (1997), among others, suggest that correspondences for the letters 'i', 't', 'p', 'n' and 's' provide a useful starting point.

To teach sound–symbol correspondences, plastic letters can be arranged in an arc so that each letter is within easy reach of the child. The letter 'a' and the letter 't', for example, can then be moved down and combined to produce the rime unit '-at'. Following this, the letter 's' can be moved down; the teacher can introduce the sound it makes, discuss its obvious articulatory features and, together with the child, establish some visual or semantic cues to link the letter shape, its name and its sound. The word produced by placing this letter in front of the letters already moved down <sat> can then be read and discussed. The child can then be asked to segment the spoken word "SAT" into its individual sounds and to simultaneously point to or touch the corresponding letter as each sound is segmented. By manipulating plastic letters in this way, the child will be learning sound–symbol correspondences, blending skills (for reading) and segmentation skills (for spelling). More letters can then be drawn down to provide onsets for the rime '-at', and the process is repeated. As a further step, the child can be asked to practise writing the words that have been constructed in this way. Thus, a multisensory and metacognitive approach to teaching will be ensured, with links made between spoken and written language and reading and spelling.

A practical scheme that is firmly based in this understanding of the developmental sequence is the *Phonological Awareness Training Programme* (*PAT*; Wilson, 1993). In the early stages, this scheme works explicitly with onset and rime, uses the concept of learning through analogy and recognizes the need for dyslexic learners to combine the skills used for reading with those used for spelling. In addition, when used following the recommended procedure, it is highly structured, provides opportunities for practice and overlearning, and promotes active participation by requiring the children to generate word lists for themselves. It is particularly useful with the older student (aged 7+ years) who has already been exposed to a basic phonic scheme, and provides a useful bridge to working at the level of the phoneme.

Teaching spelling patterns

From an early stage, it is recommended that dyslexic children be taught that sounds can be represented in more than one way. For this purpose, the *THRASS* scheme (Davies and Ritchie, 1998) provides a useful reference. Children should also be helped to appreciate consistent spelling patterns rather than simply attempting to translate individual sounds to letters. Goswami (1994) stresses the importance of encouraging a child to learn new words by analogy with those already mastered, and emphasizes the need to look for consistency in spelling patterns rather than phonic regularity. For example, a surprisingly large number of words share the ostensibly irregular spelling pattern '-ight'.

In English, the concept of regularity in spelling is by no means straightforward, and it should perhaps be thought of as a continuum. Spellings can be considered to be highly regular if they have a letter and sound sequence, or pattern, that is shared with a number of other words; conversely, they are less regular if they share their spelling pattern with relatively few words. The simplest regular patterns include CVC words, words with initial consonant digraphs (e.g. 'sh', 'ch', 'th'), final consonant digraphs ('-ng', '-ck', '-sh'), initial consonant clusters (e.g. 'sp', 'fl', 'tr') and final consonant clusters (e.g. '-nt', '-mp', '-st') (Jamieson and Jamieson, 2003). However, other letter sequences (e.g. many of the vowel digraphs) can also be viewed as relatively regular on the basis of the consistency of their pronunciation.

In words that share a spelling pattern, but in which sounds do not obviously and transparently map to symbols, the teacher can draw the dyslexic child's attention to the visual sequence of letters and encourage repetition of it (perhaps with some exaggerated intonation or stress pattern), thus leading to auditory reinforcement of the visual sequence. In this way, errors such as the spelling of NIGHT as <nihgt> are less likely to occur. The pupil can then be helped to compile a set of words that share the target spelling pattern (sometimes referred to as a 'word family') and to construct, and write, some simple sentences and stories using these words. If these are highly imageable, so much the better as the pupil can then illustrate them, further consolidating the link between the words. In this way, work on written and spoken language will be integrated, as will work at word, sentence and text level, and the pupil will be encouraged to take a multisensory approach to learning. The spelling work can then be integrated with reading by look-ing for the target pattern in simple texts, and by highlighting and naming the letter sequence.

Spelling key words

At the same time as learning how to represent sounds with symbols and to spell relatively regular words, it will be important for the dyslexic child to be learning to spell some high-frequency words that do not immediately appear to follow a regular pattern, together with vocabulary that is either topic-specific or of direct relevance (e.g. family names, address). The methods advocated for teaching such words vary, and some experimenta-tion may be necessary to establish which is the most successful for each individual learner.

Bryant and Bradley (1985) advocate the use of Gillingham and Stillman's (1956) *Simultaneous Oral Spelling* (SOS) multisensory method and emphasize its value in helping the learner to chunk words and to become familiar with sequences of letters and with patterns of movements attached to writing these sequences. Similarly, Thomson (1991) reported a study comparing teaching through SOS with teaching using a visual method ('look, cover, say, check'). He found that dyslexic children learned more effectively using SOS, whereas normal readers learned equally well with either method.

A variant of this method, devised by Brimmer and Simpson (described in Jamieson and Jamieson, 2003), which has proved popular with teach-ers and pupils, is outlined below. As a word of caution, however: this method should not generally be used for words of more than seven letters because of the memory load.

The materials required for this version of SOS are a reporter's note-book (i.e. a spiral-bound notebook with a top binding), a pencil or felt tip and a list of high-frequency words, taken for example from the National Literacy Strategy (Department for Education and Employment, 1998). The first step is to motivate the pupil to learn the words by explaining that there are some words that occur so frequently that if these can be learned and used automatically, the effect on the pupil's spelling will be signifi-cant. The next step is to identify which high-frequency words are known and which need to be learned.

Rather than subjecting the pupil to a lengthy test, one method is to compile a set of cards of high-frequency words and ask the pupil to write them to dictation. The number selected and level of difficulty will depend on the age and stage of the pupil, and confusable words (e.g. WHEN/WENT) should be tested on separate occasions. If a word is automatically spelled correctly, this is commented on and the card is put to one side in a pile of 'known words'; if it is spelled with some hesitation or incorrectly, it is allocated to the pile of 'words to be learned'. Once about three 'words to be learned' have been identified, testing is discontinued and those words become the target for teaching in that lesson. In the next lesson, a new set of words can be identified continuing the same procedure. In this way, the pupil may be encouraged to discover how many words are actually already known.

Once a set of target words for the lesson has been identified, teaching can commence. One of the target words is selected; the teacher says the word and prints it at the bottom of a page in the notebook, saying the letter names as they are written. Lower-case print rather than cursive script should be used so that the pupil is helped to focus on the sequence of the letters; letter names rather than sounds are used as, in most high-frequency words, there is no immediate relationship between the sounds and letters of the word. It may be helpful to use exaggerated intonation or to group the letters if the spelling pattern lends itself to this. The pupil then reads the word, copies it while simultaneously naming the letters, and then repeats the word and checks that the spelling is correct. If it is, the page is folded over and the pupil repeats the procedure, this time without a model to follow.

In this way, using auditory, visual and kinaesthetic channels for learning, an association is built between the word and its constituent letters. The process should be repeated at least three times for each word and practised between lessons. Words should then be reviewed regularly until the pupil is able to produce them automatically.

Not all pupils will take to the SOS method, nor do all words lend themselves to being taught and learned in this way. For others, mnemonic strategies may be helpful. This may involve making up a sentence using words that start with the letters of the word to be learned (e.g. BECAUSE – 'because eggs cause accidents, use special effort'). It is advisable to use the target word as the first word of the mnemonic, otherwise the pupil may associate it with a similar-sounding word (in this case, perhaps, BEAUTIFUL). To make the mnemonic more imageable, encourage the pupil either to draw a picture or to talk about the image it conjures up.

Brooks, Everatt and Weeks (1992) suggest that the *Words in Words* method is particularly effective for older pupils and longer words. It is also particularly suitable for pupils with considerable and persisting phonological difficulties, especially if their visual skills are relatively strong. For example, a particular student struggled with a phonic approach to spelling until she was 14 years old. The *Words in Words* approach, combined with mnemonic technique, provided the breakthrough she so badly needed. The teaching of sound–letter correspondences was abandoned in favour of using words within words, and her spelling took off quite dramatically.

Here are a few examples of words she was taught (identified initially on the basis of her own need):

- MYSTERY: I've lost MY STEREO – it's a mystery.
- PIECE: a piece of PIE.
- MINUTES: miNUTes.
- COMPARISON: comPARISon.
- HEALTH: HE, (AL) enjoys good health.
- BELIEVE: don't beLIEve a lie.

If mnemonic strategies are used, it will be important to ensure that pupils are actively involved in creating the mnemonics for themselves, as they will then be far more motivated to remember and apply them.

Using syllables for spelling

When syllable structure is accurately reflected in writing, it is almost always possible to decipher the target word. Syllable awareness is therefore a valuable skill for spelling, which can be taught to pupils with dyslexia even at the most basic stage of literacy development. The number of syllables in a word equates to the number of beats, for example CAT = one syllable, BANDIT = two syllables and ELEPHANT = three syllables. A syllable is a sound or group of sounds produced on one push of air; it may be represented by a single letter or a group of letters. In the written form, each syllable, almost without exception, contains a vowel.

Once the concept of the syllable has been grasped, the dyslexic child can be taught to clap or tap out the syllables in words of different length and to number them. The next step is to represent each syllable in writing, simply by following speech sounds. The target is not necessarily a correctly spelled word but one whose syllable structure is accurately represented. Young learners with dyslexia who have difficulty identifying the syllables in words may benefit from active strategies such as listening to a relatively long word and then jumping across a room, timing each jump to coincide with the enunciation of a syllable of the word.

A number of teaching resources refer to six kinds of *written* syllable. These are generally described as closed short vowel syllables (e.g. SIT), open syllables (e.g. BY), syllables in which the 'silent e' rule is applied (e.g. SOME), syllables containing a vowel digraph (e.g. ROAST), syllables ending with a consonant followed by the letter string '-le' (e.g. the second syllable in PEOPLE) and finally syllables in which the vowel is followed, and its sound is modified by, the letter 'r' (e.g. FIRST). These distinctions are not as helpful for spelling as they might at first appear; many words, for example, sound as though the 'silent e' convention should be applied when in fact the correct spelling is a vowel digraph (e.g. BOAT). Similarly, there can be confusion between closed syllables with a short vowel, and those with a long vowel (e.g. WAIT – a closed syllable, with a long vowel sound).

Some spelling guidelines and a suggested teaching order

Although there are more rules and conventions in the English language than may at first be appreciated, the word 'rule' should generally be avoided when talking about the spelling of English. One of the most frequently quoted rules is 'i before e except after c'. This rule is only relevant when the target sound is the long /i/ (as in the word NIECE), and even then there are exceptions (SEIZE). For this reason, the terms 'spelling conventions' or 'spelling guidelines' are preferable, and where some obvious reason for a spelling pattern can be discerned, a metacognitive approach to teaching should be adopted and the rationale for the spelling should be discussed.

Once most sound–symbol correspondences have been taught, together with some basic consonant digraphs and clusters, as described above, the teacher may find it difficult to decide which spelling pattern to teach next. There is no preordained order, especially if the teaching has been informed by individual assessment and error analysis.

The following is only a suggested order and is based on the consistency, complexity and usefulness of the patterns. It should be adapted for the individual learner as it would be frustrating to spend time on patterns that are already known; equally, there may be some unexpected gaps in knowledge. Generally, only one pattern should be introduced at a time, and patterns previously taught should be regularly reviewed and revised. Progress, and the extent to which learning has been consolidated, can be monitored in a pupil's writing in contexts other than within the spelling lesson.

Consonant digraphs

These are pairs of consonants that represent a single sound. The most useful digraphs for a child to know ('th', 'sh', 'ch', '-ng', which are the only representations for these sounds, and '-ck', which is a high-frequency and regular digraph) will be taught relatively early. One advantage of teaching consonant digraphs early is that the pupil can be taught to add some common suffixes (plural 's', '-ed', '-ing') to words ending in consonant digraphs without the complication of having to teach suffixing rules (see below). This allows the child to write a large number of longer words and is the first step in teaching about the links between spelling and morphology.

Consonant clusters

Consonant clusters are two or three consonant sounds in sequence, each represented by a letter (e.g. 'sp', 'cl', 'str'). These should be taught in the initial position before the final position, where they are more difficult for the child to hear clearly and thus to segment accurately. When they are taught in the final position, it may be helpful to teach them as part of the rime unit, for example 'h' + 'and', 'p' + 'ink'.

When teaching initial clusters, it may be helpful to group them rather than going through them alphabetically. They can be grouped into initial and final clusters.

Initial clusters are:

- those which start with the /s/ sound ('sc', 'sk', 'st', 'sl', 'sm', 'sn', 'sp', 'sw', 'scr', 'spr', 'str', 'spl', 'squ');
- those with /l/ as the second sound ('bl', 'cl', 'fl', 'gl', 'pl');
- those with /r/ as the second sound ('br', 'cr', 'dr', 'fr', 'gr', 'pr', 'tr', 'shr', 'thr');
- less frequent ones with /w/ as the second sound ('dw', 'tw').

Final clusters are:

- those which start with the /l/ sound ('-ld', '-lk' ,'-lp', '-lt', '-lth'); note that '-lk' and '-lf' are not clusters in some words, for example WALK, TALK, HALF and CALF, as the /l/ sound is not heard;
- those beginning with the /n/ sound ('-nd', '-nt', '-nch');
- those which begin with the /s/ sound ('-sk', '-sp', '-st');
- those which end with the /t/ sound ('-ct', '-ft', '-pt'; note that these are of low frequency);
- the relatively common cluster '-mp'.

As with words ending in final consonant digraphs, suffixes can be added to words ending in consonant clusters without needing to apply suffixing rules.

Common endings: '-ff', '-ll' and '-ss'

Although these double letters are frequently used to represent the final /f/, /l/ or /s/ sound in single syllable words with a short vowel, there are unfortunately a number of exceptions. Some of these relate to differences in the pronunciation of the preceding vowel, depending on dialect (e.g. the vowel in GRASS and CLASS may be pronounced as 'ah' in the south of England). The high-frequency words that are exceptions should also be taught at this stage (IF, OF, YES, BUS).

Vowel digraphs

Vowel digraphs are letter strings in which two letters represent a vowel sound, for example 'ai', 'ay', 'oa', 'ow', 'oi' , 'oy', 'ee', 'ea', 'au' and 'aw'. When teaching 'ea', be careful to distinguish between instances when it occurs as a long vowel (e.g. BEACH) and those in which it is short (e.g. DEAD). Note also that some words containing the digraph 'ai' have different pronunciations, for example '-air', and these should be taught at a later stage.

Groups of words that share both sounds and a letter sequence could be introduced together as 'word families', for example CLOWN, TOWN, BROWN, GOWN and DOWN. In addition, where a digraph generally occurs in a particular position in a word (e.g. '-ay' and '-oy' at the end of a word), this should be pointed out and discussed.

Vowel + r

These patterns ('ar', 'or', 'er', 'ir', 'ur') should be taught one at a time for vowels in the stressed position within a word (e.g. FARM, FORM, FIR, BURN); the unstressed endings (e.g. in COLLAR, VISITOR, BAKER) can be taught later. Particular attention should be paid to the patterns 'er', 'ir' and 'ur', which all represent the same sound.

Silent e

Some so-called spelling rules are actually more useful for reading. This is particularly true of the rule generally referred to as the 'silent e' or 'magic e', as in words such as LATE, BITE and HOPE. For reading, the letter-to-sound conversion is relatively consistent, and words with the 'silent e' pattern generally have a long vowel sound (high-frequency words that are exceptions being HAVE, COME and SOME). As, however, there are so very many alternative spelling patterns for vowel sounds (e.g. the vowel digraphs in the following words all representing the same sound: TRAIN, BREAK, REIN, EIGHT, STRAIGHT), this rule is not very useful for spelling. It may in fact be more useful to teach a rime unit such as '-ate', together with the words that form the '-ate' family, for example, DATE, FATE, GATE, HATE, etc.

'-tch' and '-dge' after a short vowel

Both of the spelling patterns '-tch' and '-dge' are reasonably regular. The exceptions to '-tch' are few but common: RICH, WHICH, SUCH and MUCH. The '-dge' rule can be explained almost rationally (unlike so many English spelling patterns), as follows:

- The letter 'j' is very restricted in its use (note its high value in the game of Scrabble).
- It never comes at the end of a word.
- The 'j' sound in word final position is written '-ge'.
- But '-e' (silent e) makes the previous vowel long (e.g. AGE, HUGE).

- So, after a short vowel, a final 'j' sound must be written '-dge' (distancing the letter 'e' from the vowel).

Consistent letter strings

Some letter strings have consistent pronunciations and should be introduced as such. These are spelling patterns such as '-alk', '-ight', '-ckle' and '-ttle'.

'c' followed by 'i', 'e' and 'y' sounds like /s/

This 'rule' is very reliable for reading but more complicated for spelling as it is difficult to know whether to use the letter 's' or the letter 'c'.

'k' + 'e' or 'i'

The /k/ sound followed by the sound /e/ or /i/ after it has to be represented by the letter 'k', as in KID, KENT, etc. because if the letter 'c' were used, it would give a /s/ sound.

'g' followed by 'i', 'e' and 'y' sounds like 'j' (referred to as 'soft g')

The 'rule' that 'g' followed by 'e', 'i' or 'y', sounds like 'j' parallels the 'c' rule (above) but is even less reliable because the exceptions are high-frequency words (GET, GIVE, GIRL, GIFT, GEAR, GEESE, GIDDY, GIG, GIGGLE, GIRTH).

'gu' + 'e', 'i' or 'y'

The letter 'u' keeps the /g/ 'hard' in words such as GUESS, GUEST, GUILT, GUITAR and GUIDE. This follows from the 'soft g' rule above.

'w' + a vowel

In words that start with the /w/ sound, the vowel that follows the letter 'w' is not represented as it sounds. For example, if the following sound is a short '-o-' sound, it is represented by the letter 'a' as in WASH; if the following sound is '-or-' it is represented by the letters 'ar' as in WARM. Perversely, if the following sound is '-er-', it is represented by the letters '-or-' as in WORK and WORD.

Suffixes and prefixes

Suffixes

Suffixes are word endings that change the syntactic function, tense or plurality of words. For example, '-ly' changes an adjective to an adverb (BAD ➤ badly), '-ness' changes an adjective to a noun (KIND ➤ kindness), '-ed' changes a present tense verb to past tense (WALK ➤ walked) and '-s' changes a singular noun to a plural noun (BOY ➤ boys).

The endings, plural '-s', '-ed', '-ing', '-ful' and '-ly' are a useful introduction to the concept of suffixes. At the simplest level, plural '-s' can be added to CVC words. The teaching of plurals needs to start with the basic '-s' ending, moving on to words that end in '-s', '-x', '-sh' and '-ch', in which the plural ending is '-es' (BUSES, FOXES, BUSHES, CHURCHES). The suffix '-ing' can also be introduced at a very early stage. As soon as the final consonant digraphs '-sh' and '-ng' have been taught, and some final consonant clusters are known, '-ing' can be added: 'rush' + 'ing', 'rest' + 'ing'. The past tense '-ed' suffix and the adverb '-ly' suffix can also be introduced at a basic level where there is no need to change the root word: 'rush' + 'ed', 'land' + 'ed', 'bad' + 'ly', 'loud' + 'ly'.

There are relatively few verbs whose past tense is formed by adding '-t' (e.g. CREPT, KEPT), and these usually involve a change of vowel sound, as in MEAN ➤ meant. So it is better to assume an '-ed' ending even if a /t/ is heard, as for example the final sound in the word WALKED. As '-ed' is pronounced /d/, /t/ or /id/ (PLAYED, WISHED, WANTED) depending on the root word, it is a good idea to group words of the same type together for teaching.

The next stage in teaching suffixes involves changes to the root word, and these changes depend on whether the suffix starts with a vowel or a consonant.

The doubling rule

Words of one syllable
If a word ends with one vowel letter followed by one consonant letter, double the final consonant before adding *a suffix beginning with a vowel*, for example 'clap' + 'p' + 'ing'.

So you do not double the consonant if:

- the root words has two vowels: 'read' + 'ing' = READING;
- the root word ends with two consonants: 'bend' + 'ing' = BENDING;
- the suffix begins with a consonant: 'bad' + 'ly' = BADLY.

Words of two syllables
If the stress in a two-syllable word falls on the second syllable, double the final consonant when adding a suffix beginning with a vowel, for example 'begin' + 'n' + 'ing'.

So you do not double the consonant if:

- the stress falls on the first syllable: 'gallop' + 'ing' = GALLOPING;
- the final syllable has two vowel letters: 'retreat' + 'ed' = RETREATED;

- the final syllable ends in two consonants: 'enact' + 'ed' = ENACTED;
- the suffix begins with a consonant: 'equip' + 'ment' = EQUIPMENT.

This is a relatively advanced spelling rule, and recognizing the stress patterns in words may prove too great a challenge for the dyslexic learner. One way of demonstrating how stress works in two-syllable words is to ask the learner to imagine making an animated speech, thumping the table as if to emphasize a point, while saying the chosen two-syllable word. The table will always be thumped to coincide with the articulation of the stressed syllable.

Adding suffixes to words ending in 'silent e'

- Drop the letter 'e' when adding a vowel suffix, for example MAKE ➤ making, MISTAKE ➤ mistaking.
- Keep the letter 'e' when adding a consonant suffix, for example SAFE ➤ safely.

Adding suffixes to words ending with the letter y

If the word ends in a consonant + 'y' (e.g. CARRY, BEAUTY):

- change 'y' to 'i' + suffix, for example CARRY ➤ carried; carriage; BEAUTY ➤ beautiful, beautify;
- keep 'y' after a vowel, for example STAY ➤ stayed.
- keep 'y' when the suffix begins with 'i', for example HURRY ➤ hurrying.

In order to learn and apply these rules, pupils need to have a secure knowledge of what vowels and consonants are, and what suffixes are; they must be able to distinguish between a suffix beginning with a vowel and a suffix beginning with a consonant. One metacognitive approach to teaching is to provide learners with several words to which suffixes have been added, and guide them towards eliciting the rules for themselves. They can also be encouraged to compile separate lists of vowel suffixes and consonant suffixes for reference. Only one rule should be addressed at a time, and each should be taught in a series of graded steps.

These rules can be practised through word-sums: 'clap' + 'ing', 'safe' + 'est', 'sad' + 'ness', 'hurry' + 'ed'. Teachers should, however, be aware that some learners may appear to have grasped the rules for the purpose of completing word-sum exercises but will not apply them in their own writing. It is therefore important to ensure that a metacognitive approach to teaching is adopted, in which writing is related to reading, and the spelling rules are applied at sentence and text level.

Prefixes

A key difference between suffixes and prefixes is that prefixes modify the meaning of words but do not affect syntactic function. For example, LIKE has the opposite meaning to LIKE, but both words are verbs. Once some suffixes have been mastered, prefixes such as 'un-', 'dis-', 're-' and 'pre-' can be introduced. These are best taught as detachable units having a particular effect on meaning, so that the pitfall of doubling letters in the wrong place, for example <dissappointment>, is less likely to arise. Double letters occur only when the prefix ends with the initial letter of the root word, for example ILLEGAL, UNNECESSARY and IMMOBILE. Prefixes are therefore relatively straightforward as far as spelling is concerned, but they play a significant role in the development of vocabulary.

Root words

An effective method for teaching prefixes and suffixes is to focus on root words, seeing how many different prefixes and suffixes can be added to them. For example, the word COURAGE can be combined with the prefixes 'en-' and 'dis-', and with the suffixes '-ing', '-ed', '-s' and '-ment'; the resulting words can then be used in sentences to show how meaning and syntax are affected. This approach will be particularly important for learners with dyslexia, whose links between orthographic, semantic and morphological representations are likely to be imprecise.

It is also useful to teach how the stress pattern of words sometimes changes when suffixes are added, so that vowels that are neutral in one form of the word become stressed and therefore readily identified for spelling in another form of the word, for example ECONOMY/ECONOMIC and PHOTOGRAPHY/PHOTOGRAPHIC.

Teaching homophones and silent letters

Homophones (words that are pronounced the same but have a different meaning and spelling) and silent letters generally present dyslexic learners with particular difficulties and illustrate quite clearly why a reliance on sound–symbol conversion alone is so unreliable.

The spelling of homophones can often be taught by using a mnemonic technique and encouraging the pupil to make an explicit link between the spelling of one of the words and its meaning, syntax or distinctive visual features. There is then no need to create a mnemonic for the other word as it is simply 'the other one'. For example:

- BUY/BY – Buy you (u) a present.
- FIR/FUR – Draw a fir tree round the 'i' in fir.

- THEIR/THERE – Relate THEIR to MY, HIS, HER, YOUR, using it in phrases – MY HOUSE, THEIR HOUSE.
- HEAR/HERE – You hear with your EAR.

To check that learning has taken place and been consolidated, both words should be put into sentences for dictation.

Silent letters can often be learned by actually articulating them along with or within the word, for example k̲-night, parl̲i-ament, while writing the word.

Conclusions

Spelling in English is at best complex, at worst chaotic. It is certainly not systematic, yet it is the task of the teacher to convey that there is at least some rationale underlying the hundreds of ways in which words are conventionally represented in writing.

Mastering orthography involves the application of a range of linguistic skills, all of which may prove difficult for dyslexic learners. They are likely to have particular difficulty with the initial challenge of reflecting on the sound structure of words and mapping sounds to written symbols. Consequently, whereas children who are not dyslexic are able to express their ideas in writing from a very early age, simply by following their speech sounds, children with a weakness in phonological processing are not usually able to do this. The first challenge for the teacher is therefore not to teach dyslexic children to spell but to enable them to start to write.

Unfortunately, mapping sounds to symbols, although enabling written communication, does not generally result in correct spelling. Dyslexic children very soon need to be taught that sounds may be represented by more than one letter and that groups of letters sometimes symbolize units of grammatical meaning rather than simply sounds. There is no room for approximation in spelling; there are numerous ways in which almost every sound can be written, but only one of these will be correct for a particular word.

Spelling often proves to be a persisting weakness for people with dyslexia, but a well-structured, metacognitive approach to teaching, with a focus on individual need, is the only way in which significant progress is likely to be made.

In summary:

- Spelling in English is challenging for all, but even more so for the learner with dyslexia.
- Spelling involves making links between sounds, letters, meaning and grammar.

- An awareness of morphology should be incorporated into the teaching of spelling from the earliest stages.
- The teaching of spelling should be informed by qualitative assessment.
- An analysis of errors yields information about an individual's use of strategies and highlights gaps in knowledge.
- Even the youngest dyslexic learner can benefit from a metacognitive approach to teaching.
- Learners with dyslexia need to be taught in a structured, sequential and cumulative way, with plenty of opportunity for overlearning.
- Teaching should not take place 'in a vacuum' but should encompass the integration of spoken and written language, the integration of word-, sentence- and text-level learning, and the integration of reading and writing skills.
- The cognitive strengths and weaknesses of the learner and the wider school curriculum should be taken into account.
- The SLT may play an important role in identifying which children with speech and language problems are at risk of literacy difficulties, and in providing intervention training.
- Once sound–symbol correspondence and letter name knowledge are secure, programmes for teaching spelling should include spelling patterns, key words, syllable structure, spelling rules, homophones, silent letters, suffixes and prefixes.
- Some well-known spelling rules are actually more useful for reading than for spelling. The most useful rules relate to prefixes and suffixes.

CHAPTER 11

Developing handwriting skills

JANE TAYLOR

Writing systems have been developed by mankind for communicating thoughts and ideas in a permanent way. A great variety of languages and their corresponding scripts are used in different parts of the world today, and to be able to use these effectively, the codes as well as their written forms must be mastered. Handwriting is a complex skill involving cognitive, linguistic and perceptual motor skills. The purpose of this chapter is to examine some of the difficulties experienced by children learning to write, and to suggest strategies for helping both the beginner writer and the child whose handwriting is a cause for concern.

Let us consider the information processing that is involved when writing a letter. First, it requires cognitive organization – attention, selection, analysis and integration of the components of a letter and competent gross and fine motor coordination. It involves visual, auditory and tactile acuity. It also involves memory – the knowledge of a letter and its rule elements in order to produce the trace of the letter and to check the outcome. Finally, it requires motor organization – planning how to write the letter and initiating the necessary movements to produce the trace.

Underlying deficits that cause handwriting difficulties

There are a number of reasons why a child may be experiencing handwriting difficulties, although not every child will fit neatly into a specific group. Children falling within any of the following groups should be considered 'at risk'.

Developmental coordination disorder

Pupils with developmental coordination disorder (DCD), previously referred to as 'clumsy', are children 'who experience movement difficulties out of proportion with their general development and in the absence of any known medical condition' (American Psychiatric Association, 1994). Developmental milestones may have been delayed, and children may have proprioception difficulties such as poor balance and body image. They may experience gross motor difficulties such a poor postural tone, poor eye-tracking, an inability to cross the midline, and directionality and later-ality confusion. They may find the gross motor control required to maintain a good writing posture and correct tool-hold difficult to sustain. Activities such as dressing, physical education and games are often a problem.

Children with DCD frequently have more than one area of weakness. They may have sequential and motor planning difficulties, and poor fine motor control. Poor hand–eye coordination skills may lead to difficuties in producing the correct movement pattern for each letter. In addition, the act of writing may be slow and laborious. The *Movement Assessment Battery for Children* (*Movement ABC*; Henderson and Sugden, 1992) is a helpful diagnostic tool frequently used by therapists to pinpoint the degree and precise nature of the motor impairment. Included in this battery is a check-list that teachers can use to screen 'at-risk' children. The manual provides guidelines for management and remediation, and will assist teachers to plan suitable physical education intervention programmes.

Visual-perceptual and visual-motor difficulties

Many children with DCD have poor visual perception, which makes the acquisition of handwriting skills more difficult. A child with visual-motor perceptual problems may find it difficult to recall the shape of a specific letter, the sequence of the movement pattern of a letter and the sequence of letters in a word. Such children may reverse letters or fail to see similar patterns in letters. They may have difficulty regulating the slant or appre-ciating the relative height of letters, and find it difficult in maintain an even space between letters and words.

Gardner (1996), in his *Test of Visual Perceptual Skills*, defines visual per-ception as 'the ability to give meaning to what is seen'. He suggests that seven areas can be identified:

- *visual discrimination*: the ability to match or determine the exact charac-teristics of two forms when one of the forms is among similar forms;
- *visual memory*: the ability to remember for immediate recall all of the characteristics of a given form, and to be able to find this form from an array of similar forms;

- *visual-spatial relationships*: the ability to determine, from among a number of identical forms, the one single form or part of a single form that is going in a different direction from the other forms;
- *visual form constancy*: the ability to see a form, and to be able to find that form, even though the form may be smaller, larger, rotated, reversed and/or hidden;
- *visual sequential memory*: the ability to remember for immediate recall a series of forms from among a larger set of forms;
- *visual figure–ground*: the ability to perceive a form visually, and to find this form hidden in a conglomerated ground of matter;
- *visual closure*: the ability to determine, from among a number of incomplete forms, the one that is the same as the stimulus form, i.e. the completed form.

The test is purely visual and examines each area, with the scores giving a very clear indication of a child's strengths and weaknesses. Gardner's test of *Visual-Motor Skills – Revised* (1995) is a useful short, untimed, shape-copying test of fine motor skills for children aged 3 years to 13;11 years. The test is designed to assess the child's ability or inablity to translate 'motorically' (i.e. with his or her hand) what he or she perceives. If the design is copied badly, Gardner suggests that the examiner can ask the child whether his or her drawing is the same as the stimulus. If the child thinks that the drawing is the same, he or she is very likely to have a visual-perceptual disorder. If the child thinks that the drawing is different, he or she is likely to have a visual-motor disorder.

Another useful test, which ascertains a child's ability to copy a presented form accurately, is the *Developmental Test of Visual-Motor Integration 3R* (*VMI*; Beery, 1989). A sequence of 24 geometric forms is presented to the child for him or her to copy.

Programmes to use in the classroom to strengthen specific areas of weakness need to be implemented and should be considered to be an essential part of a school's handwriting policy (see Appendix 1 for suggestions). If the child has serious problems, with either motor coordination or visual perception, it may be necessary to seek advice from a physiotherapist and/or occupational therapist.

Dyspraxia

Dyspraxia is an immaturity of the organization of movement, an immaturity in the way in which the brain processes information that results in messages not being properly transmitted. Dyspraxia affects the planning of what to do and how to do it. It is associated with problems of perception, language and thought (see www.dyspraxiafoundation.org.uk).

The terminology of DCD and dyspraxia has developed over the years. Henderson and Henderson (2003) suggest that it continues to present a problem for therapists and teachers, some using the term DCD and others referring to children as dyspraxic.

Dyslexia

Dyslexia is best described as a combination of abilities and difficulties that affect the learning process in one or more of reading, spelling and writing. Accompanying weaknesses may be identified in the areas of speed of processing, short-term memory, sequencing and organization, auditory and/or visual perception, spoken language and motor skills. It is particularly related to mastering and using written language, which may include alphabetic, numeric and musical notation (see the British Dyslexia Association website: www.bda-dyslexia.org.com). Because these children find learning to read, to spell and to express their thoughts on paper difficult; they write fewer words, which means that they have less practice than their peers. Some children have additional DCD and/or attention deficit hyperactivity disorder difficulties.

Attention deficit disorder

Attention deficity disorder is a disorder that affects those parts of the brain which control attention, impulse and concentration (see http://ADDIS. co.uk). In addition, a child can be hyperactive (attention deficit hyperactivity disorder) and may also suffer from mood swings and/or social clumsiness (see the Attention Deficit Disorder Information and Support Service website: www.addiss.co.uk). By the very nature of this underlying difficulty, these children are likely to have problems focusing sufficient attention on detail, which mastering handwriting requires in the early stages of learning to write.

Asperger syndrome

These children may have 'impaired social interaction and obsessional pursuits of repetitive or idiosyncratic interests, while at the same time emphasizing normality of cognitive and early language development' (Henderson and Green, 2001, p. 65; see also American Psychiatric Association, 1994). In additon, 'clumsy' movements are considered to be a common feature but are not considered as a defining feature. Henderson and Green go on to say that, although Asperger attached considerable weight to 'clumsiness', and more recently a number of studies have commented on handwriting being a special problem for these children, there has been no satisfactory systematic research that sheds light on the problem. Teachers still, however, need to ensure that these children are monitored carefully. Some may find handwriting so frustrating that acquiring keyboard skills may be more appropriate (see the National Autistic Society website: www.nas.org.uk).

Physical handicaps

There are other physical disabilities such as cerebral palsy and osteogenesis (brittle bones) that affect children and may make the acquisition of fluent handwriting problematical. These children may need to bypass handwriting altogether and master keyboard skills as an alternative.

Other reasons for handwriting difficulties

Some children, whether disabled or not, fail to pick up elements of handwriting for less clearly defined reasons. They may have been expected to write before they were ready. There may have been insufficient teaching, learning and practice at a vital stage in learning to write, or the standard of handwriting that a teacher expected may have been considerably lower than a child's potential ability. On the other hand, they may simply have missed handwriting instruction lessons for a variety of reasons, such as illness or change of school.

Many children with poor handwriting skills have poor self-esteem. Whatever the underlying deficit may be, children who are finding the acquisition of handwriting skills slow and laborious should be considered to be 'at risk'. An accurate diagnosis of the underlying causes is a necessary precursor to remediation.

Ergonomics

Before embarking on handwriting instruction, the teacher must be aware of the physical environment in which the child is expected to write. It is necessary to consider the following:

- *Whether the height of the table and chair fit the child.* Brown and Henderson (1989) suggest that, as a rule of thumb, the height should be half the height of the child, and the chair seat should be one third of the child's height. However, Lewis and Salway (1989) pointed out that sitting the 'small older child' on two stacked chairs produced more mature behaviour. The alternative is to use adjustable furniture or a foot stool. The present trend is to consider whether a healthy back is more efficiently maintained if the chair seat slopes slightly forward (National Back Pain Association Back, 1995; see www.backcare.org.uk). A hard foam wedge placed on the seat is an alternative.

- *The use of a sloping writing surface on which to write.* A sloping surface improves the position of the wrist, head and hand in relation to the writing surface. Strain and pressure may also be reduced when the hand is supported in this position. An angle of 20 degrees is the most comfortable (Brown and Henderson, 1989).
- *The type of tool to be used.* Children should be offered a variety of pencils and pens from which to select the one that feels most comfortable and best suits their style of writing. Pens may, for example, have shafts of different shapes and diameter, and tips with different widths.
- *The stage at which the change from pencil to pen is to be made.*
- *The size and type of paper to be used.* Lined paper should be used once the child can form letters correctly. The number of lines to be used and the width between lines are important to consider.
- *The surface on which the child writes.* This should not be too hard. Children are frequently expected to write on a single sheet of paper placed directly on the table. A large piece of card can used as a 'presser'. The presser can be used as an aide memoir for the 4Ps – presser, paper position, posture, pencil hold. The table or desk should be uncluttered.
- *The child's sitting position.* The child should be taught to adopt a good posture with feet flat on the floor, bottom well back on the chair, hips slightly flexed, a straight back and the non-writing hand stabilizing the paper.
- *The position of the paper.* The right-handed child should have the paper tilted 10–20 degrees to the right. The non-writing hand should be placed above the right hand to hold the paper still. The left-handed child should have the paper tilted to the left at an angle of about 30 degrees. The top right-hand corner should be in line with the child's navel. It is vital that children learn to place their writing hand below the writing line, which enables them to see the letters as they are written. It is essential too that the non-writing hand is placed above the writing hand as this allows the writing arm to move freely across the page. If the child has a hooked grasp, the paper should be in the right-handed position.
- *The right-handed child should sit on the right of a left-handed child* so that both children can move their writing arm freely.
- Children need to be reminded that, as they write, they should *move the paper up* rather than moving their writing arm down, thus maintaining the hand and arm in the optimum position.
- *The grasp that the child uses.* The ideal grasp is considered to be the dynamic tripod grasp – this is when the thumb, index finger and middle finger combine to form a tripod. Time should be spent learning how to

hold the pencil correctly. This activity should be reinforced whenever children are using a writing implement. Start with the point of the pencil facing the child. Ask the child to pick up the pencil between the thumb and first finger raising it to a vertical position, and then to place the middle finger under the pencil and let the pencil slowly drop back. Many pencils have triangular shafts that can assist in achieving the correct grasp. If necessary, the use of an additional shaped grip, slipped on to the shaft, may facilitate an improved grasp. The fingers control the up–down movement, the thumb the circular movement and the wrist the side-to-side to side movement.

- *The light source should ideally lie to the front of the child* – from the left for the right-hander, and from the right for the left-hander.

Children should to taught to appreciate the importance of these ergonomic principles, which are as relevant to handwriting as the specific skills required in sporting activites.

Learning to write

The task is to be able to write the 26 small and capital letters, the numerals 0–9 and basic punctuation automatically, i.e without having to conceptualize how each letter is formed. To promote the acquisition of the necessary skills, specific teaching and plenty of time for practice are required in the early stages of learning to write.

Before a child embarks on a handwriting programme, the teacher might find it helpful to observe how the child does the following:

- *Draws a person* (Naglieri, 1987). Michael (1984) suggests that the ability to draw a person should be an indicator of whether the child is ready to begin writing. He states that a child is ready to make letters when he or she can 'draw a person with details correcly placed' and is able to 'make one shape inside another' (Michael, 1984, pp. 10–11). In the author's experience, however, some children who have shown poor body concept in their drawings have learnt, with appropriate teaching, to write successfully. Nevertheless, as a rule of thumb, a child who shows inconsistency in his 'draw a person' task should be considered to be 'at risk'. Nicky was one such child; he was a right-handed child with DCD when seen at 7;3 years of age. Figure 11.1 shows that his drawing of a person was fairly rudimentary. His handwriting performance is shown in Figures 11.2 and 11.3.
- *Copies a circle, a cross, a square, a triangle and a diamond*. Sheridan (1975) states that a child should be able to copy a circle at 3 years of age, a cross at 4 years, a square at 5 years and a triangle at 5;6 years. Many of the

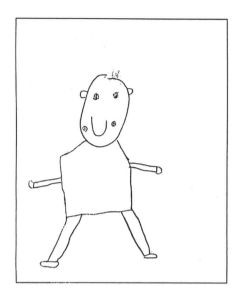

Figure 11.1 Nicky's 'Draw a person'. Nicky is 7;3 years and left-handed, and has developmental coordination disorder.

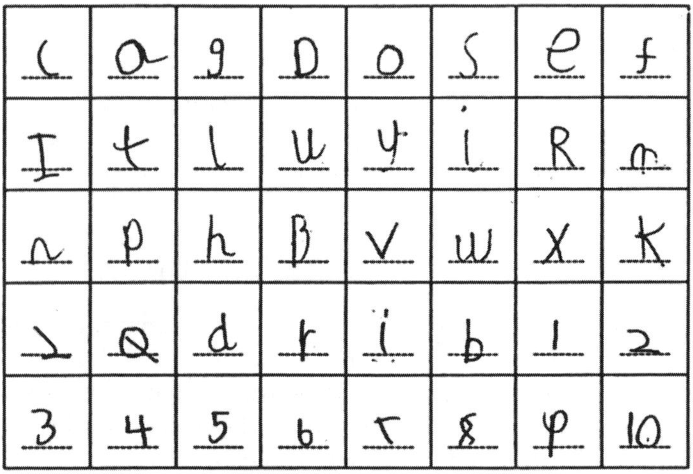

Figure 11.2 Nicky's letter formation.

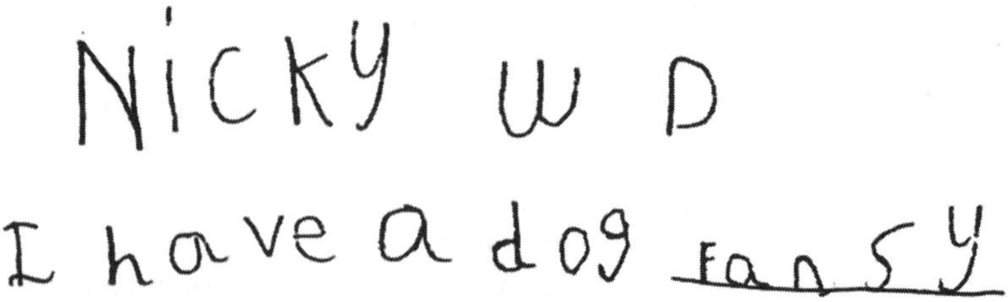

Figure 11.3 Nicky's free-written expression.

letters have movements similar to these basic shapes. For example, 'v', 'w', 'x', 'z' and 'K' have diagonal lines, so if a child is unable to draw a triangle, he or she may find these letters difficult to write.

If children can draw a person and copy the basic shapes, they are ready to write. If they are unable to do so, they will need to spend a considerable amount of time mastering prewriting skills before embarking on learning to write individual letters. Teachers are, however, under considerable pressure from the targets set in the National Literacy Strategy (Department for Education and Employment, 1998), which suggests that children should be able to write their first name by the end of year R. In a further National Literacy Strategy publication, *Developing Early Writing* (Department for Education and Employment, 2001), designed to help teachers and practitioners, it clearly states that 'until children have gained reasonable fine motor control through art and other activites formal handwriting worksheets are not appropriate'.

In addition, the child should be able to:

- understand the language of instruction, for example 'top', 'next to', 'starts with', 'ends with';
- recognize letters by matching, which is the beginning stage of internalizing the shape of letters;
- identify the names and/or sounds of the letters as this skill avoids letter confusion, although some children may initially be able to write letters without knowing their names or sounds.

Before embarking on teaching handwriting, it is desirable that the teacher identifies those children who experiencing any of the above difficulties and ensures that they are given plenty of time to acquire the above-mentioned skills. If prewriting patterns are used, these should relate to letter shapes. Colouring is a useful activity. Colouring within boundaries requires the integration of fine motor and perceptual skills, involving wrist movement as well as fine finger movements.

Learning about letters

Learning about letters and numerals can be made fun and interesting. Children should be encouraged to observe the variety of styles used for letters and numerals, for example in magazines, on advertisements or on food packets. They should learn to appreciate the similarities and differences between letters and should be taught that letters fall naturally into groups. Sets of wooden or plastic alphabet letters are an essential piece of equipment at this stage.

Letters can be divided into groups – letters with ascenders (tall letters), letters with descenders (letters with tails) and x-height letters (middle-size letters) (Figure 11.4). Alternatively, as letters with straight lines occur in more than half of the alphabet, letters with straight lines could be put into a group. Initially, the letters can be sorted into the suggested groups. In *Developing Early Writing* (Department for Education and Employment, 2001), letters are grouped into four movement groups. The suggested advantage is that aligning letters with a key letter will help children to remember the starting point and subsequent movement of the letter. The four groups are:

- down and off in another direction, exemplified by the letter 'l' (long ladder): i, j, l, t, u (v, w with rounded bases);
- down and retrace upwards, exemplified by the letter 'r' (one-armed robot): letters b, h, k, m, n, p, r; numbers 2, 3, 5 follow a clockwise direction;
- anti-clockwise round, exemplified by the letter 'c' (curly caterpillar): letters c, a, d, e, g, o, q, f, s; numbers 0, 6, 8, 9;
- zigzag letters: letters (k), v, w, x, y, z; numbers 1, 4, 7.

I prefer the letter 'k' to be taught in the one-armed robot group and letters 'v', 'w' and 'y' in the long-ladder group.

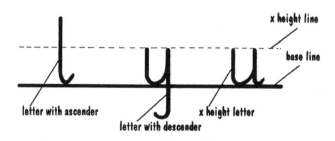

Figure 11.4 Examples of how letters can be grouped.

Every child should be able to orientate each wooden/plastic letter correctly before being expected to it to write it. Letters can initially be placed on the table. Once orientation is correct, the next stage is to learn to appreciate how letters relate to a base line. Provide the child with a long, thin piece of card with a base line drawn across it. The next stage is to learn the similarities and differences of letters. For example, the letters 'a', 'd' and 'g' are all based on the letter 'c'. An appreciation of this fact lessens the amount of information that has to be remembered. It is worth spending time familiarizing the children with the letters in this way. Some children may be able to go through the stages quickly, whereas others will need to take their time. At the learning-to-write stage, this basic letter knowledge should enable them to become self-critical and help them to monitor whether the letters they produce match the model given.

Mastering the formation of letters and numerals

The aim is for every child to write each letter using the correct movement patterns. Letters that end on the base line should be taught, from the beginning, with an exit stroke to facilitate the natural progression to a joined script. The teacher needs to spend time demonstrating exactly how each letter is formed, stressing and verbalizing the movements required. The teacher can then ask the children to demonstrate the movement patterns by writing the letter in the air, with their writing arm and index finger outstretched, repeating the verbal instructions as they do so. Once they have the movement pattern firmly established, they can then repeat the exercise without verbalization, and finally they repeat the activity with their eyes shut. Writing a letter with the eyes shut means that the correct movement pattern of the letter has been internalized, the beginings of achieving automaticity; tracing over letters does not achieve this.

The next stage is for the children to write letters with their index finger in a variety of media, such as in sand on a small tray. At this stage, children should draw a base line from left to right in the sand so that they can learn to align the letter correctly. Finally, they can use a writing implement and practise writing on a white board or a sheet of paper, again remembering to draw the base line. Some children may need paper with both the base and x-height line indicated (Figure 11.5). This type of paper should be used until a child's handwriting is consistent and completely automatic. Michael (1984) suggests that children should be able to write all the letters of the alphabet before they are expected to express themselves in writing.

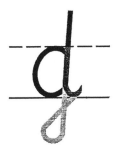

Figure 11.5 Illustration to show how the shape of the letter 'c' forms part of the letters 'a', 'd' and 'g', with base and x-height lines indicated.

Automaticity

At this stage, it is important to build automaticity into handwriting practice. The teacher dictates the letters at random from a letter group, for example the 'c' 'family'. The children check that the letters are well formed and correctly aligned. Once all the letters have been mastered, the children can practise writing out all the letters of the alphabet in a given amount of time.

Developing a cursive script

Once the child can form each letter correctly, he or she is ready to join letters. This means that some children will move to joining letters very quickly, whereas others will need more time before they are ready.

The progression from single letters to joining letters is easy if the child has learned to use appropriate exit strokes from the beginning. When the exit stroke is extended, it becomes the entry stroke of the next letter. If, however, the child does not use any exit strokes, he or she may need to practise this first before attempting to master the diagonal joins. To achieve fluency, the exit strokes should be at an angle of about 45 degrees from the base line.

There are three basic joins:

1. *Horizontal join*. The letters 'o', 'r', 'v' and 'w' can exit with a horizontal join (Figure 11.6), and the letters 'f' and 't' can exit from the cross bar (Figure 11.7).

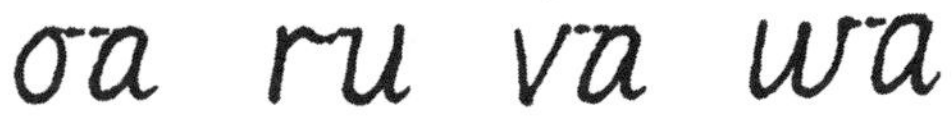

oa ru va wa

Figure 11.6 Horizontal joins.

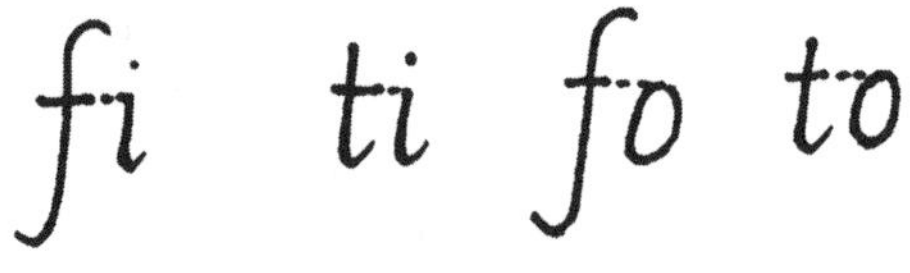

fi ti fo to

Figure 11.7 Horizontal joins from cross bar.

2. *Diagonal join*. The exit strokes of letters 'a', 'c', 'd', 'e', 'h', 'i', 'k', 'l', 'm', 'n', 't', 'u', 'x' and 'z' are extended to become the diagonal join (Figure 11.8).

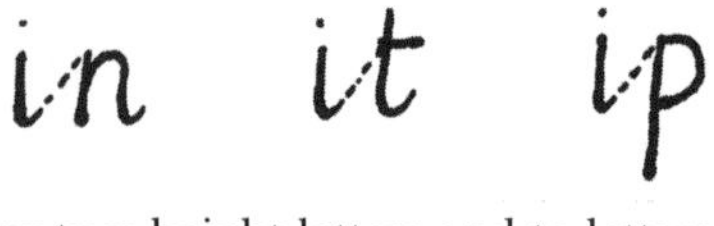

in it ip

Figure 11.8 Diagonal joins to x-height letters and to letters with ascenders and descenders.

3. *Diagonal join extended to an oval letter.* The letters 'a', 'c', 'd' and 'g' require the diagonal stroke from the preceding letter to be extended (Figure 11.9) with a curve to the right to accommodate the oval letter.

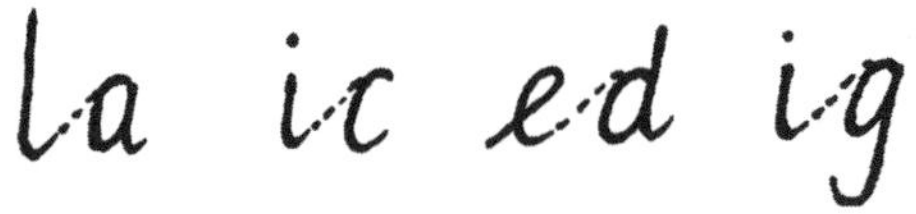

$$la\ ic\ ed\ ig$$

Figure 11.9 Diagonal joins to oval letters.

In the initial stages of learning to write, there are some letters that need not be joined. For example, the tails of the letters 'g', 'j', 'y' and 'q' can be left unjoined or can be extended to form a diagonal join (Figure 11.10). Similarly, the joins from the letters 'b', 'p' and 's' can be left unjoined or can be joined from the bottom (Figure 11.11). For those children who confuse the letters 'b' and 'p', learning to write an open 'b' and 'p' may be helpful (Figure 11.12).

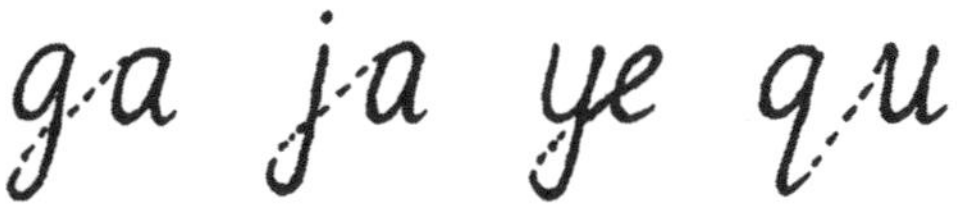

$$ga\ ja\ ye\ qu$$

Figure 11.10 Diagonal joins from letters with descenders.

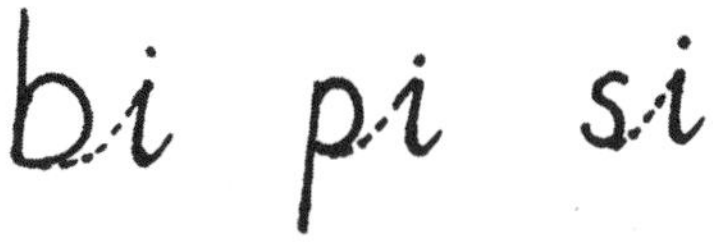

$$bi\ pi\ si$$

Figure 11.11 Diagonal joins from closed 'b', 'p' or 's'.

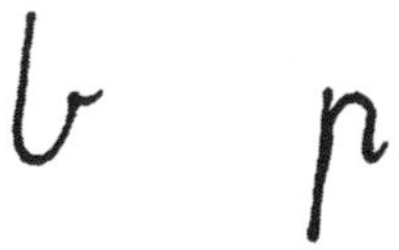

$$b\ \ \ p$$

Figure 11.12 Open 'p' and 'b'.

For children who have spatial and orientation difficulties, learning to start all letters from the base line can help with mastering spelling patterns as each word is a continuous series of movements. Once again, it is important that the entry stroke leads up to the base line at an angle of about 45 degrees.

Fluency

Fluency is essential for automatic, legible handwriting and should be incorporated into every teaching programme. Fluency can be developed by spending time on producing letters at speed. This can be achieved by asking the child to write the same letter legibly as many times as possible in a given time. A suitable period for this exercise is 10–15 seconds. The child then ticks the 'good' letters, i.e. the well-formed ones, which reinforces the child's self-critical skills. Once a number of letters have been learned, the child can be asked to write out one or two words that contain those letters and then to write a sentence using the two words, checking the letter formation at the end of the task.

Capital letters

Capital letters will need to be learned, but as there are fewer directional changes, they tend not to cause too much difficulty. For a child with severe writing difficulties who might still want to be able to write but is finding lower-case letters too difficult to master, sticking to capital letters could be an alternative.

Numerals

The correct movement patterns of the numerals 0–9 need to be taught. Numerals should be the same height as capital letters.

Monitoring progress

A self-monitoring system can be introduced to maintain a continued focus on letter formation. The young child may have an individual chart that is ticked once a letter has been mastered. The older child could use a more detailed chart to include information on letter formation, slant, alignment, the relative size of letters and spaces between letters and words. For example, having learnt the letters 'i', 't' and 'l', the child could be asked to indicate on the chart: 'My straight lines are straight and parallel?' YES/NO. This system should encourage children to become more aware of the details of handwriting that still require continued practice, and enable them to monitor their own progress.

Progress should be regularly evaluated. Evaluation might consist of checking letter formation or the child writing out the alphabet at speed. Alternatively, a free-writing test in which the child is asked to commit ideas to paper within a time limit can be given. This piece of work will provide the teacher with a good deal of information for monitoring handwriting, spelling, punctuation, grammar and use of language (see Chapter 6 in this volume).

Handwriting is assessed as part of the Standard Attainment Tests for key stages 1 and 2. The marking system is explained in *The English Tasks Teacher's Handbook* (Department for Education and Skills), which is updated every year.

To achieve legible, fluent and attractive writing produced with ease, it is essential to ensure that sufficient time is given to the practice of this skill, with an appropriate monitoring of performance.

Assessment of handwriting difficulties

In order to assess the nature and causes of a child's difficulty with handwriting, a sample of letter formation and free writing should be collected and dated. The following checklist provides a useful guide. Check for the following:

- *Posture, paper position, tool-hold and pressure.*
- *Alphabet knowledge.* The names of letters should be known. Common confusions are b/d, m/w, u/y, f/t, g/j, p/q and i/j/l.
- *Letter formation.* This can only be done by watching the child write the letters. Identify those letters which are incorrectly or poorly formed.
- *Formation of numerals.* Identify those numerals which are incorrectly formed.
- *Relative height of letters.* Letters with ascenders, letters with descenders and x-height letters should all be the correct height.
- *Slant of straight lines.* Straight lines should be straight and parallel.
- *Alignment.* Letters should sit correctly on the line.
- *Space between letters and words.* The space between letters and words should be even.
- *Size of writing.* The writing should not be too big or too small.
- *Correct use of capital letters and punctuation.* A sentence begins with a capital letter and ends with a full stop.
- *Joins.* If the letters are joined, it is important to check that the join is at about an angle of 45 degrees.

Handwriting speed

A considerable amount of time in school is spent writing. Some children are able to produce legible, attractive handwriting at speed, whereas for others, it is always a laborious task. It is useful for the teacher to know the writing speed of a child as this has implications for written tasks that the child is expected to produce. This information may be derived from an evaluation of speed-copying test. The familiar sentence 'The quick brown fox jumps over the lazy dog' can be used for this purpose. Younger children could use the phrase 'cat and dog' (Zivianni, 1998). First, the children are asked to copy the sentence in their best handwriting. This task is timed. They then copy the sentence for 3 minutes in fast writing.

There are no national norms for writing speeds in the UK, but research in New Zealand and the UK has indicated an average speed of between 77 and 82 letters per minute for 11-year-olds (Alston, 1992) Correspondence with the Dyslexia Institute suggests that, on average, 13-year-olds are writing 14–15 words per minute and 15-year-olds write closer to 16–18 words per minute. Alternatively, data can be collected from all pupils within a class to create class norms (see the website of the Centre for Reading and Language – www.york.ac.uk/res/crl – for some such 'norms'). Another possiblity is to compare an individual's performance from one time to the next, i.e. monitor a 'PB', or personal best. A useful activity is to copy a short passage for 5 minutes. The child should then count the number of words and rewrite it at speed, noting the time taken. A partner can then be asked to underline any words that are illegible.

For those children whose handwriting does not meet the demands of the writing situation, alternative methods of communication should be considered. Decisions may need to be made as early as 6 or 7.

Written expression

A free-writing sample can also be useful for establishing the normal range of performance within a class or school irrespective of national norms. Alston (1995) describes one method of evaluating written output, grammatical competence and expression. The child is requested to write about any of the following topics:

- My favourite person.
- Someone I know very well.
- Something in which I am very interested.

Figure 11.13 shows the free written expression of Luke, aged 12;1 years, with dyslexia.

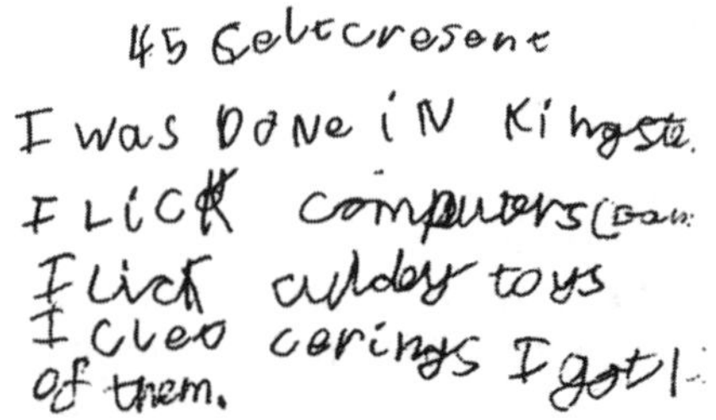

Figure 11.13 Luke's free-written expression at 12;1 years.

Children should ideally write for a 20 minute period, but the actual time should be noted if the full period of writing is not possible. Writing can be assessed under five headings:

1. handwriting;
2. spelling;
3. punctuation;
4. grammar;
5. logical, stylistic and expressive writing.

Children aged 7–10 years (86 girls and 82 boys) from a Cheshire primary school were asked to write for a 20 minute period. The mean number of words produced per minute by children in different age groups is shown in Table 11.1 (Alston, 1995). Older children have been studied by Dutton (1992). In this study, the children were asked to write 'My life history' in a 30 minute period. Writing speed was one aspect that was examined, and the results are summarised in Table 11.2. The results suggested that girls tend to perform at a better level than boys.

Table 11.1 The writing speeds of primary school children during a 20 minute free-writing exercise

Age of children (years and months)	Mean (words per minute)	Standard deviation
7;10	3.76	1.91
8;10	5.63	2.61
9;10	5.98	2.22
10;10	7.64	3.14

Table 11.2 The writing speeds of senior school children during a 30 minute free-writing exercise

Age of children (years and months)	Mean (words per minute)
13;00	12.7
14;00	14.4
15;00	15.9
16;00	17.1
17;00	18.4

The teacher should ideally examine untimed and speed samples as well as a sample of free writing to ascertain whether the child has specific difficulties such as:

- maintaining legibility when writing at speed or when involved in free-written expression;
- a slower than average writing speed;
- written expression difficulties that are affecting output.

For example, compare Figure 11.14 showing 5 minutes of Luke's written work at the age of 14 years, with Figure 11.15, showing his copying performance when he had more time to concentrate on legibility.

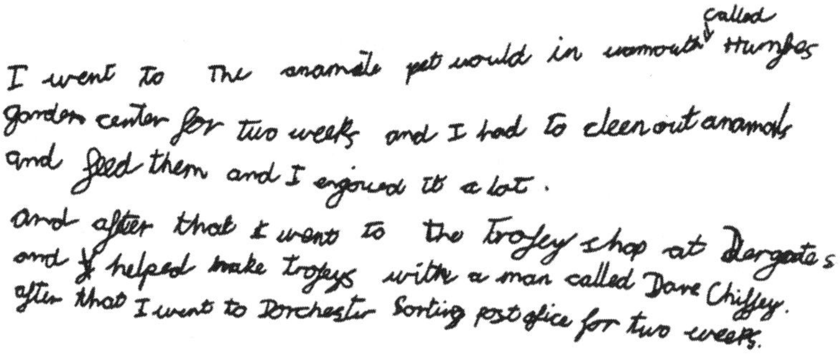

> I went to the anamale pet would in wamouth called thumbas
> gorden center for two weeks and I had to cleen out anamols
> and feed them and I enjoued it a lot.
> And after that I went to the trofey shop at Dergates
> and I helped make tropeys with a man called Dave Chiffey.
> after that I went to Dorchester Sorting post office for two weeks.

Figure 11.14 Luke's free-written expression in 5 minutes at 14 years.

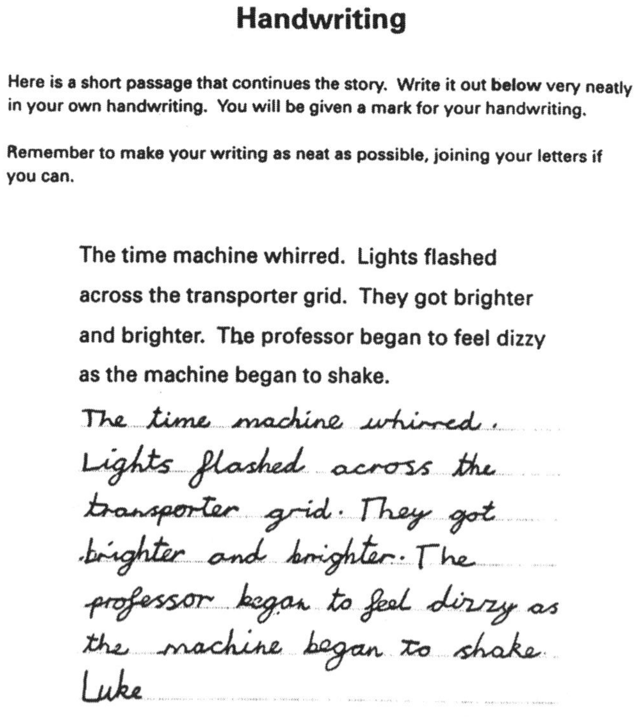

Handwriting

Here is a short passage that continues the story. Write it out below very neatly in your own handwriting. You will be given a mark for your handwriting.

Remember to make your writing as neat as possible, joining your letters if you can.

The time machine whirred. Lights flashed across the transporter grid. They got brighter and brighter. The professor began to feel dizzy as the machine began to shake.

> The time machine whirred.
> Lights flashed across the
> transporter grid. They got
> brighter and brighter. The
> professor began to feel dizzy as
> the machine began to shake.
> Luke

Figure 11.15 Luke's copying performance.

Involving children in the assessment of their own handwriting

In a survey of secondary pupils' (year 7) attitude to their own handwriting, Whitmarsh (1988) found that 85 per cent of children wished that they could write better and 88 per cent thought that being able to write was important. Children are much more likely to make an effort to improve their handwriting if the teacher does not start by criticizing what is incorrect but praises all that can be done well. Children should be asked whether they know, or have previously been told, what is problematic with their handwriting. This changes the emphasis from one of authority to one of partnership, of discovering together where the problems lie.

Handwriting can be considered to be 'rule-based'. The following rules can be presented to children for them to select the one that they think identifies a problem area for them.

1. All letters except 'd' and 'e' start at the top.
2. Oval letters should be closed and watertight.
3. Letters with straight lines should be straight and parallel.
4. The relative height of letters should be uniform.
5. Letters should be correctly placed in relation to the base line.
6. The space between letters should be even.
7. The space between words should be even.
8. Letters that end at the top join horizontally.
9. Letters that end on the base line join diagonally.
10. A sentence should begin with a capital letter and end with a full stop.

The particular difficulties that a child is experiencing should be discussed and itemized on a checklist with teaching objectives listed. Teaching is likely to be more positive if children are encouraged to identify their own errors. The teacher may have to use some discretion if there are too many faults. Children's chance of success will be greater if they are expected to work on only one, or at most two, faults at a time.

Implementing a teaching programme

Before embarking on a remedial handwriting programme, the teacher should check that there are no underlying problems with the child's vision and hearing. Indications in the medical records that the child has seen a speech and language therapist, physiotherapist or occupational therapist should alert the teacher to possible earlier difficulties with speech and language, sensorimotor or perceptual difficulties, which may still persist. The teacher may wish to seek advice of the other professionals or to liaise with them about the teaching programme.

Improving posture and paper position should be the starting point of any remedial programme. It should be explained to the child that, as handwriting is one of the most complex physical skills that we learn, attention must be paid to organizing the body to achieve maximum efficiency, just as one would in any sport.

The 'rules' of handwriting used to identify the difficulties can now form the basis of the teaching programme. The teaching approach for the child who has failed to master handwriting skills should be similar to the approach already described for the beginner writer. The use of rules should be seen as a technique to focus the child's attention on the detail and therefore to make handwriting practice more meaningful:

- Rule 1: Once the inaccuracies of letter formation have been identified, each letter must be worked on as already described.
- Rule 2: This is achieved by ensuring that the letters 'a', 'd', 'g' and 'q' are begun at approximately the 1 o'clock position and are not written as a round 'o' with an exit stroke.
- Rule 3: The child is asked to use a fine red pen to mark the straight lines on a sample of writing. He or she can then observe whether the slant is regular.
- Rule 4: The child is asked to divide a set of plastic letters into three groups: letters with ascenders, letters with descenders and x-height letters. Alternatively, the child is asked to write out all the letters of the alphabet and then to write them out again in their specific groups. This will highlight which letters are not placed correctly on the base line. The letter 'j' is often placed in the 'letters with ascenders' group. Lined paper, with the base and x-height lines indicated, will assist the child to work on improving the relative height of the letters.
- Rule 5: Discussing the purpose of the base line and how letters and words should be correctly aligned should assist the child to identify those letters which are incorrectly aligned.
- Rules 6/7: The child is asked to measure the distance he or she leaves between letters and words. The correct amount of space that should be left between letters/words is then discussed. The space between letters is often uneven because the joining stroke is irregular. The space between words should be approximately the size of two of the child's small 'o's. The child is asked to write either a word or a sentence checking the spaces between the letters or words and ticking those spaces which are even.
- Rules 8/9: See the section on developing a cursive script, earlier in this chapter.
- Rule 10: The child needs to appreciate the reasons for punctuation.

Ideas for teaching writing-related skills

The underlying deficits that often create handwriting difficulties may also mean that other skills, such as puctuation, presentation of written work and copying from a white board, are a struggle.

Punctuation and presentation

The child needs to be taught that punctuation marks are inserted immediately after the last letter of a phrase or sentence. Children who experience difficulties with the presentation of their written work, such as underlining headings, need to be given specific instructions. As they find instructions difficult to remember, one solution is to paste a model of what is expected by each subject teacher in the front of the exercise book or in a note book. Instruction on labelling techniques should also be given, for example emphasizing the need to use a ruler when drawing the indicating lines (Figure 11.16). Some children find it very difficult to write neatly without a guide line. It can be helpful to provide them with lines on a laminated piece of card that can be placed under the diagram and provide a guide line.

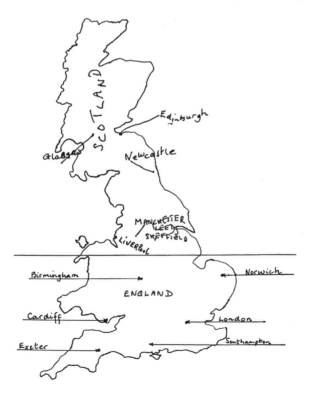

Figure 11.16 A map showing untidy and neat labelling.

Copying from a distance

If copying from a distance is a problem, alternative methods of copying should be considered. For example, a photocopied handout could be given.

Note-taking

Children should be taught note-taking skills, including a personal shorthand such as '+' for 'and' or 'posv' for 'positive'. A list could be devised by each subject teacher.

Keyboard skills

Legibility and speed may always be a problem for some children. For a child whose handwriting is painfully slow, labourious and unattractive, and does not meet the demands of the writing situation, alternative methods of communication should be considered. Decisions may need to be made when the child is only 6 or 7 years old. The computer is a great boon, with presentation being so much better than any handwritten work (see Appendix 1 for suggestions).

Keyboarding is a physical skill, so the child who needs to use word processing on a regular basis must be provided with proper instruction and given sufficient time to master touch-typing before he or she uses these skills for class work.

Conclusions

To achieve legible, fluent and attractive writing produced with ease, it is essential to ensure that sufficient time is given to the practice of this skill, with an appropriate monitoring of performance.

Each school should have a handwriting policy with clearly defined, step-by-step objectives through which each child should be able to progress at his or her own speed. Time spent on providing a meaningful teaching programme in the early stages of learning to write, together with regular monitoring of progress, should enable most children to acquire fluent, legible and attractive handwriting. For some, however, practice will not always make perfect, and competent word-processing and keyboard skills should be the alternative for the 'at-risk' child.

Appendix 1: Teaching handwriting resource list

Addy L (2004) Speed Up – A Kinaesthetic Programme to Develp Fluent Handwriting. Wisbech: LDA; a training programme focusing on movements to develop kinaesthetic awareness and sensitivity in order to improve handwriting fluency and speed.

Alston J, Taylor J (2000) Teaching Handwriting. A Guide for Teachers and Parents. (Previously published as Handwriting Helpline). Lichfield, Staffordshire: QEd.

Archibald M, Martin C (2003) Jump Ahead. Chris Sage, WSCC Learning Support Team. chris.sage@westsussex.gov.uk; a year's intervention programme focusing on gross and fine motor and perceptual skills.

Centre for Micro-Assisted Communication, www.cenmac.com; this provides a list of typing tutors.

Department for Education and Skills. English Tasks Teacher's Handbook, Key Stage 1 (levels 1–3) and 2 (levels 3–5). Updated yearly. Available from Sudbury: Qualifications and Curriculum Authority Publications; this booklet gives guidelines for assessing handwriting in the Standard Assessment Tests.

East Kent Community NHS Trust (1998) The Fizzy Training Games Programme. Canterbury, Kent: East Kent Community NHS Trust, Mary Sheriden Centre; a graded and measurable activity programme in three stages: beginners, intermediate and advanced. It works in three specific areas: balance, ball skills and body awareness.

Handwriting Interest Group (1998, revised 2004) Hands up for Handwriting. Handwriting Interest Group; a quick 'work-out' session preparing the hands for handwriting. Membership form, details of courses and publications, etc. of the Handwriting Interest Group (which is to become the National Handwriting Association) are available at www.nha-handwriting.org.uk

Handwriting Interest Group (2004) Which Handwriting Scheme?; a review of the currently available handwriting schemes. www.nha-handwriting.org.uk

Hawley G, Rae S (2004) SpLD (Specific Learning Difficulties) Resources Booklet; full of useful information for teachers and parents, for example a list of typing programmes, study skill courses and publications. Updated regularly. Available from Gillian Hawley, The King's Mill House, Great Shelford, Cambridge CB2 5EN, UK.

Nash-Wortham M, Hunt J (1997) Take Time. Stourbridge: Robinswood Press; provides numerous physical exercises.

Penso D (1999) Keyboarding Skills for Children with Disablities. London: Whurr; provides the information necessary to determine which children will benefit from learning to use word processing. Over 100 sheets provide methods of learning keyboard skills using both hands, one hand only or a limited number of fingers.

Ripley K (2001) Inclusion for Children with Dyspraxia/DCD. London: David Fulton Publishers; provides a checklist for motor skills and a motor skills training programme.

Taylor J (2001) Handwriting: A Teacher's Guide to Multisensory Approaches to Assessing and Improving Handwriting Skills. London: David Fulton Publishers; provides a comprehensive teaching system, templates for assessment, and record sheets for monitoring both the individual and whole class.

Teodorescu I, Addy L (1996) Write from the Start. Wisbech: LDA; over 400 graded, structured pencil and paper activities to develop hand–eye coordination, form constancy, spatial organization, orientation and laterality.

Therapy Services for Children (2002) Beam Movement – Towards Learning in Primary Schools (2002) Available from Therapy Services for Children, Foster Street Clinic, Foster Street, Maidstone, Kent ME15 6NH, UK; this is a 6 week programme split into three blocks of graded activites to ensure that children entering school have the opportunity to practise and improve their gross motor abilities.

Voors RO (2000) Write Dance. Bristol: Lucky Duck Publishing; a movement to music programme to develop prewriting skills.

Webb A (2004) Pegs to Paper. Available from Angela Webb, 24A Londale Square, London N1 1EN, UK; peg-board exercises to aid handwriting improvement.

CHAPTER 12

Managing the needs of pupils with dyslexia in mainstream classrooms

JANET HATCHER

Most of the chapters in this book concern the assessment and management of children as individuals, children who need individualized approaches typically delivered in one-to-one situations. Rightly, however, teachers often ask, 'How can I help the child with literacy difficulties in the classroom?' Unfortunately, there are no easy 'answers' to this question, or 'tips for teachers' that will provide a ready solution. This chapter focuses on the challenges that teachers face when responding to the diversity of pupils' needs in the mainstream classroom and offers some potential strategies that aim to overcome barriers to learning.

The most effective teaching practices are those which provide pupils with the maximum opportunity to learn (Westwood, 1997). To develop such practices, teachers need to consider how they will manage *needs* (rather than how they will manage individuals). To do this effectively, they must take an 'ecological perspective' that recognizes that the impact of a learning difficulty depends upon a combination of factors – the child, the teacher, the classroom, the school and the family – all within the prevailing national context. This chapter provides an overview of how these factors (or levels) are interrelated before suggesting how teachers might help individual pupils.

The ecological perspective

The 'ecological perspective' distinguishes between 'within-pupil' factors (e.g. their individual learning characteristics) and 'outside-pupil' factors, such as the school and the curriculum.

Within-pupil factors

One of the most basic facts that the teacher must embrace is that not all pupils with dyslexia are the same: each will present with their own 'symptom' profile and process information differently. This means that pupils will require and use different strategies and skills, and teachers will need to assess individual strengths and weaknesses to adapt their teaching approaches to meet individual needs. In addition, teachers need to be aware that reading and writing are not the only problems experienced by pupils with dyslexia. They may, in fact, present a range of other processing and learning difficulties. Indeed, commonly they may:

• have poor short-term memory;
• do poorly on tasks involving planning a strategy;
• have poor attention to the relevant aspect of a problem;
• tend not to formulate and use mediation techniques;
• not transfer learning from one task to another;
• have poor study habits.

Therefore, when working with a pupil with dyslexia, one of the most important questions that the teacher needs to ask first is 'What learning characteristics does the pupil have, and how does the pupil approach learning tasks?'

Inevitably, because they feel insecure about their skills in learning, pupils with dyslexia may feel apprehension, stress, low self-esteem or poor confidence, although many work hard to overcome these problems. Riddick (2002) describes studies of the social and emotional consequences of reading delay and concludes that, for children with dyslexia, literacy skills are their main problem, but that these can lead to secondary problems such as inattentiveness, low motivation, restlessness or disruptive behaviour.

Teachers and therapists are well aware that one of the greatest disincentives to learn is experiencing repeated failure. Pupils who are not experiencing learning success can develop a variety of work avoidance tactics, such as sharpening pencils, sorting materials or 'helping' others. Lewis (1995, p. 32) reported how 'Few children go to the lengths of one child . . . who ate the school goldfish rather than attempt, yet again, an activity he found difficult.' Examples from classroom observations show that such avoidance tactics do not have to be overtly off-task but can be disguised as 'on-task' behaviour, such as handing out work, dealing with writing implements or waiting for a response from the teacher (Hatcher, unpublished data). Teachers therefore have the task of sustaining pupils' confidence and enthusiasm for learning. The failure cycle is a hard cycle to break for 'If at first you don't succeed, you don't succeed.'

Thus, in addition to helping pupils with dyslexia to overcome their literacy difficulties, teachers may have many other, within-pupil, aspects to consider, some of which may be hard to address within the classroom situation.

Outside-pupil factors

Any discussion of how to manage the needs of pupils with dyslexia in the classroom will be highly affected by the national educational context. Where there is a national curriculum that all teachers have to follow and abide by, this will set the parameters by which teaching is delivered. In the UK, for example, teachers use the framework of the National Curriculum (Department for Education and Employment, 2000). Following a set curriculum for all pupils has, of course, great benefits. It means that all pupils have the same basic educational entitlement, no matter whether or not they have underlying difficulties. It also means that there is a clear curriculum framework for teachers to follow, and therefore a structure within which teachers can differentiate work for pupils with different abilities and needs. Where, however, the needs of the individual are concerned, there may be some reservations about the same curriculum for all pupils. There is undoubtedly a tension between ensuring that each pupil is given the same opportunities as the next while needing to adjust the provision for some pupils to cater for individual differences.

This is nowhere more evident than when considering whether pupils with dyslexia should be integrated within the classroom, thus accessing support alongside their peers, or whether more specific, targeted intervention would be more beneficial for them. It could be argued, for example, that a young pupil with dyslexia who is struggling to get on to the 'reading ladder' may make more gains by following an individualized, structured, multisensory literacy intervention rather than being fully integrated within the classroom-based 'literacy hour' (National Literacy Strategy; Department for Education and Employment, 1998). For such a pupil, the literacy hour may be providing breadth at the expense of depth.

It can be argued that there are problems with differentiating the curriculum to cater for individual needs. The ability to differentiate effectively requires teacher expertise and knowledge, together with adequate resources. It is much easier to say that teaching is being differentiated than to do it in practice. There has, however, been a change in recent years from the notion of integration to that of inclusion. The *integration* of a pupil with learning difficulties into a classroom requires that extra support be provided to help that pupil participate in the mainstream programme without its content or delivery necessarily being changed in any fundamental way. The concept of *inclusion*, on the other hand, requires significant changes to be made to the mainstream programme in terms of organization, content and delivery in order to accommodate the wide range of needs of its pupils. Furthermore, the concept of inclusion is firmly based at the school and class level, and influences such areas as:

- school ethos and provision;
- quality and type of instruction;
- teacher expectations;
- curriculum content and delivery;
- relevance of work set;
- classroom environment.

Thus not only can teachers have more control over these aspects, but they should also be more amenable to modification.

Creemers (1994), who looked at multilevel research into school effectiveness, suggests that class-level factors are as important at influencing educational outcomes as are school-level factors. He describes the three main components in classroom education as the teacher, the resources and the organization of the classroom, with an interrelationship between the three components.

Principles of inclusion

This inclusive approach stresses that pupils' needs should be supported within systems-orientated frameworks at the school and classroom level.

Peer and Reid (2001), discussing the principles, practices and challenges of inclusion, conclude that all teachers should be responsible for supporting and helping pupils with dyslexia within subject frameworks. In addition, schools should move towards a collective improvement model of provision in the classroom rather than an individualistic, needs-led model. The dilemma is how to provide for the education of all pupils while paying regard to diversity among individuals (Norwich, 1996).

From the ecological perspective, the learning problems that pupils with dyslexia experience are seen as being due to a complex combination of interacting factors. Although some of them may be more amenable than others to modification in the classroom, all these factors need attention. This means that, in addition to sufficient support systems and effective liaison between schools, parents and outside agencies, there should also continue to be specialist teaching and teaching programmes alongside access to a differentiated curriculum.

Challenges of inclusion for the teacher

The optimum way to address the learning needs of pupils is to consider both the learning and teaching perspectives. This truly inclusive approach raises implications and challenges for teachers, who will need to have an underlying theoretical knowledge base of the development of reading and spelling, and may need to increase their skills, knowledge and understanding of a range of teaching and learning strategies. This will allow them to:

- identify the individual needs of the pupil with dyslexia;
- ascertain their pupil's strengths and weaknesses;
- collate and analyse their knowledge of those individual needs and of learning approaches;
- match the pupil to the curriculum;
- modify the curriculum and/or teaching approach;
- sustain pupil confidence and enthusiasm.

The classroom teacher will probably do some of this in collaboration with the special needs coordinator or literacy adviser. The teacher, however, has the pivotal role, as he or she has to implement curricular materials, employ effective groupings within the classroom and demonstrate effective instruction, while catering for individual pupils' needs.

In the UK, the national curriculum (Department for Education and Employment, 2000) recognizes these challenges. The curriculum framework is a framework for *all* pupils, and it incorporates a statutory inclusion statement that is based on three principles:

1. setting suitable learning challenges;
2. responding to pupils' diverse needs;
3. overcoming potential barriers to learning.

The remainder of the chapter uses these three principles as a framework to discuss the practical ways in which teachers can support pupils with dyslexia in their classroom.

Setting suitable learning challenges

In order to be able to set suitable learning challenges, teachers require knowledge and understanding of the nature and characteristics of dyslexia. They also require an understanding of the developmental nature of normal reading and spelling development, so that they have a yardstick by which the progress of pupils with dyslexia can be measured. At the practical level, setting challenges requires knowledge of appropriate diagnostic assessments in order to be able to identify pupils' individual strengths and weaknesses, for example in text reading, spelling, writing and handwriting. It requires an understanding of the pupils' language profile: their relative problems with word-finding, short-term memory and phonological ability. It also requires teacher skill and expertise in setting suitable pupil targets.

Knowledge and understanding of the nature and characteristics of dyslexia

Teachers and teaching assistants should have access to training in dyslexia. Ideally, there should be opportunities for training from dyslexia specialists from both within and outside the school, and teachers should update their own knowledge through personal reading.

> **RANDOM 'system'**
> *The evidence for how children make connections and links comes from their writing attempts*
>
> 1. EARLY READING – LITTLE LETTER KNOWLEDGE
>
>   Word pronunciation   Child uses elected visual cues
>
>   *Look, dog, camel*
>
> 2. SOME LETTER KNOWLEDGE
>
>   Word pronunciation   Child uses some letter sounds and shapes
>
>   *f*-ish, *c*-at, pi-*g*
>
> 3. FULL LETTER KNOWLEDGE
>
>   Word pronunciation   Child uses all letters/letter sounds
>
> **STRUCTURED SYSTEM**
> **that**
> **supports memory**

Figure 12.1 The development of children's early word reading (based on the theory of Ehri, 1999).

Understanding the developmental nature of normal reading and spelling development

To be able to set appropriate targets, teachers need to set suitable goals that pupils can aim for. These goals should reflect the developmental nature of reading and writing. Ehri (1999), for example, focuses on the processes that children acquire as they learn to read. She explains that 'mature word reading skill is possible only if pupils acquire working knowledge of the alphabetic system' Ehri (1999, p. 102). She describes the change in these processes as word reading develops, so that children progress from using a random system to a structured phonetic system, which is then available to support memory (see Figure 12.1). With this model as a framework, Ehri outlines their implications for instruction. Thus, children need to:

• learn all the letters and how to use letters;
• be aware that words are made up of sounds (phonemes);
• learn letter–sound correspondences;
• be able to match letters to the 'spelling' of words, for example through the use of Elkonin boxes (phoneme frames) (Elkonin, 1973);
• develop word-attack strategies – decoding;
• learn how to write and spell words – letter patterns;
• consolidate units – learn about word families.

Knowledge of appropriate diagnostic assessments to be able to identify the pupils' individual strengths and weaknesses

There should be a clear process within schools for the identification and assessment of pupils with dyslexia. Class teachers should be able to seek support with assessments from a dyslexia specialist or, in UK schools, the special needs coordinator. They should, however, have some knowledge and understanding of the mechanisms by which individual pupils' strengths and difficulties can be identified and, in particular, how phonological processing skills can be assessed (Hatcher and Snowling, 2002; see also Chapter 4 in this volume).

For children in the early stages of learning to read, another skill that teachers can greatly benefit from is learning how to take a 'running record' as the child is reading (Hatcher, 2000a). Taking a running record involves recording verbatim what the child reads when presented with a text, and incorporating correct responses, errors and self-corrections. The running record not only provides a record of exactly how the child has read the text, but can also be used to identify the right level of book for reading at the 'instructional' level. Targets can then be set to help the child to develop more successful reading strategies and to monitor text reading (see

Chapter 9 in this volume). For older pupils, teachers may wish to be able to identify the learning approaches that a dyslexic pupil prefers, so that they can ameliorate their classroom instruction (see below).

Identifying a pupil's cognitive profile

Schools and teachers inevitably develop preferences for the use of particular assessment tools and procedures for the assessment of dyslexia, and it is not the purpose of this chapter to be prescriptive. It is, however, important to adopt a framework for assessment, and one such guide by Rack and Hatcher (2003) provides suggestions on how to gain a pupil profile of strengths and weaknesses through supportive diagnostic testing and guidelines on when a more in-depth assessment might be required.

Setting suitable targets for pupils

With the right knowledge about individual pupils' strengths and weaknesses, a general understanding of the nature of dyslexia, and a knowledge of available teaching strategies and resources, teachers will be well placed to produce appropriately challenging learning targets. In addition, it is important that pupils are involved in setting their targets, and that parents and carers are consulted and informed regularly of the arrangements for supporting their child.

Learning targets are often set within an individual education plan (IEP). In the UK, the Code of Practice (Department for Education and Skills, 2001b) describes an IEP as 'the provision which is "*additional to*" or "*different from*" the differentiated curriculum plan that is part of normal provision'. IEPs have been part of special educational needs teaching for 10 years in the UK and over 20 years in the USA. Tod (2002) examines the development of effective IEPs for pupils with dyslexia from a range of perspectives. Despite controversy over whether dyslexic learners are different from other learners, Tod outlines a number of teaching approaches that have been found to be effective:

- *strategies* – the need for a range of approaches that combine phonic with whole-language teaching (Adams, 1990);
- *extra teaching* – the need to provide additional focused literacy skills teaching (Office for Standards in Education, 1999);
- *different/special* – well-targeted specialist help (Department for Education and Skills, 2003a); a focus on more explicit and intense interventions (see Chapter 9 in this volume; Torgesen et al., 2001).

To this should be added the need to contextualize the IEP targets within the classroom setting, so that teachers, by offering a range of methods of support for pupils with dyslexia, can facilitate pupils' learning in the classroom.

Responding to pupils' diverse needs

If it is agreed that it is necessary to respond to pupils' individual needs, it follows that teachers have to be able to respond to a diverse range of needs. For the pupil with dyslexic difficulties, the response may need to be at a variety of levels. If a pupil's literacy difficulties are insufficient to access most written requirements in the classroom, the pupil will require a specific programme of intervention as well as support in the classroom. That is, the pupil will require the differentiation of *both* teaching goals *and* teaching approaches. If, however, the pupil has made significant progress with the mechanical skills of reading and writing, he or she may be able to continue to make progress solely with support in the classroom, i.e. through differentiation of the teaching approach.

Differentiation of teaching goals

The differentiation of teaching goals implies that pupils require a programme that is 'additional to and different from' normal teaching programmes in order to ensure they are able to develop more effective and age-appropriate literacy skills. This type of teaching programme usually takes place in a withdrawal situation and in a one-to-one or very small group setting. It is unlikely that pupils with severe difficulties will make optimum progress if they are not given individual help. Any individually tailored programmes should be carefully monitored and evaluated.

In such programmes, there should be an emphasis on using a multisensory approach to teaching and learning, and a structured cumulative approach for teaching word-attack skills. Depending on the age and literacy needs of the pupil, the programme should include some or all of the following elements.

Training in phonological awareness

In order to develop word-reading skills, it is necessary to have an awareness of the sound structure of spoken words (see Chapter 4 in this volume). Pupils therefore need explicit help in developing word- and sound-analysis skills, through verbal activities and linking sounds with letters. Phonological activities should follow the pattern of normal development, moving from identifying words as separate units in a sentence, through syllable segmentation and deletion, to emphasizing the development of phoneme skills through phoneme identification, segmentation and manipulation activities. Such a progression provides the framework for a number of teaching programmes, for example *Sound Linkage* (Hatcher, 2000a; see also Chapter 9 in this volume). In addition, suggestions for phonological activities can be found in many teacher texts such as Townend and Turner (2000), the *Active Literacy Kit* (Bramley, 1998) and *Jolly Phonics* (Wernham and Lloyd, 1993).

Some aspects to keep in mind when presenting phonological awareness activities are as follows:

- With syllables, ask the pupil to clap out or sing the syllables in words or to put a hand under the chin to 'feel' the syllables.
- When working with phonemes, always insist on the pure sounds, such as /p/ rather than "puh".
- When asking a pupil to listen for a sound, always ask the pupil to repeat the sound, so the way in which the sound is formed in the mouth can be felt.
- When listening for sounds in words, encourage the pupil to say the word very slowly so that the individual phonemes can be heard more easily.
- Dyslexic learners do not 'pick up' patterns in written language as well as other learners, so present words in sound families (e.g. GOAT, BOAT, STOAT) and show the pupil how to spot patterns in words (see Chapter 10 in this volume).

Alphabet work

Pupils with dyslexia can have sequencing and memory difficulties, so alphabetic order may be problematic for them. There may need to be much overlearning and practice to ensure fluency with letter knowledge.

There are several general suggestions when teaching the alphabet:

- Keep checking that the pupil can recite the alphabet clearly.
- Do not always ask the pupil to start reciting at the beginning of the alphabet.
- Encourage the pupil to sing the alphabet if there is difficulty in saying it.
- In the early stages, encourage the pupil to use plastic or wooden letters to physically arrange the letters. This not only helps with alphabetical order, but also helps to make the link between letter and sound explicit.
- Lay out the alphabet in an arc as this is easier to keep in the field of vision than a single row is; it also makes it easier to visualize the relative position of the letters.
- Help the pupil to develop study skills, for example dictionary skills.

(Walker, 2000, personal communication)

Letter–sound decoding

Learning how to decode unfamiliar words is essential for the development of reading skills. Word attack will include the phonic decoding of sounds, blending sounds into words and segmenting words into syllables. Programmes such as the *Dyslexia Institute Literacy Programme* (*DILP*; Walker et al., 1993) have at their core learning how to decode words following a structured, cumulative framework. The letters and letter strings are taught in an orderly sequence that mirrors the frequency with which letters occur in the language. Teaching and learning the letters and sounds encourages multisensory links so that pupils learn that each letter has a name, a sound, a shape and a 'feel'. When learning a letter or word, pupils are encouraged to link its appearance, its pronunciation and the movements needed to write it. Thus, when teaching a new letter or sound, the teacher aims to use questioning that directs pupils to discover the concept or 'rule' for themselves. Because pupils with dyslexia are generally slow to develop automatic responses, concepts need to be taught very thoroughly, and teaching needs to be intensive and explicit.

Reading books

Since the key characteristic of dyslexia is a phonological deficit (see Chapter 1 in this volume), interventions should have phonological awareness training at their core. Evidence shows, however, that the most effective interventions for children with reading difficulties combine reading with phonological awareness training (Hatcher, Hulme and Ellis, 1994; see Chapter 9 in this volume). Thus, pupils need also to learn how to use word and sentence contexts to support their reading development and develop their decoding skills. They do this by learning reading strategies as well as by learning to integrate those reading strategies so that they can check whether their decoding attempts are accurate. Teachers should therefore look for evidence that pupils are using the meaning of the text, the structure of the sentences, the visual appearance of the words and the relationship between sounds and letters in order to attempt unknown words. In short, pupils need lots of opportunities to read connected text and be exposed to a range of literature for their reading practice (Adams, 1990).

Spelling

Pupils with dyslexia need to be encouraged to use a multisensory strategy for learning new spellings. This could be the 'look, cover, write, check' approach, in which the visual representation of the word is presented to the learner. The 'echo, spell, write, check' approach does not have the visual representation of the word so is useful for confirming spelling knowledge. This entails the teacher saying the word (e.g. "bend"), the pupil repeating the word ("bend"), the pupil spelling out the names of the letters ("b-e-n-d") and then writing the word, and finally the pupil checking for the correct spelling.

Writing

The teacher needs to provide plenty of opportunities and time for writing. Through the medium of writing, the pupil will be able to practise newly acquired words and write phonetically complete spellings of words. As indicated earlier, it is through the writing attempts that evidence of how children are making links and connections can be seen.

Handwriting

Many pupils with spelling difficulties are helped by learning a cursive script (see Chapter 11 in this volume). Encouraging joined writing from the earliest stages helps to establish automatic responses to letter strings. This then helps to cut down on memory load. Joined handwriting simplifies the writing process as every letter begins in the same place and every letter has a lead-in and lead-out stroke; it also reduces the risk of capital letters appearing in the middle of words.

Linking an individualized programme to the general curriculum and to support in the classroom

In the classroom situation, it is very difficult to implement a personalized system, in which each pupil is taught the information he or she requires when he or she needs it. Nevertheless, for individualized literacy programmes that are delivered outside the classroom to have the most effect, they should be linked with curriculum delivery in the classroom. This entails establishing the roles and responsibilities of the class teacher and the 'specialist' teacher/teaching assistant, and, importantly, ensuring that time is put aside for effective liaison.

In order to support the work that the pupil is doing outside the classroom within the whole-group situation, the teaching approaches used should aim to be highly explicit. Explicit teaching includes:

- analysing, preparing and presenting new learning tasks in very clear, easy steps;
- teaching skills explicitly by providing clear modelling, demonstration and 'thinking aloud' on the part of the teacher;
- providing follow-up training in phonemic awareness, letter knowledge and decoding;
- providing ample guided, successful practice with corrective feedback – in meaningful contexts;
- re-teaching particular skills where necessary;
- teaching directly how to go about a task and how to develop pupil independence through self-monitoring strategies;
- providing frequent revision of skills and knowledge already learned.

Alongside this, reading and writing development should be directly supported in the classroom. With this objective in mind, some suggestions for reading, writing, spelling and handwriting activities are given below.

Reading

Fluent and experienced readers adapt their style of reading to suit the purpose of the reading task. This needs to be taught explicitly by:

- ensuring that the pupil's mode of reading is appropriate to the task, for example reading for detail, scanning, skimming or reading for reference;
- teaching the different types of reading if necessary and providing practice in each type of reading.

Be aware of the reading load. Develop teacher awareness of text level and match this with the individual characteristics of pupils. For some pupils, it may be necessary to:

- use video- or audiotape to ease the bulk of reading;
- pre-check the 'reading age' of any text material;
- check the clarity of presentation of text information, and prepare the pupil for text that is not presented clearly.

Because of weak memory and the need to concentrate on decoding skills, some dyslexic pupils lose the meaning of what they are reading. It may therefore be necessary to teach them how to read text in order to answer comprehension questions:

- how to answer what the question asks;
- practising answers orally before committing to paper;
- looking for clues to provide the 'big picture', for example pictures, diagrams or graphics.

Owing to some pupils' limited exposure to books, their reading experience may be minimal. The teacher may therefore need to:

- explicitly teach the language and vocabulary of literature, for example characterization and plot, ambiguity and allusion, shape, impact and styles of writing;
- provide alternative support, such as:
  - information and computer technology – text-to-speech technology, voice recognition;
  - videotapes;
  - audiotapes;

- support weak memory and organization of thoughts through clear examples of aspects of literature, such as underlying themes, characterization or the interrelation of characters.

Writing

Structuring writing is a very difficult skill for many pupils with dyslexia. For them, the planning and drafting of writing must be explicitly taught. This can be done through:

- teaching the separate skills involved in writing: planning, structuring, evaluating and revising;
- ensuring practice in a range of writing tasks to encourage the gradual development of planning, organizing and presentation of information;
- supporting pupils by:
  - *scaffolding* – showing how planning proceeds in real task situations and providing information on the thinking process as well as on the mechanics of planning;
  - *modelling* good practice;
  - *demonstrating* the pre-planning of written tasks and recording key points for the pupil to use as a guide;
- teaching the knowledge of language and language/vocabulary concepts, such as words, sentences and paragraphs, and their interrelation and interdependence;
- teaching parts of speech (e.g. active versus passive) and figures of speech (e.g. idioms and metaphors);
- reviewing examples of well- and poorly written work so that strengths and weaknesses in writing can be identified.

In addition, support in the classroom will be helped by:

- allowing sufficient time in lesson-planning for the drafting process;
- accepting that pupils with dyslexia may take longer in the drafting process;
- providing word-processing facilities where appropriate;
- clearly displaying information about writing conventions in the classroom.

Spelling

For older pupils, spelling is often a greater difficulty than reading as the skills needed for spelling tap exactly those areas in which dyslexic pupils have weaknesses. Pupils with dyslexia can be helped by:

- explicitly teaching knowledge about the English spelling system, including the reasons why words are spelt the way that they are (see Chapter 10 in this volume);
- teaching appropriate terminology (consonant, vowel, syllable, etc.);
- providing a morphological framework for spelling. For example, Henry and Redding (1996) and Tuley (1998) illustrate how teaching the changes of meanings of Latin and Greek words, by adding prefixes and suffixes, can be done following a suggested framework;
- utilising strengths:
  - visual: teaching letter patterns, mnemonics;
  - reduce memory load: teach word derivatives (affixes, root words);
  - teach spelling strategies;
  - teach how to use the ACE Dictionary (Moseley, 1998). This dictionary utilizes a different method of finding words from regular dictionaries, words being listed according to how they sound;
  - having an agreed approach to marking that provides consistency of expectations (a whole-school policy).

Handwriting

With older pupils, poor handwriting can give the wrong impression of ability. Not all pupils with dyslexia have poor handwriting skills, and difficulties can be variable. The problems could be with style, speed or letter formation. Where possible, teachers should provide opportunities to word-process work and to practise typing skills.

Differentiation of teaching approach

By differentiating the teaching approach, the teacher adjusts the teaching approach to individual learners. As already noted, pupils with dyslexia are not the same and may process information differently, so this may mean devising settings that give the best chance of success. In other words, it may be about aspirations rather than absolutes. Nevertheless, knowing the most common difficulties of pupils with dyslexia, especially among older pupils, helps to ensure that aspirations are more likely to be achieved. As pupils with dyslexia become more proficient with reading skills, the most common persisting problems are with:

- speed of reading;
- higher-order reading skills, such as skimming and scanning text for information;
- the development of spelling and writing skills;

- the use of reference materials, and the ability to extract and synthesize information;
- the planning of ideas and structuring thoughts before writing.

Teachers can differentiate their teaching and learning approach according to the pupils' interests, the approach to learning, and classroom organization and ethos.

These general approaches to differentiation are summarised in Table 12.1 and detailed below. More specifically, however, teachers can differentiate by seeking to overcome the potential barriers to pupil learning.

Table 12.1 General approaches to differentiation in the classroom

Aspect to be differentiated	Teaching approach
Interest and previous experience	• The work set is more likely to interest the pupil if the starting point is self-selected by the pupil • Provide parallel tasks so that pupils are aiming for the same target but are using materials at different interest levels
Approach to learning	• Consider learning tasks in terms of input and output so that these may vary for different pupils at different times and for different tasks • Vary the pace of teaching/learning so that pupils move through the same set of materials at varying speeds • Pupils may proceed through the sequence of tasks in a different order
Classroom organization	• Mixed ability and friendship groupings can provide peer support and result in fewer demands for help • Paired work – peer tutoring • Develop a system of 'study buddies' • Provide opportunities for pupils to sit near the front of the class • Encourage the pupils to sit near well-motivated pupils • Try to keep the background noise level and visual distraction to a minimum • Ensure ready access to classroom resources by keeping them clearly arranged and marked

Table 12.1 General approaches to differentiation in the classroom (continued)

Aspect to be differentiated	Teaching approach
Classroom ethos	• Balance high expectations for intellectual ability against achievable goals • Watch for signs of pupil tiredness or fatigue • Watch for signs of decreasing pupil self-esteem and lack of confidence • Develop an environment in which pupils feel safe and supported at the same time as being challenged. Ensure that pupils know that it is OK to say, 'I don't understand' • Provide opportunities for structured reflection

Overcoming potential barriers to pupil learning

The UK government's vision for providing pupils who have special educational needs with the opportunity to succeed is set out in the document *Removing Barriers to Achievement* (Department for Education and Skills, 2004). The vision recognizes that teachers need to respond to a wide range of needs in the classroom through providing teaching and learning experiences that 'enable children to access the whole curriculum' (Department for Education and Skills, 2004, p. 31). Putting in place more effective provision means developing continua of teaching approaches through differentiation.

The term 'differentiation' is, however, freely used but ill defined. Lewis (1995) suggests that differentiation means meeting all children's learning needs so that they can all share the same curriculum. Gross (1996, p. 27), however, applies a more practical, teacher-focused definition in suggesting that 'differentiation is the ability to adapt tasks and teaching/learning styles to meet the wide range of ability in the classroom'. The different views about differentiation relate to differences in the social values of equality and individuality (Norwich, 1996). Whether one considers differentiation to be a task or a process, the inclusive agenda requires that significant changes be made to mainstream programmes in order to accommodate a much wider range of pupil needs. Table 12.2 presents a framework for differentiation in terms of overcoming potential barriers to learning. The remainder of the chapter provides examples of alternative approaches within this framework.

Table 12.2 Differentiation framework for teaching

Input – Presentation of activities	• Curriculum delivery • Means of access to the curriculum • Modification of written presentation
Process – Approach to learning	• Use active learning approaches • Development of metacognitive skills • Opportunities for repetition, reinforcement and transfer of skills
Output – Mode of pupil response	• Alternatives to written record • Organizational supports

Presentation of activities (input)

Curriculum delivery

Importantly, the pupil should be physically comfortable, facing the teacher and able to see the board or screen easily in order to gain optimum benefit from curriculum delivery. With this in place, useful strategies include varying the level of questioning, ensuring a multisensory approach and employing explicit teaching methods (see below).

Vary the level of questioning
- Classroom instructions and explanations should be delivered clearly and slowly, with time for the meanings to penetrate.
- Allow time for the pupil to focus attention on the task before giving instructions, for example say the pupil's name before asking a question.
- Cue in specific attention that might be needed for a certain task.
- Allow pupils time to familiarize themselves with the content, and then time for processing.
- Model the right answer, for reinforcement.

Make it multisensory
A great deal of classroom teaching relies on visual and auditory input. Pupils with dyslexia need to learn how to activate all learning channels so that their learning becomes more secure. This is because using several senses gives the brain more connections and associations, and thus makes it easier to find information later. Teachers therefore need to provide a model for multisensory learning, by linking the appearance of a word, its sound, its pronunciation and the movement needed to write the word.

Employ explicit teaching methods in lesson planning
In each lesson aim to:

- *review* previous learning;

- give a clear outline or *overview* of the lesson at the beginning of the lesson;
- summarise the *main points* in logical order;
- set clear *goals/targets*;
- break the *content* down into manageable 'chunks';
- demonstrate *learning* ;
- build in *review* opportunities, so that pupils can show that they understand;
- aim for maximum productive pupil time on-task.

In order to make learning manageable for pupils:

- avoid learning confusions;
- teach learning strategies, for example mnemonics, mind-mapping and acronyms;
- link a new or difficult skill with something that the pupil can already do;
- ensure sufficient varied repetition;
- provide opportunities for learning to be generalized;
- allow for practice at demonstrating the newly acquired learning;
- ensure that the pupil can verbalize what has to be done.

Means of access to the curriculum

Ensure variety of access to curriculum materials
Pupils with dyslexia will have potentially greater access to the curriculum if information is presented through a variety of media. Thus, weak phonological skills can be linked to conceptual and pictorial strengths by means of visual associations and cues, such as flow diagrams, or linking factual information with sound or feel. There are many ways in which information can be presented, a few of which are listed in Table 12.3, which shows both means of accessing the curriculum and the varying means by which pupils can record their knowledge.

Modifying the written presentation of tasks

Pupils can be helped to access course content more effectively by teachers carefully reviewing the resources that they use.

Are class reading materials at the right reading level?
Resources need to be selected carefully to ensure that the reading level is appropriate. By using well-placed illustrations and symbols, pupils may be supported or cued in to understanding more demanding text. Alternatively, the information may need to be supplemented by teacher-produced materials that are more readily accessible.

Is printed material as clear as possible?
Worksheets can and do have a useful role to play in supporting pupils with literacy difficulties. However, great care needs to be given to the presentation of printed matter. When choosing or producing printed materials,

take into consideration the clarity and quality of the material and the use of white space, breaks, symbols and emphases. Some very useful ideas on the presentation of subject-specific worksheets, drawings and diagrams are provided in Peer and Reid (2001).

Approach to learning (process)

Employ active learning methods

Like all learners, pupils with dyslexia learn more effectively and with deeper understanding when they are actively engaged with tasks. Cottrell (1999, 2001) suggests that learners should *do* something, no matter how small, to increase active engagement with a topic. Teachers can help dyslexic pupils by ensuring that learning is as active as is practicable. Pupils with dyslexia often, for example, have strengths in oral work, and therefore spoken skills should be encouraged.

This could include providing opportunities for structured talk such as paired/group investigations, puzzles and games or role-play/dramatization. Preparation for literature tasks could be made more active by providing opportunities for pupils to discuss ideas in groups, contribute in formal and informal class discussions, or plan work through discussion. Paired homework could involve one pupil having to check with a paired pupil that he or she can explain the content or vocabulary of a topic.

Learning preferences

We all learn in an individual way, and as a result some theorists suggest that people have different learning styles, that is, they are *visual, auditory* or *kinaesthetic* learners. A number of texts that provide study-support suggestions for dyslexic pupils stress the importance of this approach. For example, Ostler and Ward (2002) provide a learning style questionnaire, and Holloway (2000) a learning style inventory. Holloway also discusses whether we have 'left-brain' or 'right-brain' learning preferences. Blakemore and Frith (2005) question whether we should use the 'left brain–right brain' differentiation in education, and argue that in fact it could act as an 'impediment to learning'. If pupils are labelled as being a certain 'type' or as having a certain 'style', they could be over-identified as that type, and there might be rigid views about the way in which pupils learn. A better way is to recognize that there are many different elements that contribute to how a pupil learns best, and that pupils have individual learning preferences.

Having said that, teachers often have their own preferred teaching approach that may focus on one or two channels. They need to be aware of different learning 'preferences' and offer activities that suit the range of learners in the classroom.

Develop metacognitive skills

Helping children to develop self-management skills

Some teachers tend to work in ways that can foster a pupil's dependence rather than independence. When pupils with dyslexia can function independently, they become more like the other pupils in the class, which is the goal of inclusion.

Teachers, therefore, need to:

- believe that teaching children to be independent is important, and that it is possible to teach self-management skills to pupils who do not possess them;
- consider precisely which skills are required in order for pupils to function independently in the classroom;
- provide modelling and specific instruction;
- use descriptive praise, so that the pupil knows precisely why he or she is being praised and can then make appropriate connections between effort and outcome.

Developing self-regulation in learning (metacognition)

Self-regulation is the learner's ability to regulate his or her own thinking processes while involved in a learning task. That is, learners play an active role in their learning and monitor closely the effects of various actions they take and decisions they make while learning. So, for example, pupils can learn when to pause, double-check, try again, weigh up possible alternatives or seek help. To help pupils to develop such strategies, teachers need to provide them with a clear modelling of the appropriate strategies, for example appropriate questions to ask themselves and strategies for self-checking. They can often do this simply by ensuring that they give clear verbal cues and corrective feedback. Once a self-regulatory strategy has been learned, the pupil can then be helped to generalize the application of the strategy to a new situation.

Provide opportunities for rehearsal and transfer of new skills

All teachers know that, after pupils have been shown something for the first time and have learned how to do it accurately, they need to be able to practise the skill until it has become second nature to them. The problem for teachers is often planning for sufficient practice time in a crowded curriculum and a busy classroom schedule. Even beyond this phase, however, pupils need to demonstrate that they can perform the skill when direct instruction is no longer continuing, and that they can use the skill that they have been taught in different contexts. Only when pupils can successfully solve a problem that requires them to adapt the skill are they demonstrating that they have fully learned and internalized that skill.

Teachers can help to support these processes by providing:

- opportunities for later stages of learning, for example techniques to develop fluency – timed exercises with the child involved in recording progress;
- ways of checking/recording whether earlier knowledge and skills have been retained or have reached fluency;
- opportunities for over-learning in usual classroom activities, for example over-learning can be incorporated into 'spare time' rules for the classroom – if a pupil completes a set piece of work before other pupils in the class, any 'spare' time can be effectively used in independent practice of words or spellings, and computer programs can be personalized to give immediate feedback so that pupils can monitor their own progress and improvement;
- new contexts for using new skills and knowledge to enable generalization and adaptation.

Mode of pupil response (output)

Alternatives to written records

When pupils are expected to produce written work, they should be provided with extra time for writing, and a high-quality finished product should always be encouraged. Teachers should, however, allow pupils to use different ways of recording information some of the time, so that they can demonstrate their understanding, knowledge and skills. This could include (see also Table 12.3):

- graphic sorting and classifying;
- concept maps, spider maps, continuum diagrams and Venn diagrams;
- organizational frames for note-taking and planning, sorting and arranging materials for writing;
- differentiated writing frames, for example suggesting opening paragraphs, sentence stems, connectives and key words;
- card layout games to illustrate the order of events;
- text-reconstruction exercises;
- peer help in planning and drafting work;
- technical support: a word processor or laptop, a spelling/grammar check and the teaching of typing skills;
- computer spelling programs with subject-based words, and key words;
- multisensory CD-ROMs.

One of the most widely used note-taking and planning tools that dyslexic pupils are encouraged to use is the mind-mapping technique (Buzan,

Table 12.3 Varying the means of access to and means of recording curriculum information

Means of *access*	Means of *recording*
Teacher – team-teaching, senior management team	Computer-assisted recording, storage and retrieval systems
Computer-assisted instruction (see British Educational Communication and Technology Agency)	Diagrams, pictures, cartoons
TV, video, radio	Displays
Tape-recorder	Typing
Language master	Dictaphone, tape-recorder
Children – peer tutoring, cross-age tutoring	Art work
Diagrams, pictures, photographs	Models, craft
Books	Maps, plans, mind maps
Worksheets	Graphs, charts
Visits, excursions	Venn diagrams
Experiments, discovery learning	Taped discussions
Drama, movement, dance, role-play	Scribe
Art	Checklist
Models, craft-work	Photographs
Visitors to classroom	Video
Group/individual presentation, discussion	Drama, role-play
Games	Written work, cloze, notes
Displays	Group work with peer scribe
	Paired work
	'Can Do' records of achievement

1993). Cogan and Flecker (2004) devote a chapter to mind-mapping. They recognize that it is very difficult to teach something that you do not use yourself and are not committed to. They therefore suggest that teachers of dyslexic pupils should 'learn about mind-mapping, recognise its value and encourage their pupils to use it' (Cogan and Flecker, 2004, pp. 43–44).

Study and oganizational skills

As well as giving pupils with dyslexia the requisite language skills, teachers also need to provide them with the tools for study and research. This can be done by helping pupils to think about and verbalize appropriate planning strategies. With some pupils, it may be necessary to explicitly teach the skills of planning and organization. There are many study skills books available, some of which (e.g. Ostler, 1996; Tuley, 1998) are specifically for dyslexic pupils.

To help pupils to develop more efficient ways of working teachers can:

- demonstrate that the pupil will manage better if he or she knows what to expect and is prepared in advance;
- emphasize routines and regular activities, for example by providing readily visible class timetables;
- discuss with the pupil the most useful external memory aids (notebooks, homework diaries, tapes, etc.);
- help in setting up organizational structures to aid more efficient working, for example offering advice on making and keeping an organized file or how to deal with multiple worksheets.

Conclusions: Towards an integrated approach to supporting pupils with dyslexia

This chapter has shown that certain elements are necessary to make learning time productive for pupils with dyslexia (Creemers, 1994). The elements that increase the effectiveness of learning in the classroom are the quality of the instruction provided, the time scheduled for learning and ensuring that there is the optimum opportunity to learn. The teacher is, of course, pivotal to the integration of these elements. We know that barriers to pupils' learning can arise as the result of an interaction between the pupils' learning characteristics and the learning provided in the classroom. Teachers therefore need to ensure that they are maximizing the opportunities for learning. One way of doing this is for teachers to reflect on their teaching approach by asking appropriate questions:

- How are different learning preferences reflected in my lesson-planning and delivery?
- How can I analyse the demands that a piece of work makes on pupils?
- What opportunities can I create to allow pupils to show their knowledge?
- In a busy classroom, how can I obtain reliable and valid information about a pupil's understanding, learning and attainment?
- How is pupils' work assessed? How helpful is the assessment in improving the pupils' understanding?
- How do I convey positive expectations?
- How can learning time be maximized and pupils encouraged to persevere with learning activities?

This chapter has set out some ways in which teaching and learning might be enhanced for pupils with literacy difficulties. In doing so, however, it stresses that teachers need to explore the ways in which pupils with dyslexia can be included in the classroom without losing the core belief in meeting individual needs.

Appendix 1: Useful websites

www.york.ac.uk/res/crl – Centre for Reading and Language, based at the Psychology Department, University of York, UK.

www.becta.org.uk – British Educational Communication and Technology Agency; information on different forms of differentiation, including information on dyslexia and ICT.

www.dyslexic.com – information on iANSYST, which deals with information technology for students with dyslexia.

www.betterbooks.co.uk – Better Books; mail-order service.

www.patoss-dyslexia.org – professional association for teachers.

www.teachingideas.co.uk

www.dyslexia-teacher.com – general teaching resources.

www.sen.uk.com – SEN Marketing; mail-order service.

CHAPTER 13

The assessment and management of psychosocial aspects of reading and language impairments

POPPY NASH

> I have never let my schooling interfere with my education.
>
> Mark Twain

Mark Twain's saying may seem a curious way to begin a chapter on the psychosocial aspects of reading and language impairments. On one hand, it could be seen as an acknowledgement of the challenge of school; on the other hand, it heralds the fact that even bad school experiences cannot stop education in its tracks – good news indeed for those whose school days are not the happiest days of their life. This chapter looks at the implications of what it is like on a daily basis for a young person to live with a reading or language impairment. It begins by exploring why psychosocial aspects must be addressed in managing such a child's needs, and proceeds to discuss issues surrounding the assessment and management of psychosocial well-being.

What is meant by 'psychosocial'?

The term 'psychosocial' refers to the combination of psychological and social factors that may influence how one thinks, behaves and feels about things. There is often confusion over terms and definitions, such as self-esteem, self-worth, self-image, self-perception, self-belief, self-concept, self-regard, self-efficacy and self-competence, some of which are used interchangeably. What all of these constructs have in common are aspects of self-evaluation that are learned rather than being innate. A crucial question for this chapter is how and why particular self-evaluations are formed.

It is helpful at this point, to highlight the three groups of learning difficulty that will be considered:

* reading difficulties (e.g. dyslexia);
* language difficulties (e.g. specific language impairment);
* reading and language difficulties (e.g. dyslexia with language problems, speech and language difficulties with literacy problems, and Down syndrome).

Although children in each of these groups undoubtedly display a distinct profile depending upon the predominant area of difficulty, it is possible to identify common psychosocial difficulties arising almost regardless of type and extent of impairment. Because reading and language impairments have an impact upon learning, they may also be referred to as learning difficulties.

The child with learning difficulties may experience any or all of the following difficulties on a daily basis:

* poor self-esteem, poor self-efficacy and poor self-perception;
* poor school attainment;
* unrewarding social and personal relationships (e.g. social withdrawal, social exclusion and bullying);
* concomitant behavioural difficulties;
* poor health;
* a negative experience and perception of school.

Poor self-esteem, poor self-efficacy and poor self-perception

Despite the extensive literature on self-esteem, self-efficacy and self-perception, there continues to be a debate over the precise nature of these constructs. Harter (1985) proposes that self-esteem lies in the balance between how children see themselves now (*actual self*) and how they would like to be (*ideal self*). The more closely these judgements correspond, the better and the healthier children's self-esteem. Brumfitt (1999) points out that problems can arise if an individual feels powerless to pursue any aspects of the ideal self. In some instances, such feelings can contribute to mental illness (e.g. depression).

Self-esteem is, however, not a matter of just being good at something as it is also determined by how much that skill is valued. As Daniel and Wassell (2002, p. 54) suggest, 'a child who would like to be good at art, but perceives that his or her drawings are poor, will have a lower esteem than a child who does not value art and whose drawings are poor'. Grantham (2000) asserts that, although for some individuals self-esteem is determined by their sense of competence, others base their self-esteem on feelings of self-worth.

Beliefs about the perceived *value* of skills are especially critical for self-efficacy, which relates to personal effectiveness. It centres on beliefs about cognitive aspects of mastery and effectiveness, rather than feelings and personal needs. Individuals' personal beliefs about their own competence (or sense of achievement) and effectiveness are considered to be integral to all three psychosocial constructs (self-esteem, self-perception and self-efficacy). That is, if an individual feels competent in an area that is personally valued (e.g. public speaking), this can enhance his or her self-esteem. If the skill is not particularly valued, this can have the opposite result and effectively lower self-esteem (Brumfitt, 1999). Elliott (2002) argues that it is important to provide young people with a sense of personal efficacy, a belief that, whatever their natural abilities, they can achieve if they are prepared to make a significant and sustained effort.

According to Kremer et al. (2003), self-perceptions comprise the two elements of self-esteem and self-competence: self-esteem is the evaluative component of the self that reflects a generalized sense of social worth, whereas self-competence is a theoretically related construct that reflects a person's sense of efficacy in a particular life domain. Although the cause-and-effect relationship between self-perception and self-esteem is unclear, one way of differentiating between them is to view self-perception as the product of the social comparison process. That is, self-perceptions are intrinsically determined by the individuals or groups with which we choose to compare ourselves (Kremer et al., 2003).

Similarly, Burns (1982) defines self-concept as the uniquely personal, evaluative and dynamic identity that a person develops in interacting with his or her psychological environment. In short, self-esteem and self-perception collectively represent:

- what we think we are;
- what we think we can achieve;
- what we think others think of us;
- what we would like to be.

Lown (2000) indicates that poor self-esteem 'appears to be rife' among children who are struggling to succeed in education. Maines and Robinson (1995) also note the tendency for children with specific language impairment to show lower levels of self-esteem and self-confidence compared with their unaffected peers (e.g. Rice, 1993).

The literature on the psychosocial difficulties associated with dyslexia is still relatively sparse. Elliott (2002, p. 38) refers to literacy as a 'sphere of activity . . . that is strongly associated with emotions of shame and inadequacy'. In a similar vein, Farmer, Riddick and Sterling (2002) note that college students with dyslexia are affected by anxiety and stress, lack of self-esteem and a lack of self-confidence (see also Lawrence, 1985). Although the debate over causal relationships continues, self-esteem, self-efficacy and self-perception are integrally linked to all of the core psychosocial difficulties. It should be emphasized at this stage that these constructs are not static and invariable as they are determined by a combination of the individuals' make-up, personal circumstances and life events. Changes in any of these influential factors can affect psychosocial functioning to a lesser or greater degree.

Poor school attainment

The child with reading and language impairments often has to cope with the implications of poor school attainment. Lindsay and Dockrell (2000) suggest that children with language impairments are likely to harbour negative self-perceptions owing to:

- the effects of failure at school and the associated negative feedback;
- the stigmatizing effects of being singled out and labelled;
- effects specific to the nature of communication difficulties.

Negative self-perception can be manifest as a lack of motivation to learn (Elliott, 2002). The common consequences of this are underachievement and a lack of perseverance as the child expects to encounter failure (Pressley and McCormick, 1995). This is especially poignant in Western society, where the ability to succeed in competition with others is closely related to human value.

Children are motivated to learn when fundamental needs are met. If these needs are not fulfilled, the children concerned may not be in a psychological position to benefit from the educational opportunities offered to them in school (Nash et al., 2002). Maslow's (1970) hierarchy of needs indicates that basic physiological, safety, love and belonging needs have to be satisfied before an individual's self-esteem can flourish. Those responsible for the welfare of the learning-impaired child (e.g. parents and teachers) have an important role in meeting these primary needs.

Unrewarding social and personal relationships

Social competence, especially the quality and quantity of social and personal relationships, is another aspect of development often adversely affected by learning impairments. Harter (1985) indicates that relationships with friends, classmates and teachers all to some extent affect a child's self-esteem. Individuals' identities are partly determined by how others treat and behave towards them (Erwin, 1998). In this, a self-fulfilling prophecy operates, whereby other people's expectations of how a person is going to behave somehow determine how he or she actually does behave (Kremer et al., 2003). This is what Cooley (1902) described as 'the looking-glass self'. Thus, if learning-impaired children feel different from others, they may feel alienated, behave as if they are being alienated and will before long become alienated, socially excluded and even bullied.

A vicious circle can develop whereby a child with learning difficulties may possess inadequate social skills, become aggressive and consequently experience difficulty in making and keeping friendships. As a consequence, the individual has less experience of socializing and less opportunity to learn and develop these vital skills (Daniel and Wassell, 2002). In highlighting this vicious circle, Nash et al. (2002) propose the VOS cycle of disadvantage (Figure 13.1), in which the individual is collectively *victimized* (e.g. bullied), *ostracized* and *stigmatized*. Without appropriate management and intervention, this cycle can become progressively distressing for the child concerned and prove hard to reverse.

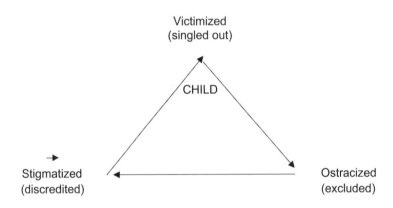

Figure 13.1 The VOS cycle of disadvantage (adapted from Nash et al., 2002).

In characterizing the classroom experiences of the socially impaired child, Rustin and Kuhr (1999) describe the tendency for the individual to be on the periphery of the social system within the class. The child is perceived as passive or isolated and rejected by his or her peers, as opposed to being actively involved in group activities (see also Horne, 1985). These adverse experiences have potentially damaging effects upon the child at school. For example, Knox and Conti-Ramsden (2003) suggest that any negative social experience, such as bullying, may interfere with a child's ability to learn and perform in the classroom. In similar vein, Mooney and Smith (1995) note that if schoolchildren are preoccupied with anxiety about being bullied during the next break time, it is likely that both their self-esteem and their school work will suffer. However, as Daniel and Wassell (2002) emphasize, the ability to make friends is only part of the equation – the types of friendship established are also important, and positive relationships with peers (rather than socialization with delinquent peers) are reported to be protective, especially in adolescence (Fergusson and Lynskey; 1996; Quinton et al., 1993).

Behaviour difficulties

Children with reading and language impairments also commonly experience behaviour problems (Lown, 2000). The prevalence of behavioural difficulties is not surprising if one considers the levels of frustration and anger that a child with learning difficulties can experience on a daily basis at school. Add to this the constant sense of failure and under-achievement that some children experience, and behaviour difficulties can be an understandable manifestation of their psychosocial dysfunction. As Cross (2004) highlights in the subtitle of her book addressing children's emotional and behavioural difficulties: 'There is always a reason.' Instances of problematic behaviour can manifest themselves in a variety of ways, including aggressiveness towards others and disruptive behaviour in the classroom.

Poor health

Unless the wider psychosocial aspects of reading and language impairments are addressed, the most vulnerable individuals continue to display signs and symptoms of stress-related illness, such as headaches, inadequate sleep and irritability (among others). In more serious cases, the individual may develop some form of psychopathology (e.g. depression, school phobia or even suicide).

Mruk (1999, p. 92) offers an explanation of the association between stress and self-esteem: 'stress can certainly tax our sense of worthiness as a person, especially if it comes from a negative source and is prolonged'. Self-esteem can, however, serve as an effective buffer in reducing the adverse effects of stress. It is thought that those with high self-esteem are at an advantage as they are better protected from the sense of rejection, failure and low self-worth that is so often associated with stress. Frey and Carlock (1989) indicate that the lower the self-esteem, the more likely it is to be damaged by the mildest of life events, and the greater the resistance to healthy development.

Asher and Coie (1990) highlight the relationship between peer rejection, social exclusion and an enhanced risk of psychosocial and psychiatric difficulties in later life (Schaffer, 1996). Figure 13.2 documents the potential consequences of unresolved psychosocial difficulties related to reading and language impairments.

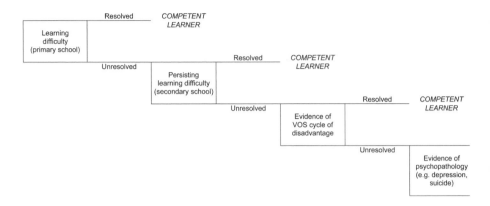

Figure 13.2 Potential consequences of unresolved psychosocial difficulties related to reading and language impairments (adapted from Nash et al., 2002). VOS, victimized, ostracized, stigmatized.

Negative experience and perception of school

To appreciate the collective impact of psychosocial difficulties on an individual's everyday life at school, both the classroom and the playground context need to be considered as each contributes to the child's experience and perception of school. In the classroom, children with learning difficulties may feel inadequate, incompetent and different from their peers. The impact of these experiences is often carried into the playground, where children can continue to feel stigmatized and socially excluded by their peers and be the target of school bullying.

In profiling the most vulnerable children in psychosocial terms, it is necessary to explore further the interface between the child's classroom and playground experiences. Figure 13.3 is a schematic representation of the interface between experiences in the classroom and in the playground, children falling into one of the four quadrants (Nash, 2003). For the purpose of this matrix, *positive (+ve) classroom experiences* refer to rewarding, enjoyable, stimulating learning experiences rather than academic success and achievement. On the other hand, *negative (–ve) classroom experiences* refer to the opposite of these, namely confusing, demotivating and overwhelming experiences. Not only do perceptions of constant failure reinforce the child's negativity, but also self-fulfilling prophecies held by teachers concerning underperformance are likely to be realized.

Positive (+ve) playground experiences allude to enjoyable recreation time spent with friends that offers a rich means of developing communication and interpersonal skills. *Negative (–ve) playground experiences* are, however, often characterized by social isolation and exclusion from games, during

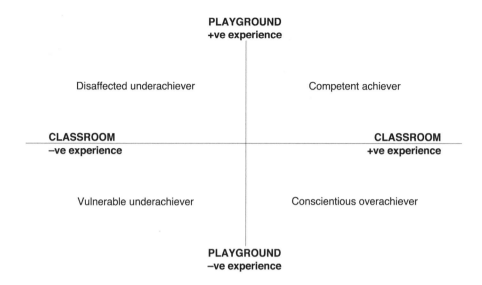

PLAYGROUND
+ve experience

Disaffected underachiever

Competent achiever

CLASSROOM
–ve experience

CLASSROOM
+ve experience

Vulnerable underachiever

Conscientious overachiever

PLAYGROUND
–ve experience

Figure 13.3 Interface between classroom and playground – what influences what? (Nash, 2003).

which the individual spends much time alone and lonely. Opportunities to build friendships and practise social skills are therefore lost and are replaced by perceptions of dread, anxiety and even intimidation. It is important not to forget that, for most school children, nearly one third of the school day is spent in the playground, which equates to approximately 2 hours when divided between the usual morning, lunch and afternoon break times. This is a considerable amount of time, especially if the playground spells fear for the individuals concerned.

The four quadrants shown in Figure 13.3 can be characterized as follows:

- *Positive classroom + positive playground experiences*: 'competent achiever', characterized by the following:
  - happy at school;
  - popular with other children;
  - enjoys learning;
  - achieves as expected.

- *Positive classroom + negative playground experiences*: 'conscientious over-achiever', characterized by the following:
  - sometimes happy and sometimes unhappy at school;
  - few friends, often a loner, and a potential target for bullying as regarded a 'swot' by his or her peers;
  - enjoyment of learning hampered by anxiety and the need to excel;
  - achieves more than expected for age and stage of development.

- *Negative classroom + positive playground experiences*: 'disaffected under-achiever', characterized by the following:
  - happiness at school determined by popularity with others;
  - popular with other children as a ring leader; a potential bully figure;
  - not interested in learning;
  - underachievement largely owing to indifference, lack of motivation and/or limited ability.
- *Negative classroom + negative playground experiences*: 'vulnerable under-achiever', characterized by the following:
  - school is a constant struggle;
  - few, if any friends (most susceptible to the VOS cycle);
  - difficulties encountered in learning that reinforce the sense of failure;
  - underachievement associated with learning difficulties and related psychosocial dysfunction.

Although many of those with reading and language impairments experience some degree of psychosocial dysfunction, some children show remarkable resilience, as we will discuss later.

Assessment of psychosocial aspects of reading and language impairments

The assessment of psychosocial functioning should be seen as part of the management process of a child with a reading or language difficulty. Indeed, it is only when a child has been adequately assessed that optimum management can be planned. The assessment of psychosocial adjustment may also form an important component of the school's monitoring and review of learning-impaired children, and may be conducted by the class teacher or special educational needs coordinator at school.

What psychosocial aspects need to be assessed?

The aspects of a child's psychosocial functioning most conducive to measurement, and therefore most commonly assessed, are self-esteem and self-perception (or self-concept). In assessing psychosocial aspects, the practitioner needs to ensure that self-esteem and self-perception are being assessed both adequately and accurately. In this context, 'adequately' refers to obtaining sufficient information in the time available, and 'accurately' alludes to the fact that a child's anxiety levels can mask genuine areas of difficulty. For example, care must be taken to enable the child to feel comfortable and safe during assessment. In some instances, anxious children can feel so intimidated by the whole process that they do not give an accurate presentation of their capabilities, or are so distracted that the full extent of their difficulties is hard to estimate.

When should psychosocial aspects be assessed?

In developmental terms, a child's self-perception and self-esteem may not be sufficiently stable and reliable to obtain an accurate measure until the age of approximately 7 years (e.g. Harter, 1985). Assessment before this age may therefore reflect an unstable self-concept. In view of this, Harter and Pike (1983) have developed a pictorial version of self-perception scales. Although it is still debatable whether such young children can respond in a consistent and reliable way, such scales can give an indication of notable psychosocial dysfunction at this age. It is also important not to underestimate the value of informal observations and anecdotal information given by the carers of the child to supplement other measures.

What form should psychosocial assessments take?

In undertaking an assessment of the individual's psychosocial functioning, the particular advantages and disadvantages of the following methods should guide the choice of measures used:

- formal – usually quantitative, standardized measures (e.g. tests, questionnaires and scales);
- informal – usually qualitative, non-standardized assessments (e.g. semi-structured interview, observations and checklists);
- a combination of both formal and informal methods.

Whereas the use of formal measures (e.g. tests, questionnaires and scales) has the advantage of providing a discrete score or set of scores, which can be compared with age norms, they are limited in the amount of information about the individual concerned that they can elicit, and the value of informal assessment must not be underestimated. Methods include semi-structured interviews with the individual (and family members), based on key questions. By recording and then analysing the interviewee's responses to the largely open-ended questions, this form of assessment yields invaluable anecdotal information about the individual. Observing the child's behaviour in different settings offers another means of gathering important information about psychosocial functioning. Kaplan (1991) proposes that useful indicators of self-esteem are facial expressions and the degree to which the individual reproaches or congratulates him- or herself. For example, poor self-esteem could be manifest in those who rarely smile or display happiness.

Some children have been undergoing informal assessment by the class teacher long before being formally assessed by a specialist (e.g. psychologist). The teacher (or classroom assistant) is the ideal person to undertake these largely observational classroom assessments. One of the challenges of doing so is being aware of the defensive strategies used by the less able children to disguise the extent of their reading and language difficulties, for fear of losing face with their classmates, teachers and families. Elliott (2002) identifies four such strategies often adopted in school by those with low self-esteem and those who are uncertain of what others think of them:

- making little or no effort so that ability cannot be used to explain low performance;
- procrastination (leaving the task so late that poor performance is unavoidable);
- self-handicapping (an emotional or physical cause being used to explain performance);
- a selection of tasks either so difficult that the child cannot be blamed for failure, or so easy that success is guaranteed.

Thompson (1999) points out that these strategies court further failure for those concerned as they exacerbate feelings of incompetence, hopelessness, anger and emotional burn-out.

Which measures should be used in assessing psychosocial aspects?

Ideally, a combination of both formal and informal assessment elicits the richest source of information about the child's psychosocial functioning. With regard to formal measures, it is difficult to obtain a single measure that accurately represents a child's psychosocial functioning. The current trend is to gain as comprehensive a picture as possible of the child being assessed, by using a variety of measures. For example, Harter's (1985) *Self-Perception Profile for Children* comprises six subscales, or domains, that together offer a multidimensional assessment of the child's self-perception in different domains, as follows:

- Scholastic Competence;
- Social Acceptance;
- Athletic Competence;
- Physical Appearance;
- Behavioural Conduct;
- Global Self-worth.

The following measures have also been found useful in deriving a comprehensive profile of a child's psychosocial adjustment.

Pictorial Scale of Perceived Competence and Social Acceptance for Young Children *(Harter and Pike, 1983)*

There are two age bands for this measure: the Preschool-Kindergarten (4–5 years) and the First and Second Grade forms (6–7 years). Unlike the children's profile, these scales contain no self-worth scale as, developmentally, young children are not able to make such judgements until the age of around 8 years old. The pictorial format focuses upon four domains: Cognitive Competence, Physical Competence, Peer Acceptance and Maternal Acceptance.

Self-Perception Profile for Adolescents *(Harter, 1988)*

The adolescent version of Harter's Self-Perception Profile for those aged 14 years and over comprises the same question format as the children's scale. However, more domains are tapped to reflect the youngsters' greater psychosocial maturity at this stage. For example, in addition to the six domains outlined above, additional subscales allude to Job Competence, Romantic Appeal and Close Friendship.

Self-Image Profiles for Children (SIP-C, and for Adolescents, SIP-A; *Butler, 2001a, 2001b)*

Butler's profiles for children (7–11 years) and adolescents (12–16 years) are brief self-report measures that elicit a useful visual display of the individual's self-image and self-esteem. Both versions comprise 25 age-appropriate self-descriptions: 12 positive and 12 negative characteristics, with one neutral item.

Strengths and Difficulties Questionnaire (SDQ; *Goodman, 1997)*

The SDQ is a quick behavioural screening questionnaire for use with 3 to 16-year-olds. It comprises 25 items about positive and negative attributes, which subdivide into five scales: Prosocial, Hyperactivity, Emotional, Conduct and Peer Problems. There are versions for children, parents and teachers, which enable the comparison of the total difficulties score in each instance.

Sentence Completion for Depression (SCD-15, Short Form; *Barton, 2003)*

The SCD-15 is a sentence completion measure for depression. The individual is asked to complete 15 sentences following the given prompt (e.g. 'My friends . . .'). The responses are then coded according to their negative, neutral or positive thought content. Five or more negative responses suggests a clinically depressed mood.

Life at School Profile (LASP; *Nash and Latham, in preparation*)

The LASP is a 56 item questionnaire for 8 to 13-year-olds in which the individual is requested to make a series of 'Like me' or 'Not like me' choices. The scale taps two domains, which focus on perception of self as a learner and in relation to peers (i.e. classroom and playground contexts). The second of these domains also provides an indication of the child's emotional vulnerability at school.

Me-As-A-Learner Scale (MALS; *Burden, 2000*)

MALS provides a simple 20 item measure of children's perceptions of themselves as learners and problem-solvers. It is designed for use with 11–13-year-olds. A version of the scale for younger children is currently being developed.

Management of psychosocial aspects of reading and language impairments

Having established the nature and severity of the individual's psychosocial difficulties, careful consideration should be given as how best to manage those difficulties. Depending upon the level of need, 'management' might constitute giving teachers and parents guidance regarding a plan of action, with an opportunity to monitor and review progress over a period of time. Alternatively, individuals might be offered some form of psychosocial intervention as part of the overall management of their learning difficulties.

What is the aim of intervention – what are we seeking to achieve?

Before mounting an intervention programme, the aim of the exercise must be clear to all concerned. The primary aim of intervention is to motivate vulnerable learners, who long ago may have decided that effort does not produce results. Care must be taken to ensure that the intervention complements and does not replace an intervention directly focusing on the language and reading needs of the child. However, as Dockrell and Messer (1999, p. 151) state: 'When children believe they can tackle a task, they will learn, given time and appropriate educational opportunities.'

A key factor in this process is the extent to which the child believes in his or her own capabilities and self-worth. By engaging in activities that reinforce individuals' self-perception and self-esteem, it is anticipated that there will be concomitant improvements in their motivation to learn and in their personal and social relationships with others. Daniel and Wassell (2002, p. 54) among others assert that 'Self-esteem can change and is amenable to improvement. During the school years the potential for boosting self-esteem . . . is great.'

Intervention offers a unique means of facilitating self-esteem and equipping those who are struggling at school with a means to self-respect. This can be pursued by focusing upon developing positive feelings about oneself and one's particular abilities (e.g. feeling proud of achievements, newly learned skills and competencies), rather than heaping non-contingent praise upon the individual in the hope that the 'message' will get through. Indeed, Elliott (2002, p. 42) cautions: 'Those who experience greater difficulties with their learning may find unconditional praise untrustworthy or demeaning and, as a result, are likely to become even more defensive in how they present themselves to others.'

This thinking taps into Erikson's (1963) fourth stage of psychosocial development, 'Industry versus inferiority'. Kaplan (1991, p. 65) explains that, during middle childhood, youngsters are required to master the skills of reading, writing and mathematics in addition to social skills, which society considers necessary for adult life. Most children develop a sense of *industry* and pride in mastering these skills (positive self-perception). Some children, however, harbour a sense of *inferiority* instead as they are frequently and unfavourably compared with those who are achieving more than they are (Hamachek, 1988).

Erikson's work has direct implications for intervention, in explaining the child's fundamental psychosocial needs during childhood. These needs are echoed by Santrock (1994), who stipulates four components of psychosocial intervention:

1. identifying the causes of low self-esteem and the domains of competence important to the individual concerned;
2. emotional support and social approval;
3. achievement (to develop a sense of industry);
4. coping skills (to meet daily challenges).

How should intervention be undertaken?

There are various options regarding how intervention should be undertaken:

- Should the child participate in a group programme or receive individual attention?

- Should the intervention programme be run in or out of school?
- Should the intervention programme be residential or non-residential?
- Should the intervention programme be run on an intensive or regular (e.g. weekly) basis?

The nature of the young person's psychosocial needs will determine whether he or she will benefit most from group or individual attention. For example, whereas one individual could benefit from discussing an issue about being bullied in the context of a supportive group, another child might gain more from talking about their painful experiences in a one-to-one situation. Given that psychosocial difficulties tend to revolve around relationships with other people, small-group work (involving 4–6 participants) is often the best context for intervention. Larger groups of up to 12 participants can also work well when addressing less sensitive issues and as a vehicle for introducing topics that can be explored further in small-group work.

The setting for the intervention programme requires careful thought as the implications for a school or external base will differ. If the programme is to be run within school hours, there is the question of withdrawing the child from lessons, perhaps on a regular basis (see below), or requiring the child to miss break or lunchtime. The advantages and disadvantages of each option need to be carefully thought through. For example, forgoing break times is not the obvious choice as it means that the individual does not have a 'break' (and all that that implies), and it robs the child of further opportunities to socialize with his or her peers.

Who should offer intervention?

An intervention programme that focuses on the psychosocial aspects of learning difficulties can be mounted by a member of the school staff (e.g. a teacher or classroom assistant) or by a specialist who may or may not be attached to the school (e.g. a psychologist or speech and language therapist). In the latter case, it can be beneficial for the specialist to work closely with the school staff and perhaps involve a classroom assistant in the programme. In this way, skills and training can be passed on to the school and become a part of the school's portfolio. The decision concerning who should offer the intervention is partly determined by where the programme is to be undertaken.

Where should intervention be undertaken?

The primary decision regarding venue is whether or not the programme should be based in or out of school. The latter can be further divided into local or further afield, for example if the course is to be run on a residential basis. Whereas a residential programme run on an intensive basis over a period of a week or fortnight offers a unique opportunity to work on psychosocial difficulties, special attention needs to be given to the generalizability and maintenance of progress after the course has finished. Unless arrangements are made (e.g. with school staff or the child's speech and language therapist) beforehand regarding the reinforcement and continuation of progress made during the intervention programme, such progress can unfortunately regress, or at best plateau. Different venues offer different advantages, as shown in Table 13.1.

Table 13.1 The advantages and disadvantages of different venues for mounting an intervention programme

Venue	Advantages	Disadvantages
School-based	Familiar environment Regular sessions/non-residential After-school activity School staff involvement Able to use school facilities No cost to parents/caregivers	Associations of school Missed lessons or break times Child may be tired from the school day Child may prefer non-school staff Limited space Cost to school budget
Out of school	Neutral environment Residential or non-residential After school/during holiday times Child may prefer non-school staff Sufficient space guaranteed Tailor-made facilities available	Unfamiliar environment Transport could pose a problem Withdrawn from school to attend Staff not connected to school May incur expenses Possible cost to parents/caregivers

Which intervention programme should be used?

Rather few psychosocial intervention programmes have been specifically designed for children and young people with reading and language impairment. A notable study was undertaken by Lawrence (1985), who developed the *Distar* programme, which combines reading tuition and enhancing self-esteem. On the basis of his findings, Lawrence concluded that remedial teachers could be more effective in their efforts to help the retarded reader if they systematically paid attention to the child's self-concept. McKissock (2001) also highlighted the value of counselling adults with dyslexia. In line with Lawrence (1985), she also reported that extra reading tuition was far more effective when combined with work on increasing self-esteem.

Place et al. (2002) have devised a resilience package for vulnerable children with learning difficulties, and Nash et al. (2002) have produced a programme for children with persistent communication impairment. Research findings from each of these programmes endorse the need to incorporate work on enhancing the individual's psychosocial functioning alongside their reading and language skills.

Case profiles: Assessing and managing children with reading and language difficulties

In appreciating how assessment and management considerations need to dovetail, it is useful to look briefly at two profiles of children – Helen and Simon – both of whom have dyslexia. This exercise also highlights the importance of selecting assessments that directly tap into the content of the intervention programme. For this purpose, attention is drawn specifically to the assessments that measure psychosocial functioning.

Helen

Cognitive assessment has shown Helen (aged 10;3 years) to be of above-average intelligence, with an IQ score of 116. She has a specific learning deficit in phonological skills (speech processing) consistent with a diagnosis of dyslexia. Helen is very aware of her difficulties, which cause her a great deal of anxiety and frustration over her school work.

Psychosocial assessment has identified Helen's particular psychosocial difficulties:

- a negative perception of herself and her academic abilities;
- anxiety about her school work and a sense of underachievement;
- negative emotions of frustration and anger associated with her specific learning difficulty.

Simon

On assessment Simon (aged 8;6 years) gained an IQ score of 88, which is indicative of low-average intelligence. He has a specific learning difficulty characterized by phonological deficits and consistent with a diagnosis of dyslexia. Although he is a happy and well-adjusted child out of school, Simon lacks confidence in many areas of the school curriculum and tends to find school work a constant struggle.

Psychosocial assessment has identified Simon's particular difficulties:

- a negative perception of himself and his academic abilities;
- anxiety about school, especially relating to school work;
- anxiety about how his peers perceive his abilities in view of his difficulties.

Following assessment, it was thought that Helen and Simon would benefit from psychosocial intervention to help them to gain a more positive view of themselves, to reduce their frustration and to increase their motivation and interest in their school work. A 1 week intensive intervention programme in which literacy tuition was integrated with confidence-boosting activities during large- and small-group work aimed to meet these aims by:

- enabling the children to identify negative and positive thoughts and feelings, and when these were likely to arise;
- equipping the children with coping strategies to replace unhelpful negative thoughts with more helpful, positive ones;
- enhancing the children's self-confidence and self-respect as learners, through focusing on their strengths rather than their difficulties;
- mastering simple relaxation techniques for reducing the tension associated with reading, writing and spelling activities.

Helen and Simon made some notable improvements following their participation on the intervention programme. These are evident in Tables 13.2 and 13.3, which compare assessment scores obtained before (pre-) and after (post-) the programme. Although an increase in scores over time is desirable for some of the assessments (MALS and SIP-C Positive Self-Image), a decrease in scores is sought for others (e.g. LASP Vulnerability and SIP-C Negative Self-Image), depending upon the nature of the items. In the case of the SIP-C Self-Esteem measure, the score is obtained by calculating the sum of discrepancies that exist between how the child sees him- or herself

Table 13.2 Pre- and post-intervention assessment

Assessment (and desirable direction of change in scores)	Helen Pre-	Post-	Simon Pre-	Post-
LASP (vulnerability – decrease desirable)	5/27	2/27	7/27	1/27
MALS (increase desirable)	69/100	74/100	60/100	76/100
SIP-C (Positive Self-Image – increase desirable)	45/72	54/72	62/72	71/72
SIP-C (Negative Self-Image – decrease desirable)	29/72	25/72	12/72	6/72
SIP-C (Self-Esteem – decrease desirable as score shows discrepancy between actual and ideal self)	15	15	15	0

LASP, Life at School Profile (Nash and Latham, in preparation); MALS, Me-As-A-Learner (Burden, 2000); SIP-C, Self-Image Profile for Children (Butler, 2001b).

now (actual self) and how he or she would like to be (ideal self). The higher the discrepancy, the lower individuals' self-esteem, as this reflects their dissatisfaction with how they perceive themselves now. Therefore, a decrease in scores over time indicates an increase in self-esteem.

A closer look at the breakdown of scores on the SIP-C according to different dimensions, or Aspects of Self (Table 13.3), indicates where the greatest changes have been made following reassessment. Aspects of Self scores are derived from responses made to the Positive and Negative Self-Image items on the SIP-C assessment. For example, the aspect named 'Behaviour' relates to behaviours associated with a negative self-image, such as 'lazy', 'moody' and 'bossy', whereas 'Social' represents characteristics indicative of a positive self-image, such as 'kind', 'happy' and 'friendly'.

Table 13.3 Aspects of Self (SIP-C) mean scores

Aspects of Self (SIP-C) (and desirable direction of change in scores)	Helen Pre-	Post-	Simon Pre-	Post-
Behaviour (decrease desirable)	2.25	2.13	1.13	0.75
Social (increase desirable)	4.00	4.50	5.00	6.00
Emotional (decrease desirable)	2.75	2.25	1.50	0
Outgoing (increase desirable)	3.67	5.00	6.00	6.00
Academic (increase desirable)	3.50	4.00	4.00	5.50
Resourceful (increase desirable)	3.00	2.00	3.00	0
Appearance (increase desirable)	3.00	4.00	6.00	6.00

At post-intervention assessment, the improvement in scores (as indicated in Tables 13.2 and 13.3) was borne out by Helen and Simon's greater confidence in talking about their literacy difficulties, a more relaxed attitude towards school in general and a sense that they had some degree of control over their situation. Both children mentioned that they had remembered and put into practice the simple relaxation techniques that they had mastered during the intervention programme, particularly before starting their school homework. Simon's mother commented on her son's willingness to read at home since attending the programme, Helen's mother mentioned that her daughter was now experiencing notably less anger and frustration when she encountered difficulties with her school work. As with all programmes, the effectiveness of intervention lies in the maintenance of progress over time.

The relationship between assessment and management should be a very close one, in that information gleaned from the assessment should inform the direction and nature of the management of the child's difficulties. On this occasion, 'management' took the form of participation on an intervention programme run during the school summer holidays. On other occasions, assessment may indicate that the child would benefit from a programme of individual sessions. It is always desirable to keep in close contact with the child's school regarding assessment and management decisions.

The concept of resilience

In assessing young people with reading and language impairments, it soon becomes evident that although many of them report some degree of psychosocial difficulty, a minority of them exude an appetite for life despite its challenges. This desirable and advantageous quality is resilience, which Rutter (1985) believes comprises three fundamental components: a sense of self-esteem and confidence, a belief in one's own self-efficacy and ability to deal with change and adaptation, and a repertoire of social problem-solving approaches. The close association between resilience and self-esteem, self-efficacy and social competence is noted by various authors (e.g. Daniel and Wassell, 2002; Gilligan, 1997; Luthar, 1991). The irony is, of course, that resilient children are less susceptible to being bullied because their peers perceive their resilience, and they are therefore not seen as 'soft and easy' targets. By identifying what it is that makes some children so resilient, it should be possible to help more vulnerable youngsters to develop the fundamental qualities (Nash, 2002). Cooper (2000, p. 31) endorses the need for these qualities, which she describes as 'the ability to take hard knocks, to weather the storm and to continue to value oneself whatever happens'.

With respect to the aim of effective intervention, Grotberg (1997) describes the resilient individual as one who is able to say in positive tones:

- I AM, for example 'I am a likeable person and respectful of myself and others';
- I CAN, for example 'I can find ways to solve problems, and I can control myself';
- I HAVE, for example 'I have people who love me and people to help me'.

It is interesting to note that, in discussing resilience, Cooper (2000) pinpoints three manifestations of resilience that directly map onto Grotberg's descriptions:

- *cognitive resilience* ('I AM'), i.e. the capacity to talk to oneself in a supportive and positive way;
- *behavioural resilience* ('I CAN'), i.e. the capacity to interact successfully with others and manage their reactions;
- *emotional resilience* ('I HAVE'), i.e. the capacity to feel good about oneself and one's ability to cope successfully with difficulties.

A further dimension of resilience, noted by Brooks (1994), is the importance of an internal locus of control, especially in coping with success and failure. Children with high self-esteem tend to have a realistic sense of their own abilities and view any successes as the result of their own efforts, over which they have control. On the other hand, youngsters with low self-esteem are much more likely to ascribe favourable outcomes to chance. As they are often driven by an external locus of control, failures are seen as evidence of their low intelligence or lack of ability. In this way, they display both hopelessness and helplessness, and anticipate that failure is inevitable.

Figure 13.4 depicts potential relationships between learning difficulties and psychosocial functioning. The matrix suggests that the vulnerable group are actually disadvantaged by their psychosocial dysfunction, to the extent that they present an 'at-risk' group (maladaptive dysfunctional). The 'resilient copers', on the other hand, may have severe learning difficulties but are able to cope with them in a remarkable way (adaptive dysfunctional). These individuals seem to be driven by positive feelings about their self-worth and their capabilities. They often have a keen sense of humour and the conviction that they can cope with whatever they may encounter (Nash et al., 2002).

Positive Psychosocial Status
*(e.g. high self-esteem, positive self-perception,
adaptive coping style, therefore high motivation to achieve)*

Adaptive-dysfunctional: • Positive self-esteem • Positive self-perception • Social competence hampered by learning difficulties • Sense of self-efficacy • Adaptive coping style The 'resilient copers'	**Adaptive-competent:** • Positive self-esteem • Positive self-perception • Socially competent • Sense of self-efficacy • Adaptive coping style The non-impaired norm

(+) ——————————————————————————— (−)

Learning Difficulties (left)   **Learning Diffculties** (right)

Maladaptive dysfunctional: • Disadvantaged by negative self-esteem • Disadvantaged by negative self-perception • Socially incompetent due to constellation of disadvantages • Little sense of self-efficacy • Maladaptive coping style The 'at-risk' group	**Maladaptive-competent:** • Negative self-esteem • Negative self-perception • Potential to be socially competent but lacks confidence • Little sense of self-efficacy • Maladaptive coping style The hampered competent

Negative Psychosocial Status
*(e.g. low self-esteem, poor self-perception,
maladaptive coping style, therefore low motivation to achieve)*

Figure 13.4 Matrix showing potential relationships between learning difficulties and psychosocial status (adapted from Nash et al., 2002).

Daniel and Wassell (2002) have suggested that the way in which children cope with their difficulties can be 'plotted' on a continuum with 'resilience' at one end and 'vulnerability' at the other end (Figure 13.5). They indicate that the individual's intrinsic qualities (e.g. temperament and coping skills) and extrinsic factors (family and community environments) largely determine where they are located on the continuum. These factors can be either protective (supportive) or adverse (antagonistic or indifferent), that is, they can help to 'rescue' the child or can exacerbate his or her difficulties further, as evidenced by the 'at-risk' group. The wide range of individual differences that these factors represent should be at the forefront of any management decisions made on behalf of the learning-impaired child.

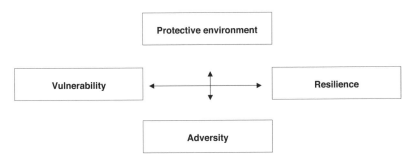

Figure 13.5 Framework for the assessment of resilience factors (Danie, Wassell and Gilligan, 1999, cited in Daniel and Wassell, 2002).

Place et al. (2002) note that examination of underlying risk and protective factors is crucial in promoting resilience in a therapeutic way. Whereas risk factors increase the likelihood of mental health problems, protective factors reduce this likelihood (Rutter and Rutter, 1993). Their resilience package for vulnerable learners seeks to enhance specific protective factors in the child, especially positive self-esteem, social skills and problem-solving skills.

In fostering resilience, Brooks (1994) emphasizes the importance of capitalizing upon any special interests or talents that the individual may show. The challenge for those working with young people is to explore ways of enabling them to experience success by identifying their 'islands of competence'. In identifying their strengths and abilities, they can be encouraged to develop empowering strategies such as relaxation and coping with bullying.

The focus upon resilience in addressing psychosocial difficulties is gaining popularity. It is being heralded as a means of offering young people an alternative framework for intervention, with its emphasis upon assessing potential areas of competence. As yet, however, there have been few attempts actively to promote resilience (Daniel and Wassell, 2002). Luthar (1991) offers a word of caution, noting that some apparently resilient youngsters may be internalizing their distress. With careful and sensitive assessment, such instances can be recognized by the practitioner.

The importance of self-talk in effective management of reading and language impairments

One explanation for the apparent difference between resilient and vulnerable learners may lie in the nature of their self-talk, that is, the type of self-instruction they engage in. Self-talk reinforces the positive or negative feelings that individuals have about themselves, and may be largely determined by self-esteem and self-perception. Nash (1998) describes the nature of self-talk as a continuous patter going on in one's head, which can persist throughout the day. This patter often echoes the voice of the parent, urging the child on, or it can resemble the protesting child being asked to do something he or she does not wish to do.

By listening carefully to the nature of self-talk, it is possible to break these habitual and sometimes maladaptive circling thoughts. With appropriate help, the unhelpful thoughts can be replaced by more constructive ones, which work for rather than against the individual and others concerned. Where the child's self-talk is negative and undermining, it can operate as a self-fulfilling prophecy. For example, children who constantly feel that they are failing at school may habitually tell themselves by means of self-talk that they are 'no good at . . .' or that they 'can't do . . .'. Such perceptions fuel expectations of failure and lower their motivation to try; in doing so, they can actively make further failure more likely. Figure 13.6 shows how a self-fulfilling prophecy is reinforced by self-talk.

An obvious application of training in self-talk (or 'self-instructional training'; Meichenbaum, 1975) is in coping with being bullied. Frances (2000, pp. 179–80) provides an example of 'good self-talk' as:

> something you say to yourself silently or under your breath e.g. 'One, two, three ... ten' when you are feeling unbearably provoked. Self-talk is an important strategy, especially as children get older. Good self-talk acts as a form of 'inner self-defence' and can help a child or teenager to cope calmly.

As all individuals engage in self-talk and negative self-talk can be a clear manifestation of psychosocial difficulties, practitioners need to incorporate this dimension into any intervention programme that they are able to offer those with reading and language impairments.

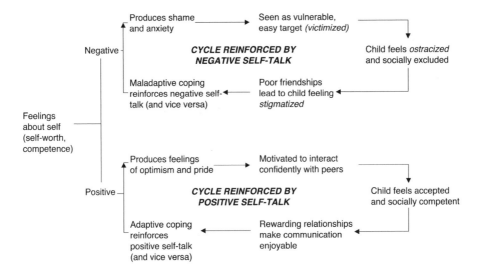

Figure 13.6 How a self-fulfilling prophecy is reinforced by child's negative or positive self-talk (adapted from Nash et al., 2002).

Conclusions

This chapter has looked at the nature, assessment and management of psychosocial difficulties associated with reading and language impairments. It is important to end it by emphasizing the crucial roles that can be played by the local and wider communities in helping the individuals concerned, not least in building a protective network around them. These communities comprise a range of experiences and environments:

- immediate and extended family members (e.g. grandparents);
- friends and peers;
- school staff;
- the wider community in which the child lives.

A belief in oneself and one's abilities as an adult are firmly established in childhood experiences. Enabling children to foster a positive self-belief is therefore an investment for them now and for their future adult lives. In view of this, there is a great need for further research that focuses on not only the identification of those who are struggling at school (despite the various guises to suggest the contrary), but also effective interventions.

CHAPTER 14

Supporting language and literacy in the early years: interdisciplinary training

JANNET A. WRIGHT AND JANET WOOD

In a book about dyslexia and speech and language, the importance of children's language development in the early years cannot be underestimated. Children's spoken language abilities can influence their educational and social development. A number of researchers have shown that spoken language skills underpin reading and writing abilities (Catts et al., 1994; Snowling, 2000; Stackhouse and Wells, 1997). If children have difficulties acquiring their speech and language skills, they may also have difficulties in developing their literacy abilities. For example, normally developing children acquire phonological awareness skills as part of their developing speech and language abilities. Phonological awareness appears to be a key oral skill for literacy development as it will help children to 'crack' the phoneme–grapheme correspondence code that they need in order to be able to read. If children have difficulties with their speech and language acquisition, they may have problems with developing phonological awareness, and this can have an impact on their literacy development. If they have problems with understanding spoken language, this can influence their understanding of the written word.

If language development is so crucial for literacy development, it is important that attention is paid to the types of activity and experience that children have which help them to develop their linguistic abilities. Many young children spend time not only with their parents, but also with carers in preschools and nurseries. Their experiences in such settings provide opportunities for interaction with adults as well as the opportunity to practise language skills with their peers. During this time, young children are developing and extending the language skills that underpin literacy development. Other practitioners from a range of agencies also have opportunities for supporting development in this area.

In this chapter, the ways in which early-years practitioners can help children to develop their speech, language and literacy skills prior to school entry will be explored. The factors that influence the work of early-years practitioners will also be considered, as will interdisciplinary training and the ways in which this is experienced by early-years practitioners.

The early-years setting

What is meant by the term 'early years'?

Throughout this chapter, the term 'early years' will be used when referring to children in the period up to and including 5 years of age. These children may be spending time in preschools, nurseries or reception classes in schools. Included within this early-years period are children from 3 to 5 years old who, in England, are following the Foundation Stage of the UK'S national curriculum (www.surestart.gov.uk).

Who works with children in the early years?

From birth onwards, children come into contact with a range of people other than their immediate family members, all of whom may be seen as early-years workers. The health-surveillance programme in the UK is organized within the National Health Service (NHS) so that children are seen by health visitors at specific ages to check on their development. Thus, the contact that children have with health visitors may be infrequent but will occur at specifically timetabled points.

If there are concerns about children's health or general development, they and their families may be brought into contact with doctors. Children who are identified as having difficulty with speech and language development in the early years may be referred to speech and language therapists. In addition, occupational therapists and physiotherapists may be involved with children where there are concerns about motor development. Children with difficulties in their general development or with sensory problems such as hearing or visual impairment may have contact with psychologists and specialist teachers. Day nurseries, nursery schools and nursery classes bring many young children into contact with education and/or social work staff on a very regular basis.

The practitioners who might be involved with children in the early years could therefore include:

- health visitors;
- GPs/family doctors;
- clinical medical officers;
- paediatricians;

- early-years educators, including playgroup staff;
- nursery staff;
- nursery teachers;
- learning support assistants;
- teachers of the deaf/ visually impaired;
- nursery nurses;
- librarians;
- volunteers;
- speech and language therapists;
- portage workers;
- social workers;
- educational/clinical psychologists;
- occupational therapists;
- physiotherapists.

In order to obtain a holistic view of the children whom they see, practitioners strive to liaise or work with colleagues from other disciplines. In the UK, they are encouraged to do this by the NHS, the Department for Education and Skills (DfES) and the Department of Health.

Influences on the ways in which early-years practitioners work together

The NHS

There is clear evidence that attempts have been made in the NHS to create an environment in which families receive a 'seamless service' and health practitioners work together through, for example, the introduction of the Health Action Zones (HAZs). The role for the HAZs is to tackle inequalities in health in the most deprived areas of the country through health and social care programmes. These were first established in 1998 and are multiagency partnerships between the NHS, local authorities (including social services), voluntary and business sectors, and local communities. Practitioners are encouraged to focus on health issues as well as factors that influence health, such as education.

Education service

As with the HAZs, the introduction of Education Action Zones (EAZs) focused on disadvantaged urban and rural areas. The aim is to raise standards through local partnerships. Each EAZ consists of a cluster of two or three secondary schools with feeder primary schools and local special schools. They work in partnership with Local Education Authorities (LEAs), parents, business and other representatives from the local community. An Education Action Forum, made up of the main partners, manages the EAZ and has to raise a certain amount each year from the private sector in addition to the funding they receive from the DfES.

The EAZs focus on four main themes:

1. improving the quality of teaching and learning;
2. social inclusion;
3. family and pupil support;
4. working with business and other organizations.

Before the introduction of EAZs, the government encouraged practitioners in education to work together for a number of years through the *Code of Practice* (Department for Education and Employment, 1994), *Excellence for all Children* (Department for Education and Employment, 1997) and the *Special Educational Needs Code of Practice* (Department for Education and Skills, 2001b). In the revised edition of the SEN Code of Practice, there is a clear focus on providing support for children with difficulties in learning in the early years.

The language development of young children was highlighted when the foundation stage was introduced into the National Curriculum in September 2002 (Education Act, 2002). This gave practitioners a clear directive to focus on communication, language and literacy, and meant that they needed the 'knowledge and skills to assess, monitor and promote spoken language' (Locke, Ginsborg and Peers, 2002, p. 14).

Social services

In social services, Early Excellence Centres are being developed to provide high-quality early-years education, alongside childcare, family support and learning, adult education, childminder support and parenting education. The aim is for the Early Excellence Centres to demonstrate how care and education can be integrated to provide services for children aged 0–5 years. These centres are to be open all day and throughout the year.

There have been many government initiatives that influence practitioners working in the early years. There has been a focus on working together in order to develop children's communication. It is, however, not always easy for people to work together.

Interagency collaboration

Professionals often believe that one of the benefits of working collaboratively across agencies is that children receive a holistic approach. For teachers and speech and language therapists who work together, this means that they can provide each other with professional support and an opportunity to share concerns about specific children. Teachers and therapists have reported that, when they work together, they learn from each other (Wright, 1996; Wright and Kersner, 2004).

An example of collaboration between health and education can be found in the Bookstart project (www.bookstart.co.uk). Here, health visitors have become involved in providing babies in the UK and their parents/carers with a Bookstart pack of free books and guidance materials. The project, which involves the library services, focuses on the parents and carers of 7–9-month-old babies. Health visitors see parents and children at this age and are able to talk to families about the desirability of an early focus on literacy and language activities.

Speech and language therapists, employed by the NHS, have been encouraged to work with educational staff, and there is evidence in the UK that supports such working partnerships (Law et al., 2000b; McCartney and van der Gaag, 1996; Popple and Wellington, 1996, 2001; Reid et al., 1996). It may be that service-level agreements can be used to clarify roles and ensure that joint working can be monitored in a meaningful way. For a period from 2000, the DfES encouraged LEAs and speech and language therapy services to join together to bid for funding through the Standards Fund for projects related to speech and language therapy. This provided new opportunities for services within LEAs and the NHS to work together (Law, Luscombe and Roux, 2002).

Sure Start (Department for Education and Employment, 1999; www.surestart.gov.uk), a UK government initiative, has brought together practitioners such as nursery staff, health visitors and speech and language therapists to provide programmes for children and their families. Sure Start aims to enhance and extend services available for families and has been established to tackle 'child poverty and social exclusion'. Children living in areas of socioeconomic deprivation are at risk of language delay, and research has established clear links between language delay and low socioeconomic status (Locke, Ginsborg and Peers, 2002).

The government has also introduced, through Sure Start, the framework of *Birth to Three Matters* (Department for Education and Skills, 2002), which is aimed at those registered with Ofsted to care for children up to 3 years old. Local authorities are now looking at ways in which to use the framework to support the training of practitioners working with this age group. This will enable social services and the NHS to work together when offering training to newly appointed staff.

Despite the influences described above, collaboration can be affected by a range of factors when professionals are employed by different agencies. Each agency is likely to have its own ethos, structures and terminology, which can become a barrier to collaboration. The expectations placed on professionals working together will also be influenced by the settings in which they work.

In the early years, there may be greater flexibility available to teachers such that they can more easily incorporate therapy targets into classroom activities. In later years, teachers and therapists report increasing tension between the curricular demands of the school and speech and language therapy targets (Wright and Kersner, 2004).

Developing children's language and literacy skills in the early years

Identifying children who are 'at risk': what do early-years practitioners know?

If early-years practitioners are expected to identify children who might have speech, language and literacy difficulties and/or to support the development of these skills, they need to have the resources to be able to do this. In 1998 in the UK, a project was set up by the charities the Association for all Speech Impaired Children (AFASIC) and the British Dyslexia Association (BDA), in collaboration with the Department of Human Communication Science, University College London (UCL). One of the aims of this project was to conduct a survey of early-years practitioners' knowledge and training needs in relation to children's speech, language and literacy development. A postal questionnaire was sent to nearly 300 early-years practitioners from a wide range of disciplines. Response rates varied between the practitioner groups and ranged from 12 per cent to 80 per cent, with an overall response rate of 38 per cent, representing responses from 113 practitioners. The disciplines represented within the responses were doctors (family doctors and paediatricians), health visitors, speech and language therapists, teachers, preschool/playgroup staff and portage home visitors.

Some of the questions within the survey related to the identification of children who either had or were at risk of having speech, language or literacy difficulties. It is evident from the literature that there are many factors that might put a child at risk of language difficulties; these include a family history of such difficulties (Tomblin and Buckwater, 1994), hearing impairment (Shriberg et al., 2000b), low birth weight (Gallagher and Watkin, 1998) and deprivation/lack of language stimulation (Skuse, 1991).

The early-years practitioners' awareness of these 'at-risk' factors was investigated within the survey by asking them to write down up to five factors that might hinder a child's language development. Just over two-thirds of the respondents were able to identify three or more relevant factors, and 19 factors were suggested overall. The three most frequent responses were 'hearing impairment' (mentioned by 82 per cent of the respondents), 'home environment' (mentioned by 76 per cent of the respondents) and 'developmental delay' (mentioned by 29 per cent of the respondents). Some practitioners were not able to list three or more relevant factors, whereas others focused on factors that were only likely to have a small impact, for example lack of confidence, an excessive use of dummies and siblings talking for the child.

The survey also investigated the respondents' awareness of factors that would support or hinder a child's early literacy development. As has been discussed in earlier chapters of this book, it is not possible to predict exactly which preschool children will go on to have literacy difficulties, but it is possible to list factors that are important in determining literacy outcome. These factors include speech and language skills (Nathan et al., 2004a; Stackhouse, 2000; Stothard et al., 1998), phonological awareness and alphabetic knowledge (see Chapter 4 in this volume) and the knowledge of how books work (Wade and Moore, 1998). The practitioners who responded to the survey were asked to list the knowledge and skills that preschool children might have that would help them to read when they started school. The most common response was alphabetic knowledge (62 per cent of respondents mentioned this), followed by a knowledge of how books work (33 per cent of respondents). Speech and language skills were mentioned by only 24 per cent of respondents and phonological awareness by just 11 per cent. Other skills that were mentioned included experience of books, attention control and the ability to match shapes and letters.

In a different question, respondents were asked to list factors that might hinder a child's reading and spelling development. The most popular answers related to relatively general factors such as hearing impairment (48 per cent), visual impairment (45 per cent) and home environment (45 per cent). Language difficulties were not mentioned at all, although speech delay or disorder was mentioned by 25 per cent of respondents. Phonological awareness was mentioned by 10 per cent of respondents and poor alphabetic knowledge by just 4 per cent. This is surprising considering the fact that alphabetic knowledge was the most popular response to the question about skills and knowledge that would help a child to read.

Overall, it seems that many early-years practitioners have some understanding of the factors that influence speech, language and literacy difficulties. This is encouraging in view of the important role that they play in identifying children with difficulties in these areas. For some practitioners, however, their knowledge was based on what could be described as common sense rather than on a knowledge of the findings from relevant research. This suggests that new research findings are not easily accessible to many practitioners working within the early years.

How do early-years practitioners work with children in relation to language and literacy?

As has been suggested, encouraging language development facilitates later literacy development. The respondents to the survey referred to earlier in this chapter were asked about the ways in which they worked with children in the early years to develop their language and literacy skills. The practitioners were given a list of activities and asked to indicate which ones they did as part of their job. The list of activities was as follows:

- painting;
- teaching children the names of things;
- assessing their development;
- developing pencil control (e.g. tracing patterns and lines);
- cutting and sticking;
- collecting things that start with the same sound (e.g. making a 'p' table);
- singing songs and nursery rhymes;
- teaching children to use correct word endings (e.g. walk*ing*)
- playing games (e.g. picture lotto);
- looking at books together;
- exploring letters and words (e.g. matching plastic letters);
- doing jigsaws;
- reading a story to a group of children;
- collecting things with a shared feature (e.g. collecting yellow things);
- clapping out children's names/other words;
- watching TV/videos;
- working on the computer;
- getting children to follow specific instructions;
- dressing up;
- teaching the child to listen to the difference between sounds in words (e.g. "key" versus "tea");
- making models;
- singing the alphabet.

The activities listed above are all examples of common activities carried out with children in the early years. Among the list, there are 13 activities that could be divided into categories related to language and literacy development. The five categories and the activities that fall into each one are given in Table 14.1.

Table 14.1 Categories of common activities carried out with children in the early years

1. Speech and language development activities
Teaching children the names of things
Teaching children to use correct word endings (e.g. walk*ing*)
Collecting things with a shared feature (e.g. yellow things)
Teaching children to listen to the difference between sounds in words (e.g. "key" versus "tea")

2. Phonological awareness activities
Collecting things that start with the same sound
Singing songs and nursery rhymes
Clapping out words or children's names

3. Alphabetic knowledge activities
Singing the alphabet
Exploring letters and words (e.g. matching plastic letters)

4. Book knowledge activities
Looking at books together
Reading a story to a group of children

5. Other
Assessing children's development
Getting children to follow specific instructions

When the responses from the practitioners were analysed, it was no surprise to find out that preschool/nursery staff and teachers carried out many of the activities related to speech and language development, phonological awareness and book knowledge. This was done as part of the curriculum in early-years settings. These activities were also carried out by those practitioners who worked with children who had been identified as having difficulty with their development. These practitioners included portage home visitors and speech and language therapists.

Family doctors and paediatricians did not carry out activities related to speech and language development, phonological awareness and book knowledge. This is as might be expected given that their role in the early years is seen mainly as one of health surveillance and prevention of illness. However, one group of health service practitioners, the health visitors, indicated that, as part of their work, they carried out some of the same activities as the nursery and teaching staff. This involvement by the health visitors in such activities is probably due to their role in assessing children's development at specific ages. At these times, they may be required to provide advice and recommendations to parents about activities to carry out with young children.

The fact that practitioners from both the health and the education services were carrying out activities related to language and literacy development is encouraging given the importance of collaboration between different agencies.

Published approaches

Practitioners may also use books and published programmes when planning language-based activities for their work with children in the early years. Rees (2002) reviews a number of approaches used by different professionals working with children in the early years. These range from the use of activity books such as *Early Listening Skills* (Williams, 1995), which is designed for preschool children with delayed listening skills, to organizing a course based on a published programme.

It Takes Two to Talk (Manolson, 1992) is one such programme that was the first parent–child interaction programme developed by the Hanen Centre (www.hanen.org) in Canada. Hanen courses have become popular in the UK, and to run an official Hanen programme, the trainer must attend a course and be certified by the Hanen Centre. Many professionals in the UK incorporate ideas and resources from parts of the Hanen programmes into their own work. The Hanen programme *You Make the Difference* (Manolson, Ward and Dodington, 1995) focuses on preschool children and is sometimes used in the UK as part of Sure Start programmes.

The *Living Language* programme (Locke, 1985), developed in the UK, remains a popular and useful approach for practitioners who are working with children who are finding it difficult to develop language spontaneously. Living Language includes assessment procedures that help practitioners to identify the areas of language on which to focus when planning activities for children. Following on from this programme, Locke and Beech developed *Teaching Talking* (1991), which is aimed at teachers working in mainstream nursery and primary schools. The strategies that the authors suggest relate to modifying the learning environment and can be easily used in the classroom.

Early-years practitioners have also drawn on the ideas and activities suggested by Layton and Deeny (2002) in *Sound Practice: Phonological Awareness in the Classroom*. Stuart and colleagues have been working with teachers of preschool children in inner-city schools to facilitate the children's language development in order to help future literacy development (Stuart, Dockrell and King, in press).

Interdisciplinary training

Whether practitioners use published programmes or approaches they have developed themselves, these will rarely work in isolation with children in the early years. It is therefore necessary to look for working practices that help practitioners to collaborate. One of these practices is joint training. As Freeth et al. (2002) point out, it seems reasonable to suggest that learning together helps people to work together more effectively.

Interdisciplinary training: opportunities and barriers

Opportunities for interdisciplinary training are available, although there is a great deal of variability in what is on offer. A series of seminars were held in cities around England in 2001 in order to discuss this issue (BDA/AFASIC/UCL, 2001). Most of the seminar participants could describe interdisciplinary courses that were run locally. However, these courses did not necessarily relate specifically to children's language and literacy development, and in many cases the courses were run for just two or three disciplines at a time. The practitioners who were already working within multiagency teams were those which were most likely to be able to access interdisciplinary training, for example practitioners working within Sure Start projects or EAZs.

The seminar participants were also asked about factors that might influence the future provision of interdisciplinary training. There was widespread agreement that it would be important to establish interdisciplinary networks in order to plan and organize such training. A number of people also highlighted the importance of gaining commitment from the managers of the relevant services. Other issues included organizing publicity effectively, making sure that the course fitted in with other training already on offer, talking to the intended participants about the aims and benefits of the course and finding an accessible venue.

In terms of barriers to interdisciplinary training, most of the comments were related to two key issues: attitudes and resources. This relates to the barriers referred to in professional working. In relation to attitudes, a number of seminar participants felt that it would be difficult to overcome the different agendas and priorities that were held by the different professional groups. Some suggested that it would be hard to pitch the training at the right level for everyone because each professional group had a different knowledge base, whereas others felt that they would struggle to convince managers that such training was appropriate. A fear of losing professional boundaries and the difficulties associated with the use of profession-specific jargon were also mentioned.

In relation to resources issues, problems with both funding and time were frequently highlighted. More specifically, seminar participants reported difficulties around cover for staff to attend courses and participants from some disciplines having to attend training in their own time. The timing of an interdisciplinary course was also seen as being a potential area of difficulty as practitioners from different disciplines often have different working patterns.

Benefits of interdisciplinary training

Once any barriers to providing interdisciplinary training have been overcome, the potential benefits are vast. This is demonstrated in a review of 217 studies that reported the outcomes of what was referred to as interprofessional learning (Freeth et al., 2002). Of the 217 studies, 53 were categorized as being 'higher quality' and were reported in more detail. Of the higher-quality studies, 76 per cent related to post-qualification training, the majority of these reporting positive outcomes, only 23 per cent reporting mixed or neutral outcomes, and none reporting wholly negative outcomes.

The positive outcomes that were reported included:

- a positive reaction to the training by participants, for example a positive rating of the educational experience and enjoyment of the interdisciplinary interaction (reported in 51% of studies);
- changes in attitude and perception, such as changes in attitude towards teamwork and perception of the competence of other professionals (reported in 31 per cent of studies);
- changes in knowledge and skills relating to interdisciplinary collaboration, for example an increased understanding of the roles of other professionals, increased knowledge regarding the nature of interdisciplinary teamwork and the development of interpersonal communication skills (reported in 45 per cent of studies);
- changes in practitioner behaviour, for instance improved interdisciplinary communication (reported in 25 per cent of studies);
- changes in organizational practice (reported in 48 per cent of studies);
- benefits to clients (reported in 25 per cent of studies).

Given the reported benefits from interdisciplinary training described above, the development of one such training pack will be described in the following section.

Language and literacy: Working together – an early-years training package

Designing the course

Following the questionnaire referred to earlier in the chapter, a training pack was developed (Wood, Wright and Stackhouse, 2000; Wright, Wood and Stackhouse 2004). One of the findings of the questionnaire indicated that the range of practitioners working with children in the early years have different:

• levels of knowledge about the relationship between speech, language and literacy difficulties;
• roles in working with these children;
• perceived training needs;
• levels of qualification and experience.

In addition to these findings, it was assumed that different practitioners were also likely to have a range of learning styles, for example active learners who like dealing with problems that relate to everyday life, reflective learners who like to consider new information from all perspectives, logical learners who like to know the reasons for things, and pragmatic learners who are keen to try out new ideas in practice (Honey and Mumford, 1992).

Despite, or perhaps because of, these differences, the majority of practitioners who were asked about their training needs (83 per cent) stated that they would like any training that related to children's language and literacy development to be of an interdisciplinary nature. This presented the project team with a significant challenge, namely to devise a single, interdisciplinary course that addressed the different learning needs of each professional group. In addition, the team felt that it was desirable to devise a course that would bring about changes in practice among the participants, as well as changes in knowledge.

A number of options were considered in order to meet these challenges. One such option was to have designated 'basic' and 'higher' level sessions within the course so that some practitioners could choose to attend only 'higher-level' sessions. It was, however, felt that this design did not fully meet the challenge of providing an interdisciplinary course and, furthermore, that it could actually hinder the development of joint working, by emphasizing stereotyped views of the roles of each discipline.

The course that was eventually designed encompassed four 2 hour sessions with the following session titles (Wood, Wright and Stackhouse, 2000):

- Getting started with language.
- Language and literacy.
- Fostering good practice.
- Working together – building links.

The methods that were used to address the challenges when designing the course could prove useful to readers who intend to organize interdisciplinary training, so these methods are described below.

Overcoming potential barriers to interdisciplinary training

Ensuring that participants are able to identify and work towards personal learning objectives

It was acknowledged that, for each topic area being covered, there would be some practitioners who were already familiar with the theoretical content. The practitioners to whom this applied would vary from one session of the course to another, but it was felt that everyone should get something out of each session, however familiar they were with the theoretical content. Similarly, it was acknowledged that some practitioners worked directly with children and would welcome a discussion of practical activities, whereas others had more of an assessment/monitoring role. For these reasons, it was decided that there should, in each session, be an equal emphasis on developing skills and knowledge in interdisciplinary working, developing theoretical understanding, and developing familiarity with practical activities that could be carried out with children. This was explained to participants at the start of the course, and they were given time to think about and record their personal learning objectives in light of the overall learning objectives for the course.

Presenting theoretical information in both summary and detailed form

All the participants received a pack of handouts in which the theoretical content of the course was presented at two levels. First was a summary format, i.e. copies of overhead transparencies with key points listed. This was intended to be useful for quick reference and for those practitioners who only needed or wanted to engage with a given topic at this level. Second, the information was presented in full-text handouts, with references for further reading, for participants who wanted to learn about a topic in more detail.

Presentation of the course

In each session of the course, a variety of teaching methods were used in order to appeal to a range of participant learning styles and to enable a transfer of new skills to the workplace, for example, small-group problem solving, whole-group discussion, mini-lectures and practical assignments. Video clips were used as stimuli for some activities, as were quizzes, role-plays and problem solving. All of the activities involved small-group work, such that the participants were able to talk through their thought processes and learn from each other. Handouts were provided in advance so that participants did not need to make detailed notes; some of the handouts contained diagrams or tables for the participants to fill in during group activities. This practice enabled participants to keep a record of the information they had learned during group discussion. Additionally, the handouts were designed to be 'dyslexia friendly', with a specified minimum font size and a left-justified text.

The activities that were used had a variety of functions. Some of them were designed to encourage participants to reflect on their current knowledge (e.g. labelling statements about children's language development as 'true' or 'false') or to examine their knowledge in light of material that had been presented (e.g. matching brief job descriptions to job titles for a range of early-years practitioners). Other activities were used to support participants in applying what they had learnt to real and/or hypothetical cases such as analysing the early literacy skills of two children in a video clip. Finally, some of the activities were designed to encourage participants to share their knowledge and information across disciplines (e.g. discussing the types of record that each discipline kept). Participants were also given workplace assignments to carry out between sessions. This provided an opportunity for them to apply what they had learnt to their own work setting. At the start of the following session, there was an opportunity for participants to report back on how they had managed the assignments.

Enabling participants to share knowledge and skills

Enabling participants to share knowledge and skills was, perhaps, the most important element of the course design. As has already been stated, there was an emphasis on small-group activities that encouraged participants to find out more about what other practitioners knew and did.

In order to ensure that all participants were able to work with a wide range of other practitioners during the course, the seating arrangements were carefully organized. For each session, participants were seated around small tables in groups of five or six. Each discipline was allocated a different colour, and coloured stickers were then placed on each table to denote which mix of disciplines should sit at that table. Coloured dots were also put on each participant's name badge so that everyone could easily see which discipline other people worked in. Each week, a different combination of dots was put on each table, and participants were asked to try to sit with as many different people as they could during the course. It became apparent that this system could break down if people arrived late for the course and then sat in the nearest available seat. For this reason, one tutor always stayed at the back of the room to greet any late-comers and to guide them to an appropriate table. This system was successful and was perceived positively by the participants. It meant that the aims of mixing people from different disciplines could be achieved without being dogmatic about where each person had to sit in the room.

Participants were, of course, sharing knowledge and skills in all the activities by virtue of the fact that they were working collaboratively. Included in the activities, however, were some that had a specific focus on sharing knowledge and skills, with specially designed handouts on which the participants could record the roles of people from each discipline in relation to a particular issue. One example of this was a handout on which each participant was asked to record the opportunities that each discipline had for identifying children at risk of having speech and language impairment.

Another method that was used to ensure that skills and knowledge were shared among the group was to encourage participants to answer each other's questions rather than all questions being answered by the course tutors. This enabled participants to get to know who they could go to in the future to find out more about particular issues or topics. The course tutors acted purely as facilitators in this process by ensuring that all questions were answered in one way or another.

Finally, it was suggested at the end of the course that some participants might want to form an interdisciplinary working group to move forward the process of collaborative working in that locality, tackling any issues that had been highlighted as being potential problems during the course.

Evaluation of the course

Once the course had been designed and written, it was run three times in order to evaluate its outcomes. Outcome measures included participant evaluation forms and semi-structured interviews. The following section reports some of the findings within the first four categories used in Freeth et al.'s (2002) review.

Reaction to the training by participants

Overall, the course was well received by participants. For example, 93 per cent of the participants indicated that the course aims were either mostly or fully relevant to them, and 99 per cent said that they would make use of at least some of what they had learnt on the course.

Most of the participants who were interviewed after the course felt that the course had been well organized and presented. The course was described as having 'a nice balance of theory and practice', and there were numerous positive comments that related to the multidisciplinary nature of the course.

Changes in attitude and perception

One of the benefits of such a course was that it enabled people to feel less isolated. One participant stated: 'it's really beneficial to see everybody else's point of view because you do become very isolated if you're just thinking one way'.

The course also helped to change some stereotyped perceptions about others' roles. One preschool worker, for example, felt that others had initially thought 'What do you know about it [children's language and literacy skills] if you only mix paint?', but by the end of the course she felt that others 'valued you for what you did'.

Similarly, one of the health visitors commented that she had been pleased to be able to highlight the fact that she did not 'just weigh babies'.

Nearly all the participants who were interviewed reported an increase in confidence in working within this area. For at least one participant, this included the confidence to be open about what she did and did not know: 'It gave me the confidence to say, "Hang on a minute, what does that mean?".'

Changes in knowledge and skills

The course enabled participants to develop their knowledge and skills in a number of ways. Some participants developed their awareness of the links between language and literacy development: 'it was linking the literacy to the language which I obviously knew but . . . hadn't really thought about'.

Others developed their understanding of referral routes: 'I know that I can ring straight to the speech and language therapist. I thought I always had to go through the health visitor.' Still others gained knowledge that could be used to develop their practice. A family doctor said:

> I'm more aware of the breadth of questions that I could ask to get information rather than being more medically orientated in my approach, which might have been the case before.

A health visitor stated that the course:

> raised my awareness of the nursery teachers to actually think of going to them . . . often we just talk to parents direct and then refer to speech therapists which sort of cuts out the nursery. But it is nice to be more aware that I can actually say, 'Oh well hang on a minute let's see what the nursery think.'

Changes in practitioner behaviour

One outcome that was particularly positive was evidence that, for some participants, the course had resulted in changes in collaborative practice. It would seem that increased confidence helped to remove professional barriers. For example, one early-years practitioner stated, 'I feel less, perhaps, nervous or worried. When the health visitors come in or phone up I do now actually . . . I can now actually speak to them.' Improved knowledge of others' roles also had an impact on practice. One speech and language therapist said:

> if I'm actually working with a child from a nursery placement I might ring them up now and say, 'what are you doing?' and I might actually give advice to the nursery, which I might not have done previously.

Overall, then, it is apparent that this particular course, and interdisciplinary courses in general, are effective at increasing the amount and nature of interdisciplinary working. The actual outcomes relate to changes in attitudes and knowledge as well as some changes in actual working practice.

Conclusions

This chapter has highlighted many of the potential difficulties associated with developing and organizing interdisciplinary working, but it has also indicated ways of overcoming some of the challenges. It is always likely to be the case that practitioners from different disciplines will have different levels of knowledge and skill and different areas of specialism. It is therefore suggested that any interdisciplinary training makes a feature of this within the course design. Interdisciplinary training should be seen as an opportunity for practitioners to share their skills and knowledge. An increased understanding of the roles of others supports interdisciplinary working, which in turn helps to ensure that children with speech, language and literacy difficulties are identified and supported as early as possible.

Acknowledgement

We would like to thank the early-years practitioners and managers who took part in the project. This work was supported by a grant from GlaxoSmithKline.

CHAPTER 15

Current themes and future directions

MAGGIE SNOWLING AND JOY STACKHOUSE

In this book, we have primarily been concerned with children's written language difficulties. A recurring theme has been that the manifestations of these difficulties are diverse: they may be obvious, they may be hidden; they may be specific or reflect more general learning difficulties; they may occur in isolation or in combination with language or visuospatial problems. In all cases, however, these difficulties can, if left unattended, cause significant educational underachievement and untold damage to children's confidence and self-esteem. We reflect here upon four main questions. First, what is the relationship between spoken and written language difficulties?; second, which children are at risk of literacy problems?; third, how can such children be supported?; and fourth, who should deliver interventions?

What is the relationship between spoken and written language difficulties?

Reading this book should leave the practitioner in no doubt that oral language skills are the foundation of reading and writing. However, the relationship between spoken and written language difficulties is not straightforward. As all who practise clinically will know, pure reading disorders are rare: different language skills interact to produce a spectrum of reading outcomes. Moreover, bidirectional links between oral and written language mean that literacy can itself transform spoken language. On a positive note, learning to spell can improve speech perception and production; on the down side, the oral vocabulary of poor readers may fail to keep pace with their development.

We have seen that, at the very least, we must consider spoken language abilities as comprising three sets of subskills. For simplicity, we will refer to these as speech, understanding and expressive language. In the same way, we can consider written language as comprising at least three subskills, namely reading as a 'decoding' process, reading for meaning, and writing, in particular spelling. Arguably, these spoken and written language processes have reciprocal links with one another. In particular, adequate speech seems necessary for the development of decoding and spelling skills, language comprehension feeds reading comprehension, and expressive language will be intricately linked with the development of writing ability.

There is no doubt that when individual children are considered, these relationships can be complex and difficult to decipher. The current manifestation of a 'reading' problem, sometimes referred to as a reading profile, will depend upon the interaction of a number of factors including:

- the age of the child and the developmental 'stage' that he or she has reached;
- the precise nature and pervasiveness of the child's speech or language difficulty;
- the severity of the child's phonological processing difficulties, including his or her current levels of phonological awareness;
- the extent to which the child has been able to compensate using intact skills;
- the amount and type of intervention the child has received.

It follows that, among children with reading difficulties, there is considerable heterogeneity, although usually without clear subtypes. It is essential to bear in mind that the ways in which the different language skills combine and interrelate is not clear cut, and there can be many modifying factors at the level of individual children. Figure 15.1 is an elaboration of the 'spectrum' discussed in Chapter 1 (p. 13). In this figure, we aim to show in more detail how the spectrum of literacy disorders relates to spoken language difficulties.

In the model, the horizontal axis represents phonology and the extent to which it is intact, from left (intact) to right (impaired). The vertical axis, in contrast, represents a dimension of meaning – semantics – from high (intact) to low (impaired). We propose that a child's position in this two-dimensional space determines the nature of the literacy difficulties that he or she experiences.

Normal readers occupy the centre portion of the model, individual variation in normal populations being associated with differing levels of phonological and semantic skills. Moving from the left, children have been described who have good phonology for their age and exceptional reading

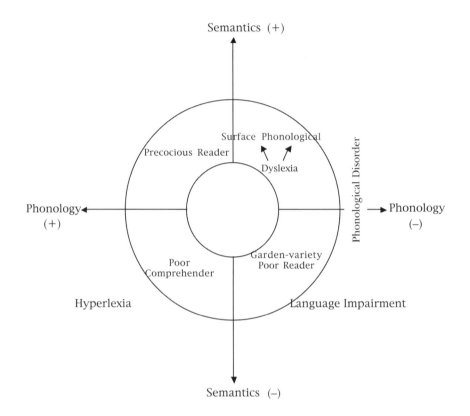

Figure 15.1 Dimensional classification of reading and language abilities.

talent; these children have been referred to as precocious readers (Stainthorp and Hughes, 1995). In contrast, children who have good phonology but difficulties with the semantic aspects of language occupy the lower part of the figure and are referred to in this book as 'poor comprehenders'. In extreme form, such children are described as 'hyperlexic'; they have a disorder of reading that is seen most commonly in children with autism-spectrum disorders (Nation, 1999).

On the right of the model are the reading disorders that most commonly attract the term 'dyslexia'. The core of these problems is poor phonology, be it obvious, as in children with persisting speech difficulties, or hidden, as in the classic child with dyslexia who may also have subtle and unidentified speech difficulties. In our view, the phonology dimension is continuous, and the severity of the phonological processing problem will determine whether the child falls at the extreme end (where we expect children with specific speech difficulties, such as developmental verbal dyspraxia), to the left, as in developmental 'phonological' dyslexia, or more centrally, as in children with the reading profile often described as 'surface' dyslexia. Finally, the lower portion of this space is occupied by children with general reading problems (sometimes referred to as 'garden-variety poor readers'). In addition to their phonological problems, these children have semantic processing impairments: they experience problems both with decoding and with reading comprehension skills.

We must emphasize however, that we are not committed to the view that children can be easily subgrouped or that they will show stable patterns of reading impairment. Their position in this two-dimensional classification is prone to change with development and as a consequence of intervention.

Which children are at risk of literacy problems?

The causal relationships between children's underlying cognitive and linguistic abilities and their reading and spelling skills have been the subject of a great deal of research, much of which has been discussed in the foregoing chapters. It is not our purpose to review the findings here. However, what practitioners cannot afford to ignore are vulnerability factors, both intrinsic and extrinsic to the child.

We have not had much to say about the role of environmental factors in relation to reading failure. It is well recognized that there is a relationship between socioeconomic status and reading skill, and that the mother's educational level is a particularly potent factor in explaining between-child differences in reading achievement (Phillips and Lonigan, 2005). Children from disadvantaged families often need support with the development of oral language as a prerequisite to learning to read (Locke, Ginsborg and Peers, 2002), as well as more direct support with literacy. More often than not, their parents also benefit from support (Hannavy, 1993). Support with family literacy may include encouragement to parents to read with their children, to instill an interest in books, as well as more direct help, if appropriate, to improve their own reading skills (Hannon, 1995). Notwithstanding this, even children who are socially advantaged may be 'at risk' of reading difficulties, particularly if they have one or more of the following :

- a family history of reading, speech or language problems;
- a history or presence of speech problems;
- spoken language difficulties;
- poor phonological awareness for their age.

Such children need an assessment of their language-processing difficulties, as well as their strengths, in order to set up individualized educational plans to support their needs.

What kinds of support and intervention do these children need?

The majority of children with speech and language impairments are now educated in mainstream schools. The move towards inclusive education has been associated with a decline in the practice of withdrawing individual children for 'therapy' or the 'remediation' of reading problems in favour of a more 'consultative model' of working by specialist teachers – speech and language therapists and educational psychologists whose role is to advise and train others, for example assistants, to work with children in the classroom or in small groups (Law et al., 2002). Research suggests, however, that it is essential for some children to receive direct and intensive help if they are to make progress. This is particularly the case for children with persisting speech difficulties (Law et al., 1998) and for children with severe reading difficulties.

A speech and language therapy service to a school will ideally combine the consultative model of working with direct but collaborative hands-on intervention with children most in need. This is a complex process that requires both expertise and careful planning. This book has brought together many examples of good practice in the field and offers those working within the 'consultancy model' and/or a direct-intervention model a variety of ways of supporting children's reading and language needs; these include techniques for supporting children in the classroom and in small-group interventions, as well as more individualistic approaches.

On the face of it, a 'staged' approach to intervention makes good sense – first try to accommodate the child's needs in the classroom, and then provide support in a small group, before moving to one-to-one teaching or therapy. Clinicians should, however, bear in mind that this approach is not always appropriate; if a child's difficulties are severe, or very complex, it may be best to begin with one-to-one input and later aim to phase this out as the child progresses through small-group to mainstream support. There are no formulaic answers – indeed, every child is different. As this book makes clear, establishing a child's current educational needs requires:

- detailed assessment;
- observation of the child in a range of settings;
- an analysis of the response to intervention(s);
- monitoring of progress;
- regular review.

With regard to more specific approaches, this book has emphasized the powerful influence of training in phonological awareness on subsequent reading achievement. Following a great deal of research, the combination of training in phoneme awareness with systematic reading instruction has proven the most effective approach to the development of basic reading and spelling skills. However, the type of intervention that works best will inevitably depend on:

- the age of the child;
- the child's current levels of phonological processing;
- whether speech and language difficulties persist and, if these are being managed, whether the child has ongoing speech and language therapy needs and whether these are being met;
- the integrity of the other skills that contribute to reading, namely visual and semantic skills;
- the persistence of spelling and writing difficulties;
- the child's self-perception, behaviour and attention;
- the child's network of support and carry-over to the home environment.

The research literature cannot yet tell us precisely which of a number of related interventions work best with individual children. It is perhaps over-optimistic to expect it to do so. In general, it is known that children with better phoneme skills and better letter knowledge at the outset of reading intervention tend to respond best to such interventions when progress is defined in terms of gains in reading accuracy. However, verbal IQ is a stronger predictor of progress in reading comprehension in such programmes. But this should not surprise us: approaches that focus on the development of decoding and spelling can be expected to have a relatively small effect on reading comprehension (except in so far as improvements in decoding free up attentional capacity to the benefit of comprehension). Nor will such approaches be sufficient to help children in the classroom if they also have memory problems or problems of organization. It is important for professionals to consider all the areas in which a child experiences difficulty and to plan support in each of these along the lines suggested in this book.

Taking stock of the evidence, both empirical and clinical, it is our firm belief that a mix of approaches is best, with different types of input needed to address different issues. We cannot envisage an intervention programme that does not include one-to-one text reading, that does not encourage language interaction between children, and that does not expect children also to have classroom 'survival' skills! We also favour highly structured, cumulative, multisensory approaches to the teaching of reading, spelling and writing skills that follows phonetic-linguistic principles (e.g. *Alpha to Omega* by Hornsby and Shear, 1976), with book reading being an essential part of the practice to ensure that links made between print and phonology are reinforced but not overemphasized, and that the child has access to language beyond single words.

In a similar vein, children with language needs are best taught to write words not just in isolation, but also in sentences to dictation; the sentences should initially be simple in structure, only later including more complex grammatical forms such as negatives, questions and passive voice. Finally, good programmes embody the idea of 'distributed practice' – children should be encouraged to do a little practice each day, maybe two or three times, and 'errorless learning' – children should never be expected to know anything that has not already been taught.

All of these features of an intervention programme can help to ensure its success, but the role of skilled teachers and therapists in delivering the programme must not be underestimated. Indeed, systematic research on the teaching of literacy shows that differences between teachers have more powerful effects on children's learning than do the programmes they teach (Snow and Juel, 2005). Professionals have an important role not only in helping the children in their care, but also in training others in the multiprofessional team to identify, assess and, where appropriate, intervene to support children's oral and written language development.

Who should deliver intervention?

It is not coincidental that the contributors to this book cover a range of disciplines: teachers, speech and language therapists, educational and clinical psychologists, and researchers. Reference is also made to occupational therapists, physiotherapists, paediatricians, ear, nose and throat surgeons, audiologists, linguists and various assistants. All have their role to play alongside parents and carers in the management of children with spoken and written language difficulties. Who is involved and when depends on the child's age and presenting symptoms. The management team changes over time depending on how the child's difficulties unfold. Inevitably, however, the face-to-face delivery of a language and literacy intervention programme will fall to the teacher, the therapist and their assistants.

It has traditionally been educationists who have been most responsible for the management of children with specific learning difficulties at school. However, the emphasis on the centrality of phonological processing skills to the normal and atypical development of literacy has led to a closer working relationship between teachers and speech and language therapists (Popple and Wellington, 1996). Together, they can investigate the causes of a child's speech and language difficulties, assess the child's communication skills in the classroom/school setting and observe the impact of any spoken language difficulties on access to the curriculum and on literacy development in particular.

The role of the speech and language therapist however, does not include *teaching* reading and spelling, which is traditionally and rightly the teacher's domain. Rather, the therapist's role is one of ensuring that the underlying oral language skills that contribute to literacy development are in place and, if not, in promoting these. Speech and language therapists are well placed to work on the prerequisites for literacy development. Arguably, this is particularly true as they are likely to encounter the future, but yet undiagnosed, dyslexics in their preschool groups. These groups provide an ideal opportunity for early identification and training of children at risk of later literacy problems. Similarly, speech and language therapists involved in Sure Start programmes or 'language enrichment' programmes have an ideal opportunity to influence the literacy development of a wide range of children, many with multilingual backgrounds, who may be disadvantaged when starting school if not supported in the early years.

Traditional speech and language therapy activities designed to improve a child's intelligibility can easily be adapted to target spoken and written language skills simultaneously. Sound–letter matched picture cards and activities, such as found in the *Nuffield Dyspraxia Programme* (Williams, 2004), can be used for a range of activities involving both speech production and letter–sound matching. There is a wealth of phonological awareness activities that can be linked to more explicit literacy activities (e.g. *Metaphon*; Howell and Dean 1994; and see Gillon, 2004, for a useful review). Therapy techniques that comprise a gesture to remind the child of how a sound is produced (e.g. *Cued Articulation*; Passy, 1993a, 1993b), can be linked with the written letter and can help to promote phonological awareness in some children with speech difficulties. Other techniques using segmentation blocks, beads or colour coding have also been incorporated successfully into therapy and teaching programmes (Lindamood and Lindamood, 1998). The emphasis in all these approaches is clearly to provide multisensory scaffolding opportunities for the child to compensate for specific processing weaknesses.

However, not all future dyslexia will be 'caught' by the speech and language therapy service in the early years. Subtle speech and language difficulties may go unnoticed or not be considered a priority for referral when there are children with more severe language and behaviour problems to deal with. Speech and language therapists have an important role here in training staff and carers in what to look out for and when to refer. Collaborative working with early years staff on promoting speaking, listening, communication and basic phonological awareness is a worthwhile aim for any speech and language therapy service for this age group.

Once at school, children are in the hands of the teacher, but the role of the speech and language therapist continues to be one of promoting communication skills and identifying underlying speech and language processing weaknesses that are interfering with educational progress. The child's spoken and written communication skills (including social skills training and self-esteem development) are a key part of the speech and language therapist's work and can be linked directly with the aims and objectives of the school curriculum. Programmes and approaches such as those described in this volume fit well with speech and language therapy activities, and there should not be a divide between what and how materials are used by professionals.

The success of a child's teaching and therapy programme clearly hinges on collaborative working between individuals and increasingly on how well trained and supported assistants are to deliver an intervention programme on an intensive basis. When working with children with spoken and written language difficulties together, professionals should aim to:

- *identify*, through a knowledge of developmental norms and recent research, children who are at risk of literacy problems;
- *analyse* a child's speech, language and literacy difficulties, using phonetic and linguistic tools as appropriate;
- *explain* why a child presents with speech, language and literacy difficulties, with reference to theoretical, processing and social models;
- *understand* a child's difficulties in the context of any medical conditions;
- *plan* an effective literacy intervention programme, taking into account any speech and language difficulties that are contributing to the child's educational progress;
- *advise* parents, carers and colleagues on how a child's difficulties might best be managed in a range of contexts;
- *collaborate* with parents, carers and colleagues on the implementation and practicalities of a child's intervention programme;
- *train* others to identify children at risk as early as possible and throughout the school years;
- *support* assistants and others to work effectively and intensively with individual or groups of children with persisting speech, language and literacy difficulties in and out of the classroom setting;
- *research* into the nature, identification and remediation of spoken and written language difficulties to ensure that children receive the appropriate support and intervention to meet their needs.

This book represents the collaborative work of a range of professionals working with children with speech, language and literacy difficulties. It reflects a growing knowledge-base on the relationships between spoken and written language difficulties, the impact of genetic and environmental factors, the identification of at-risk children, and the importance of structured and intensive teaching and therapy. More than ever before, the research agenda now needs to focus on evaluating the best ways of delivering intervention programmes and on who can do this most effectively.

References

Adams C, Cooke R, Crutchley A, Hesketh A, Reeves D (2001) Assessment of Comprehension and Expression (ACE). Windsor: NFER-Nelson.

Adams MJ (1990). Beginning to Read: Learning and Thinking about Print. Cambridge, MA: MIT Press.

AFASIC Checklists, 2nd edn (1995) Wisbech: Learning Development Aids.

Alston J (1992) Assessing writing speeds. Handwriting Review: 102–6.

Alston J (1995) Assessing and Promoting Writing Skills. Stafford: NASEN.

American Psychiatric Association (1994) Diagnostic and Statistical Manual of Mental Disorders, 4th edn. Washington, DC: American Psychiatric Association.

Armstrong S, Ainley M (1988) South Tyneside Assessment of Phonology (STAP). Ponteland, Northumberland: STASS Publications.

Asher SR, Coie JD (eds) (1990) Peer Rejection in Childhood. Cambridge: Cambridge University Press.

Baddeley A (1990) Human Memory: Theory and Practice. Hove: Lawrence Erlbaum Associates.

Baddeley A (1996) Exploring the central executive. Quarterly Journal of Experimental Psychology 49A: 5–28.

Baddeley A, Hitch GJ (1974) Working memory. In: Bower GA (ed.) The Psychology of Learning and Motivation, Vol 8. New York: Academic Press, pp. 47–90.

Baddeley AD, Wilson BA, Watts FN (1996) Handbook of Memory Disorders. Chichester: John Wiley.

Badian N (1994) Pre-school prediction: orthographic and phonological skills, and reading. Annals of Dyslexia 44: 3–25.

Ball EW, Blachman BA (1991) Does phoneme awareness training in kindergarten make a difference in early word recognition and developmental spelling? Reading Research Quarterly 26: 49–66.

Barton S (2003) Sentence Completion for Depression (SCD-15 Short Form). Version 2.2. University of Leeds: Academic Unit of Psychiatry.

BDA/AFASIC/UCL (2001) Joining Together in the Early Years: A Case Study. www.teachernet.gov.uk

Beery KE (1989) The VMI-Developmental Test of Visual-Motor Integration. Cleveland: Modern Curriculum Press.

Benson DF (1979) Aphasia, Alexia, and Agraphia. New York: Churchill Livingstone.

Bernhardt B, Major E (2005) Speech, language and literacy skills 3 years later: a follow up of early phonological and metaphonological intervention. International Journal of Language and Communication Disorders 40: 1–28.

Bernstein Ratner NE (1997) Stuttering: a psycholinguistic perspective. In: Curlee R, Siegel G (eds) Nature and Treatment of Stuttering: New Directions, 2nd edn. Boston: Allyn & Bacon, pp. 99–127.

Bird J, Bishop DVM, Freeman NH (1995) Phonological awareness and literacy development in children with expressive phonological impairments. Journal of Speech and Hearing Research 38: 446–62.

Bishop DVM (1983) Test for the Reception of Grammar. Manchester: Age and Cognitive Performance Research Centre, University of Manchester.

Bishop DVM (2003) Test for Reception of Grammar (TROG2). London: Psychological Corporation.

Bishop DVM, Adams C (1989) Conversational characteristics of children with semantic-pragmatic disorders. What features lead to a judgement of inappropriacy? British Journal of Disorders of Communication 24: 107–21.

Bishop DVM, Adams C (1990) A prospective study of the relationship between specific language impairment, phonological disorders and reading retardation. Journal of Child Psychology and Psychiatry 31: 1027–50.

Bishop DVM, Snowling MJ (2004) Developmental dyslexia and specific language impairment: same or different? Psychological Bulletin 130: 858–88.

Blachman BA (ed.) (1997) Foundations of Reading Acquisition and Dyslexia: Implications for Early Intervention. Mahwah, NJ: Lawrence Erlbaum Associates.

Blachman B, Tangel DM, Ball EW, Black R, McGraw CK (1999) Developing phonological awareness and word recognition skills: a two-year intervention with low-income, inner-city children. Reading and Writing 11: 239–73.

Blakemore S-J, Frith U (2005) The Learning Brain: Lessons for Education. Oxford: Blackwell.

Borkowski JG (1992) Metacognitive theory: a framework for teaching literacy, writing, and math skills. Journal of Learning Disabilities 25: 253–7.

Botting N (2002) Narrative as a tool for the assessment of linguistic and pragmatic impairments. Child Language Teaching and Therapy 18: 1–22.

Bowey J (1986) Syntactic awareness in relation to reading skill and ongoing comprehension monitoring. Journal of Experimental Child Psychology 41: 282–99.

Bowyer-Crane C, Snowling MJ (2005) Assessing children's inference generation: what do tests of reading comprehension measure? British Journal of Educational Psychology: 75: 189–201.

Bradley L (1984) Assessing Reading Difficulties: A Diagnostic and Remedial Approach, 2nd edn. London: Macmillan Education.

Bradley L, Bryant PE (1983) Categorising sounds and learning to read: a causal connection. Nature 30: 419–21.

Bradley L, Bryant PE (1985) Rhyme and Reason in Reading and Spelling. IARLD Monograph No. 1. Ann Arbor, MI: University of Michigan Press.

Brady HV, Richman LC (1994) Visual versus verbal mnemonic training effects on memory-deficient and language deficient subgroups of children with reading disability. Developmental Neuropsychology 10: 335–47.

Brady SA (1991) The role of working memory in reading disability. In: Brady SA, Shankweiler D (eds) Phonological Processes in Literacy: A Tribute to Isabelle Y. Leiberman. Hillsdale NJ: Erlbaum Associates, pp. 129–51.

Brady S, Shankweiler D, Mann V (1983) Speech perception and memory coding in relation to reading ability. Journal of Experimental Psychology 35: 345–67.

Bramley W (1998). Active Literacy Kit: Essential Foundations for Literacy. Cambridge: Learning Development Aids.

Brimer MA, Dunn LM (1973) Series of Plates for the English Picture Vocabulary Test, Full Range Edition. Gloucester: Education Evaluation Enterprises.

Bristow J, Cowley P, Daines B (1999) Memory and Learning: A Practical Guide for Teachers. London: David Fulton.

Brooks P, Everatt J, Weeks S (2002) Differences in learning to spell: relationships between cognitive profiles and learning response to teaching methods. Educational and Child Psychology 19: 47–62.

Brooks RB (1994) Children at risk; fostering resilience and hope. American Journal of Orthopsychiatry 64: 545–53.

Broomfield H, Combley M (1997) Overcoming Dyslexia. A Practical Handbook for the Classroom. London: Whurr.

Broomfield J, Dodd B (2004) The nature of referred subtypes of primary speech disability. Child Language Teaching and Therapy 20: 135–51.

Brown A (1996) Look What I've Got! London: Walker.

Brown B, Henderson SE (1989) A sloping desk? Should the wheel turn full circle? Handwriting Review: 55–9.

Bruce LJ (1964) The analysis of word sounds by young children. British Journal of Educational Psychology 34: 158–74.

Bruck M (1992) Persistence of dyslexics' phonological awareness deficits. Developmental Psychology 28: 874–86

Bruck M, Treiman R (1990) Phonological awareness and spelling in normal children and dyslexics: the case of initial consonant clusters. Journal of Experimental Child Psychology 50: 156–78.

Brumfitt S (1999) The Social Psychology of Communication Impairment. London: Whurr.

Brunswick N, McCrory E, Price CJ, Frith CD, Frith U (1999) Explicit and implicit processing of words and pseudowords by adult developmental dyslexics. A search for Wernicke's Wortschatz? Brain 122: 1901–17.

Bryant PE, Bradley L (1985) Children's Reading Problems. Oxford: Blackwell.

Burden R (2000) Me-As-A-Learner Scale (MALS). London: NFER-Nelson.

Burns RB (1982) Self-Concept Development and Education. Austin, TX: Holt, Rinehart & Winston.

Butler RJ (2001a) The Self-Image Profile Adolescents (SIP-A). London: Psychological Corporation.

Butler RJ (2001b) The Self-Image Profile for Children (SIP-C). London: Psychological Corporation.

Buzan T (1993) The Mind Map Book. London: BBC Books.

Buzan T (2003) Use Your Head. London: BBC Books.

Byrne B (1998) The Foundation of Literacy: The Child's Acquisition of the Alphabetic Principle. Hove: Psychology Press

Byrne B, Fielding-Barnsley R (1989) Phonemic awareness and letter knowledge in the child's acquisition of the alphabetic principle. Journal of Educational Psychology 81: 313–21.

Byrne B, Fielding-Barnsley R (1995) Evaluation of a program to teach phonemic awareness to young children: a 2- and 3-year follow-up and a new preschool trial. Journal of Educational Psychology 87: 488–503.

Byrne B, Fielding-Barnsley R, Ashley L, Larsen K (1997) Assessing the child's and the environment's contribution to reading acquisition: what we know and what we don't know. In: Blachman B (ed.) Foundations of Dyslexia and Early Reading Acquisition. Hillsdale, NJ: Erlbaum Associates, pp. 265–85.

Cain K, Oakhill JV (1999) Inference making and its relation to comprehension failure. Reading and Writing 11: 489–503.

Cain K, Oakhill JV, Bryant P (2000) Phonological skills and comprehension failure: a test of the phonological processing deficit hypothesis. Reading and Writing 13: 31–56.

Cain K, Oakhill J, Bryant P (2004) Children's reading comprehension ability: concurrent prediction by working memory, verbal ability, and component skills. Journal of Educational Psychology 96: 31–42.

Cain K, Oakhill JV, Barnes MA, Bryant PE (2001) Comprehension skill, inference-making ability, and their relation to knowledge. Memory and Cognition 29: 850–9.

Caravolas M (2005) The nature and causes of dyslexia in different languages. In: Snowling MJ, Hulme C (eds) The Science of Reading: A Handbook. Oxford: Blackwell, pp. 336–56.

Caravolas M, Hulme C, Snowling MJ (2001) The foundations of spelling ability: evidence from a 3-year longitudinal study. Journal of Memory and Language 45: 751–74.

Carroll JM, Snowling MJ (2004) Language and phonological skills in children at high-risk of reading difficulties. Journal of Child Psychology and Psychiatry 45: 631–40.

Carver C (1970) Word Recognition Test. London: Hodder & Stoughton.

Castles A, Coltheart M (1993) Varieties of developmental dyslexia. Cognition 47: 149–80.

Catts HW (1993) The relationship between speech–language impairments and reading disabilities. Journal of Speech and Hearing Research 36: 948–58.

Catts HW, Hu C-F, Larrivee L, Swank L (1994) Early identification of reading disabilities. In: Watkins RV, Rice M (eds) Specific Language Impairments in Children. Communication and Language Intervention. Series 4. London: Paul H. Brookes, pp. 145–60.

Clark-Klein S, Hodson B (1995) A phonologically based analysis of misspellings by third graders with disordered-phonology histories. Journal of Speech and Hearing Research 38: 839–49.

Clay M (1985) The Early Detection of Reading Difficulties, 3rd edn. Tadworth: Heinemann.

Clegg J, Hollis C, Mawhood L, Rutter M (2005) Developmental language disorders – a follow-up in later adult life: cognitive, language and psycho-social outcomes. Journal of Child Psychology and Psychiatry 46: 128–49.

Cogan J, Flecker M (2004) Dyslexia in Secondary School: A Practical Handbook for Teachers, Parents and Students. London: Whurr.

Compton DL, Olson RK, DeFries JC, Pennington BF (2002) Comparing the relationships among two different versions of alphanumeric rapid automatized naming and word level reading skills. Scientific Studies of Reading 6: 343–68.

Constable A (2001) A psycholinguistic approach to word-finding difficulties. In: Stackhouse J, Wells B (eds) Children's Speech and Literacy Difficulties, Vol. 2: Identification and Intervention. London: Whurr, pp. 330–65.

Conti-Ramsden G, Botting N (1999) Characteristics of children attending language units in England: a national study of 7 year olds. International Journal of Language and Communication Disorders 34: 359–67.

Cooley CH (1902) Human Nature and the Social Order. New York: Scribner's.

Cooper C (2000) Face on: discovering resilience to disfigurement. New Therapist 7: 31–3.

Cossu G (1999) Biological constraints on literacy acquisition. Reading and Writing 11: 213–37.

Cottrell S (1999) The Study Skills Handbook. Basingstoke: Palgrave.

Cottrell S (2001) Teaching Study Skills and Supporting Learning. Basingstoke: Palgrave.

Cowan N (1997) The development of working memory. In: Cowan N (ed.) Development of Memory in Childhood. Hove: Psychology Press/Erlbaum, pp. 163–201.

Cragg L, Nation K (in press) Exploring written narrative in children with poor reading comprehension. Educational Psychology.

Craik FIM, Tulving E (1975) Levels of processing: a framework for memory research. Journal of Verbal Learning and Verbal Behaviour 11: 671–84.

Creemers BPM (1994) School Development Series: The Effective Classroom. London: Cassell.

Cross M (2004) Children with Emotional and Behavioural Difficulties and Communication Problems: There is Always a Reason. London: Jessica Kingsley.

Cunningham AE (1990) Explicit versus implicit instruction in phonemic awareness. Journal of Experimental Child Psychology 50: 429–44.

Daniel B, Wassell S (2002) The School Years: Assessing and Promoting Resilience in Vulnerable Children, 2. London: Jessica Kingsley.

Daniel BM, Wassell S, Gilligan R (1999) Child Development for Child Care and Protection Workers. London: Jessica Kingsley.

Davies A, Ritchie D (1998) THRASS Teachers' Manual, and Word Chart. Chester: THRASS (UK).

De Jong P (1998) Working memory deficits of reading disabled children. Journal of Experimental Psychology 70: 75–96.

Deavers R, Solity J (1998) The role of rime units in reading. Educational and Child Psychology 15: 6–17.

Denckla MB, Rudel RG (1976) Rapid automatised naming (RAN): dyslexia differentiated from other learning disabilities. Neuropsychologia 14: 471–9.

Dennis M, Barnes MA (1993) Oral discourse after early-onset hydrocephalus: linguistic ambiguity, figurative language, speech acts, and script-based inferences. Journal of Pediatric Psychology 18: 639–52.

Dennis M, Lazenby AL, Lockyer L (2001) Inferential language in high-function children with autism. Journal of Autism and Developmental Disorders 31: 47–54.

Department for Education and Employment (1994) Code of Practice on Identification and Assessment of Special Educational Needs. London: HMSO.

Department for Education and Employment (1997) Excellence for All Children – Meeting Special Educational Needs. London: Stationery Office.

Department for Education and Employment (1998) The National Literacy Strategy: Framework for Teaching. London: DEE.

Department for Education and Employment (1999) Sure Start: Making a Difference for Children and Families. London: Stationery Office. www.surestart.gov.uk

Department for Education and Employment (2000) The National Curriculum Programmes of Study and Attainment Targets. London: DEE.

Department for Education and Employment (2001) National Literacy Strategy: Developing Early Writing. London: Stationery Office.

Department for Education and Skills (1999) Progression in Phonics. Nottingham: DfES Publications.

Department for Education and Skills (2001a) The National Literacy Strategy Early Literacy Support Programme. London: DfES Publications.

Department for Education and Skills (2001b) Special Educational Needs Code of Practice. Nottingham: DfES Publications.

Department for Education and Skills (2001c) Inclusive Schooling: Children with Special Educational Needs. Nottingham: DfES Publications.

Department for Education and Skills (2002) Birth to Three Matters: A Framework to Support Children in their Earliest Years. London: Stationary Office.

Department for Education and Skills (2003a) The National Literacy Strategy: Targeting Support: Choosing and Implementing Interventions for Children with Significant Literacy Difficulties. London: DfES.

Department for Education and Skills (2003b) Aiming High: Raising the Achievement of Minority Ethnic Pupils. Consultation Paper. London: DfES.

Department for Education and Skills (2004) Removing Barriers to Achievement. Nottingham: DfES Publications.

Department for Education and Skills. English Tasks Teacher's Handbook Key Stage 1 (levels 1–3) and 2 (levels 3–5). London: DfES.

Dewart H, Summers S (1988) Pragmatics Profile of Early Communication Skills in Children. Windsor: NFER-Nelson.

Dockrell J, Messer D (1999) Children's Language and Communication Difficulties: Understanding, Identification and Intervention. London: Cassell Education.

Dodd B, Hua Z, Holm A, Ozanne A (2002) Diagnostic Evaluation of Articulation and Phonology (DEAP). London: Psychological Corporation.

Duncan LG, Seymour PHK, Hill G (1997) How important are rhyme and analogy in beginning reading? Cognition 63: 171–208.

Dunn LM, Dunn LM, Whetton C, Burley J (1997) The British Picture Vocabulary Scale, 2nd edn. Windsor: NFER-Nelson.

Dutton K (1992) Writing under Examination Conditions: Establishing a Baseline. Handwriting Review, pp. 80–101.

Eckert MA, Leonard CM, Richards TL, Aylward EH, Thomson J, Berninger VW (2003) Anatomical correlates of dyslexia: frontal and cerebellar findings. Brain 126: 482–92.

Edwards J, Lahey M (1999) Non-word repetitions of children with specific language impairment: explosion of some explanations for their inaccuracies. Applied Psycholinguistics 19: 279–309.

Ehri L (1985) Sources of difficulty in learning to spell and read. In: Wolraich ML, Routh D (eds) Advances in Developmental and Behavioural Paediatrics, Vol. 7. Greenwich, CT: Jai Press, pp. 121–95.

Ehri LC (1999) Phases of development in learning to read. In: Oakhill J, Beard R (eds) Reading Development and the Teaching of Reading. Oxford: Blackwell, pp. 79–108.

Ehri L, Nunes SR, Willows DM, Schuster BV, Yaghoub-Zadeh Z, Shanahan T (2001) Phonemic awareness instruction helps children learn to read: evidence from the National Reading Panel's meta-analysis. Reading Research Quarterly 36: 250–87.

Elbro C, Borstrom I, Petersen D (1998) Predicting dyslexia from kindergarten: the importance of distinctness of phonological representations of lexical items. Reading Research Quarterly 33: 39–60.

Eliez S, Rumsey JM, Giedd JN, Schmitt EJ, Patwardhan AJ, Reiss AL (2000) Morphological alteration of temporal lobe gray matter in dyslexia: an MRI study. Journal of Child Psychology and Psychiatry 41: 637–44.

Elkonin DB (1973) USSR. In: Downing J (ed.) Comparative Reading: Cross-national Studies of Behaviour and Processes in Reading and Writing. London: Collier-Macmillan.

Elliott C (1992). British Abilities Scale Reading Test. Windsor: NFER-Nelson.

Elliott CD, Murray DJ, Pearson LS (1983) British Abilities Scales. Windsor: NFER-Nelson.

Elliot CD, Smith P, McCulloch K (1997) British Ability Scales, 2nd edn. Windsor: NFER-Nelson.

Elliott J (2002) Could do better? The risks of cultivating positive self-esteem. Human Givens 9: 38–43.

Erikson EH (1963) Childhood and Society, 2nd edn. New York: Norton.

Erwin P (1998) Friendship in Childhood and Adolescence. London: Routledge.

Farmer M, Riddick B, Sterling C (2002) Dyslexia and Inclusion: Assessment and Support in Higher Education. London: Whurr.

Fawcett AJ, Nicolson RI (1999) Performance of dyslexic children on cerebellar and cognitive tests. Journal of Motor Behaviour 31: 68–79.

Fawcett AJ, Nicolson RI, Dean P (1996) Impaired performance of children with dyslexia on a range of cerebellar tasks. Annals of Dyslexia 46: 259–83.

Fawcett AJ, Singleton CH, Peer L (1998) Advances in early years screening for dyslexia in the United Kingdom. Annals of Dyslexia 48: 57–88.

Fergusson DM, Lynskey MT (1996) Adolescent resiliency to family adversity. Journal of Child Psychology and Psychiatry 37: 281–92.

Flavell JH, Wellman HM (1977) Metamemory. In: Kail RV, Hagan JW (eds) Perspectives on the Development of Memory and Cognition. Hillsdale, NJ: Lawrence Erlbaum Associates, pp. 3–33.

Flowers DL, Wood FB, Naylor CE (1991) Regional cerebral blood flow correlates of language processes in reading disability. Archives of Neurology 48: 637–42.

Flynn J (1997) Literacy Screening Battery. LaCrosse, WI: LaCrosse Area Dyslexia Research Institute.

Flynn JM (2000) From identification to intervention: improving kindergarten screening for risk of reading failure. In: Badian N (ed.) Prediction and Prevention of Reading Failure. Timonium, MD: York Press, pp. 133–52.

Flynn JM, Rahbar M (1993) Effects of age of school entrance and sex on achievement: implications for paediatric counselling. Developmental and Behavioural Paediatrics 14: 304–7.

Foorman BR, Francis DJ, Shaywitz SE, Shaywitz BA, Fletcher JM (1997) The case for early reading intervention. In Blachman BA (ed.) Foundations of Reading Acquisition and Dyslexia: Implications for Early Intervention. Mahwah, NJ: Lawrence Erlbaum Associates, pp. 243–64.

Frances J (2000) Providing effective support in school when a child has a disfigured appearance: the work of the Changing Faces School Service. British Journal of Learning Support 15: 177–82.

Frederickson N, Frith U, Reason R (1997) Phonological Assessment Battery (PhAB). Windsor: NFER-Nelson.

Freeth D, Hammick M, Koppel I, Reeves S, Barr H (2002) A Critical Review of Evaluations of Interdisciplinary Education. London: Learning and Teaching Support Network, Centre for Health Sciences and Practice.

Frey D, Carlock CJ (1989) Enhancing Self-esteem, 2nd edn. New York: WW Norton.

Frith U (1980) Unexpected spelling problems. In: Frith U (ed.) Cognitive processes in Spelling. London: Academic Press, pp. 495–515.

Frith U (1985) Beneath the surface of developmental dyslexia. In: Patterson KE, Marshall JC, Coltheart M (eds) Surface Dyslexia. London: Routledge & Kegan Paul, pp. 301–30.

Galaburda AM (1992) Neurology of developmental dyslexia. Current Opinion in Neurology and Neurosurgery 5: 71–6.

Galaburda AM, Kemper TL (1979) Cytoarchitectonic abnormalities in developmental dyslexia. A case study. Annals of Neurology 6: 94–100.

Galaburda AM, Livingstone M (1993) Evidence for a magnocellular defect in developmental dyslexia. Annals of the New York Academy of Sciences 682: 70–82.

Galaburda AM, Sherman GF, Rosen GD, Aboitiz F, Geschwind N (1985) Developmental dyslexia: four consecutive patients with cortical abnormalities. Annals of Neurology 18: 222–33.

Gallagher A, Frith U, Snowling MJ (2000) Precursors of literacy delay among children at genetic risk of dyslexia. Journal of Child Psychology and Psychiatry 41: 203–13.

Gallagher TM, Watkin KL (1998) Prematurity and language developmental risk: too young or too small? Topics in Language Disorders 18: 15–25.

Gardner MF (1995) Test of Visual-Motor Skills – Revised. Burlingame, CA: Psychological and Educational Publications.

Gardner MF (1996) Test of Visual Perceptual Skills (non-motor). Hydesville, CA: Psychological and Educational Publications. Belford, Northumberland: Ann Arbor Publishers.

Gathercole SE (1999) Cognitive approaches to the development of short-term memory. Trends in Cognitive Sciences 3: 410–19.

Gathercole S, Baddeley A (1989) Development of vocabulary in children and short-term phonological memory. Journal of Memory and Language 28: 200–13.

Gathercole SE, Baddeley AD (1993) Working Memory and Language. Hove: Psychology Press/Lawrence Erlbaum Associates.

Gathercole S, Baddeley A (1996) CNRep: Children's Nonword Repetition Test. London: Psychological Corporation/Harcourt.

Gathercole SE, Hitch GJ (1993) Developmental changes in short-term memory: a revised working memory perspective. In Collins AF, Gathercole SE, Conway MA, Morris PE (eds) Theories of Memory. Hove: Lawrence Erlbaum, pp. 189–209.

Gathercole S, Baddeley A, Willis C (1991) Differentiating phonological memory and awareness of rhyme: reading and vocabulary development in children. British Journal of Psychology 8: 387–406.

Gathercole SE, Willis CS, Baddeley AD, Emslie H (1994) The children's test of nonword repetition: a test of phonological working memory. Memory 2: 103–27.

Gentry JR (1982) An analysis of developmental spelling: GNYS at WRK. Reading Teacher 36: 192–200.

German DJ (1989) Test of Adolescent/AdultWord finding (TAWF). London: Psychological Corporation.

German DJ (2000) Test of Word Finding (TWF), 2nd edn. London: Psychological Corporation.

Gilligan R (1997) Beyond permanence? The importance of resilience in child placement practice and planning. Adoption and Fostering 21: 12–20.

Gillingham AM, Stillman BU (1956) Remedial training for children with specific disability. In: Reading, Spelling and Penmanship, 5th edn. New York: Sackett & Wilhelms.

Gillon G (2002) Follow-up study investigating the benefits of phonological awareness intervention for children with spoken language impairment. International Journal of Communication Disorders 37: 381–400.

Gillon GT (2004) Phonological Awareness: From Research to Practice. London: Guildford Press.

Goodman KS (1967) Reading: a psycholinguistic guessing game. Journal of the Reading Specialist. May: 126–35.

Goodman R (1997) The Strengths and Difficulties Questionnaire: a research note. Journal of Child Psychology and Psychiatry 38: 581–6.

Goswami U (1994) The role of analogies in reading development. Support for Learning 9: 22–5.

Goswami U, Bryant P (1990) Phonological Skills and Learning to Read. Hove: Lawrence Erlbaum.

Goulandris N (ed.) (2003) Dyslexia in Different Languages: A Cross-Linguistic Comparison. London: Whurr.

Goulandris NK, Snowling MJ (1991) Visual memory deficits: a plausible cause of developmental dyslexia? Evidence from a single case study. Cognitive Neuropsychology 8: 127–54.

Grantham P (2000) How to Build Clients' Self Esteem. Seminar Notes. Wirral: Skills Development Service.

Griffiths YM, Snowling MJ (2002) Predictors of exception word and nonword reading in dyslexic children: the severity hypothesis. Journal of Educational Psychology 94: 34–43.

Grigorenko EL (2001) Developmental dyslexia: an update on genes, brains, and environments. Journal of Child Psychology and Psychiatry 42: 91–125.

Grigorenko EL, Klin A, Pauls DL, Senft R, Hooper C, Volkmar F (2002) A descriptive study of hyperlexia in a clinically referred sample of children with developmental delays. Journal of Autism and Developmental Disorders 32: 3–12.

Grogan S (1995) Which cognitive abilities at age four are the best predictors of reading ability at age seven? Journal of Research in Reading 18: 24–33.

Gross J (1996) Special Educational Needs in the Primary School: A Practical Guide, 2nd edn. Buckingham: Open University Press.

Grotberg E (1997) The international resilience project. In: John M (ed.) A Charge Against Society: The Child's Right to Protection. London: Jessica Kingsley.

Grunwell P (1985) Phonological Assessment of Child Speech (PACS). Windsor: NFER-Nelson.

Hagley F (1987) Suffolk Reading Scale. Windsor: NFER-Nelson.

Hamachek DE (1988) Evaluating self-concept and ego development within Erikson's psychosocial framework: a formulation. Journal of Counseling and Development: 354–60.

Hannavy S (1993) The Middle Infant Screening Test (MIST) and Forward Together Programme. Windsor: NFER-Nelson.

Hannon B, Daneman M (2001) A new tool for measuring and understanding individual differences in the component processes of reading comprehension. Journal of Educational Psychology 93: 103–28.

Hannon P (1995) Literacy, Home and School: Research and Practice in Teaching Literacy with Parents. London: Falmer.

Hansen J, Bowey JA (1994) Phonological analysis skills, verbal working memory and reading ability in second grade children. Child Development 65: 938–50.

Harter S (1985) Self-perception Profile for Children. Denver, CO: University of Denver.

Harter S (1988) The Self-Perception Profile for Adolescents. Denver, CO: University of Denver.

Harter S, Pike R (1983) The Pictorial Scale of Perceived Competence and Social Acceptance for Young Children. Child Development 55: 1969–82.

Hatcher J (2001) Classroom Observation of Children with Literacy Difficulties. Unpublished manuscript.

Hatcher J, Snowling MJ (2002) The phonological representations hypothesis of dyslexia: from theory to practice. In: Reid G, Wearmouth J (eds) Dyslexia and Literacy: Theory and Practice. Chichester: Wiley, pp. 69–83.

Hatcher PJ (1992) Learning To Read: The Value of Linking Phonological Training with Reading. Unpublished doctoral thesis, University of York, UK.

Hatcher PJ (2000a) Sound Linkage: An Integrated Programme for Overcoming Reading Difficulties, 2nd edn. London, Whurr.

Hatcher PJ (2000b) Predictors of reading recovery book levels. Journal of Research in Reading 23: 67–77.

Hatcher PJ (2000c) Reading intervention need not be negligible: response to Cossu (1999). Reading and Writing 13: 349–55.

Hatcher PJ (2000d) Sound links in reading and spelling with discrepancy-defined dyslexics and children with moderate learning difficulties. Reading and Writing 13: 257–72.

Hatcher PJ, Hulme C, Ellis AW (1994) Ameliorating early reading failure by integrating the teaching of reading and phonological skills: the phonological linkage hypothesis. Child Development 65: 41–57.

Hatcher PJ, Hulme C, Snowling MJ (2004) Explicit phonological training combined with reading instruction helps young children at risk of reading failure. Journal of Child Psychology and Psychiatry 45: 338–58.

Hatcher PJ, Götz K, Snowling MJ, Hulme C, Gibbs S, Smith G (in press) Evidence for the effectiveness of the Early Literacy Support Programme. British Journal of Educational Psychology.

Henderson SE, Green D (2001) Handwriting problems in children with Asperger Syndrome. Handwriting Today, Vol. 2. Handwriting Interest Group

Henderson SE, Henderson L (2003) Toward an understanding of developmental coordination disorder: terminological and diagnostic issues. In Gramsbergen A, Hadders-Algra M (eds) The clumsy child. Special Issue of Neural Plasticity 10: 1–15.

Henderson SE, Sugden DA (1992) The Movement Assessment Battery for Children, Checklist. Sidcup: Psychological Corporation.

Henry MK, Redding NC (1996) Patterns for Success in Reading and Spelling. Austin, TX. Pro-Ed.

Hesketh A, Conti-Ramsden G (2003) Risk markers for SLI: a study of young language-learning children. International Journal of Language and Communication Disorders 38: 251–63.

Hitch GJ, Halliday S, Schaafstal AM, Schraagen JM (1988) Visual working memory in young children. Memory and Cognition 16: 120–32.

Holligan C, Johnston RS (1988) The use of phonological information by good and poor readers in memory and reading tasks. Memory and Cognition 16: 522–32.

Holloway J (2000) Dyslexia in Focus at Sixteen Plus: An Inclusive Teaching Approach. Tamworth: NASEN.

Honey P, Mumford A (1992) The Manual of Learning Styles. www.peterhoney.co.uk

Horne MD (1985) Attitudes Towards Handicapped Students: Professional, Peer and Parent Reactions. Hillsdale, NJ: Lawrence Erlbaum.

Hornsby B, Shear F (1976) Alpha to Omega, 2nd edn. London: Heinemann Educational.

Hornsby B, Shear F (1980) Alpha to Omega, 3rd edn. London: Heinemann.

Howard SJ (2004) Connected speech processes in developmental speech impairment: observations from an electropalatographic perspective. Clinical Linguistics and Phonetics 18: 407–17.

Howell J, Dean E (1991) Treating Phonological Disorders in Children: Metaphon, Theory to Practice. San Diego, CA: Singular Publishing.

Howell J, Dean E (1994) Treating Phonological Disorders in Children: Metaphon – Theory to Practice, 2nd edn. London: Whurr.

Hulme C, Roodenrys S (1995) Verbal working memory development and its disorders. Journal of Child Psychology and Psychiatry 36: 373–98.

Hulme C, Maughan S, Brown GDA (1991) Memory for familiar and unfamiliar words: evidence for a long-term memory contribution to short-term memory span. Journal of Memory and Language 30: 685–701.

Hulme C, Snowling M, Quinlan P (1991) Connectionism and learning to read: steps towards a psychologically plausible model. Reading and Writing 3: 159–68.

Humphreys P, Kaufmann WE, Galaburda AM (1990) Developmental dyslexia in women: neuropathological findings in three patients. Annals of Neurology 28 727–38.

Iversen S, Tunmer WE (1993) Phonological processing and the Reading Recovery program. Journal of Educational Psychology 85: 112–26.

Jamieson C, Jamieson J (2003) Manual for Testing and Teaching English Spelling. London: Whurr.

Jastak S, Wilkinson GS (1984) The Wide Range Achievement Test Revised (WRAT-R. Jastak Associates.

Johnston RS, Anderson M (1998) Memory span, naming speed, and memory strategies in poor and normal readers. Memory 6: 143–63.

Joyner MH, Kurtz-Costes B (1997) Metamemory development: In: Cowan N (ed.) Development of Memory in Childhood. Hove: Psychology Press/Lawrence Erlbaum, pp. 275–300.

Kaplan PS (1991) A Child's Odyssey: Child and Adolescent Development. St Paul, MN: West Publishing Co.

Katz RB, Healy AF, Shankweiler D (1983) Phonetic coding and order memory in relation to reading proficiency: a comparison of short-term memory for temporal and spatial order information. Applied Psycholinguistics 4: 229–50.

Knox E, Conti-Ramsden G (2003) Bullying risks of 11-year-old children with specific language impairment (SLI): does school placement matter? International Journal of Language and Communication Disorders 38: 1–12.

Kremer J, Sheey N, Reilly J, Trew K, Muldoon O (2003) Applying Social Psychology. Basingstoke: Palgrave Macmillan.

Lake M, Steele A (2000) Improving memory skills. Birmingham: Question Publishing.

Larivee LS, Catts HW (1999) Early reading achievement in children with expressive phonological disorders. American Journal of Speech–Language Pathology 8: 118–28.

Larsen JP, Høien T, Lundberg I, Ødegaard H (1990) MRI evaluation of the size and symmetry of the planum temporale in adolescents with developmental dyslexia. Brain and Language 39: 289–301.

Law J, Luscombe M, Roux J (2002) Whose standards? Using the Standards Fund for children with speech and language needs – a survey of allocation of resources in England. British Journal of Special Education 29: 136–40.

Law J, Boyle J, Harris F, Harkness A (1998) Child health surveillance: screening for speech and language delay. Health Technology Assessment 2: 1–180.

Law J, Boyle J, Harris F, Harkness A, Nye C (2000a) Prevalence and natural history of primary speech and language delay: findings from a systematic review of the literature. International Journal of Language and Communication Disorders 35: 165–88.

Law J, Lindsay G, Peacey N, Gascoigne M, Soloff N, Radford J, Band S (2000b) Provision for Children with Speech and Language Needs in England and Wales: Facilitating Communication Between Education and Health Services. London: DfEE/DoH.

Law J, Lindsay G, Peacey N, Gascoigne M, Soloff N, Radford J, Band S (2002) Consultation as a model for providing speech and language therapy in schools: a panacea or one step too far? Child Language Teaching and Therapy 18: 145–63.

Lawrence D (1985) Improving self-esteem and reading. Educational Research 27: 194–200.

Layton L, Deeny K (2002) Sound Practice: Phonological Awareness in the Classroom, 2nd edn. London: David Fulton.

Leather CV, Henry LA (1994) Working memory span and phonological awareness tasks as predictors of early reading abiliity. Journal of Experimental and Child Psychology 58: 88–111.

Leitao S, Fletcher J (2004) Literacy outcomes for children with speech impairment: long term follow up. International Journal of Language and Communication Disorders 39: 245–56.

Leitao S, Hogben J, Fletcher J (1997) Phonological processing skills in speech and language impaired children. European Journal of Disorders of Communication 32: 91–113.

Levine M (1990) Keeping a Head in School. Cambridge MA: Educators Publishing Service.

Lewis A (1995) Primary Special Needs and the National Curriculum. London: Routledge.

Lewis C, Salway A (1989) Are you sitting comfortably? Handwriting Review: 51–4.

Liberman IY, Shankweiler D, Fischer FW, Carter B (1974) Reading and the awareness of language segments. Journal of Experimental Child Psychology 18: 201–12.

Lindamood C, Lindamood P (1998) The Lindamood Phoneme Sequencing Program for Reading, Spelling and Speech: The LIPS program. Austin, TX: Pro-Ed.

Lindsay G, Dockrell J (2000) The behaviour and self-esteem of children with specific speech and language difficulties. British Journal of Educational Psychology 70: 583–601.

Lindsay G, Soloff N, Law J, Band N, Peacey N, Gascoigne M, Radford J (2002) Speech and language therapy services to education in England and Wales. International Journal of Language and Communication Disorders 37: 273–88.

Lloyd S, Wernham S (1994) Jolly Phonics. Chigwell, Essex: Jolly Learning.

Locke A (1985) Living Language. Windsor: NFER-Nelson.

Locke A, Beech M (1991) Teaching Talking: A Screening and Intervention Programme for Children with Speech and Language Difficulties. Windsor: NFER-Nelson

Locke A, Ginsborg J, Peers I (2002) Development and disadvantage: implications for the early years and beyond. International Journal of Language and Communication Disorders 37: 3–15.

Lown J (2000) A Critical Review of the Literature on Self-esteem and its Application to Educational Psychology Practice. Unpublished essay.

Lundberg I, Frost J, Peterson O (1988) Effects of an extensive program for stimulating phonological awareness in pre-school children. Reading Research Quarterly 23: 263–84.

Luthar SS (1991) Vulnerability and resilience: a study of high-risk adolescents. Child Development 62: 600–12.

McCartney E, van der Gaag A (1996) How shall we be judged? Speech and language therapists in educational settings. Child Language Teaching and Therapy 12: 314–27.

McCormick M (1995) The relationship between the phonological processes in early speech development and later spelling strategies. In: Dodd B (ed.) Differential Diagnosis and Treatment of Children with Speech Disorder. London: Whurr Publishers.

McDougall S, Hulme C, Ellis AW, Monk A (1994) Learning to read: the role of short-term memory and phonological skills. Journal of Experimental Child Psychology 58: 112–33.

McGuinness D (1998) Why Children Cannot Read. London: Penguin.

McKissock C (2001) Dyslexia: A Psychosocial Perspective. London: Whurr.

MacMillan B (2002) Rhyme and reading: a critical review of research methodology. Journal of Research in Reading 25: 4–42.

McNamara DS, Scott JL (2001) Working memory capacity and strategy use. Memory and Cognition 29: 10–17.

Magnusson E, Naucler K (1990) Reading and spelling in language disordered children – linguistic and metalinguistic prerequisites: report on a longitudinal study. Clinical Linguistics and Phonetics 4: 49–61.

Mahon M, Crutchley A, Quinn T (2003) Editorial: New directions in the assessment of bilingual children. Child Language Teaching and Therapy 19: 237–43.

Maines B, Robinson G (1995) You Can ...You KNOW You Can! Bristol: Lame Duck Publishing.

Manis F, Seidenberg M, Doi L (1999) See Dick RAN: rapid naming and the longitudinal prediction of reading subskills in first and second graders. Scientific Studies of Reading 3: 129–57.

Mann VA, Liberman IY, Shankweiler D (1980) Children's memory for sentences and word strings in relation to reading ability. Memory and Cognition 8: 329–35.

Manolson A (1992) It Takes Two to Talk. Toronto: Hanen Centre.

Manolson A, Ward B, Dodington N (1995) You Make the Difference. Toronto: Hanen Centre.

Marshall J, Stojanovik V, Ralph S (2002) 'I never even gave it a second thought': PGCE students' attitudes towards the inclusion of children with speech and language impairments. International Journal of Language and Communication Disorders 37: 475–89.

Maslow AH (1970) Motivation and Personality, 2nd edn. New York: Harper & Row.

Meichenbaum D (1975) Enhancing creativity by modifying what subjects say to themselves. American Educational Research Journal 12: 129–45.

Metsala J (1999) Young children's phonological awareness and nonword repetition as a function of vocabulary development. Journal of Educational Psychology 91: 3–19.

Michael B (1984) Foundations of writing. Child Education January: 10–11.

Miller GA (1956) The magical number seven, plus or minus two: some limits on our capacity for processing information. Psychological Review 63: 81–97.

Mitchell JE (1988) Student Organiser Pack. London: Communication and Learning Skills Centre.

Mitchell JE (1994) Enhancing the Teaching of Memory using Memory Bricks. London: Communication and Learning Skills Centre.

Mitchell JE (2000) Time To Revise. London: Communication and Learning Skills Centre.

Mitchell JE (2001). Mastering Memory, 3rd edn. London: Communication and Learning Skills Centre.

Moely BE, Hart SS, Leal L, Santulli KA (1992) The teacher's role in facilitating memory and study strategy development in the elementary school classroom. Child Development 63: 653–72.

Mooney S, Smith PK (1995) Bullying and the child who stammers. British Journal of Special Education 22: 24–7.

Moseley D (1998) ACE Dictionary, 2nd edn. Wisbech: Learning Development Aids.

Mruk CJ (1999) Self-esteem: Research, Theory, and Practice, 2nd edn. London: Free Association.

Muter V (2003) Early Reading Development and Dyslexia. London: Whurr.

Muter V, Diethelm K (2001) The contribution of phonological skills and letter knowledge to early reading in a multilingual population. Language Learning 51: 187–219.

Muter V, Snowling M (1998) Concurrent and longitudinal predictors of reading: the role of metalinguistic and short-term memory skills. Reading Research Quarterly 33: 320–37.

Muter V, Hulme C, Snowling M (1997) The Phonological Abilities Test, PAT. London: Psychological Corporation.

Muter V, Hulme C, Snowling M, Taylor S (1998) Segmentation, not rhyming predicts early progress in learning to read. Journal of Experimental Child Psychology 71: 3–27.

Muter V, Hulme C, Snowling MJ, Stevenson J (2004) Phonemes, rimes and language skills as foundations of early reading development: evidence from a longitudinal latent variable study. Developmental Psychology 40: 665–81.

Naglieri JA (1987) Draw-a-Person. Sidcup: Psychological Corporation.

Nagy WE, Anderson RC (1984) How many words are there in printed school English? Reading Research Quarterly 19: 304–30.

Nash P (2002) Managing Persistent Communication Difficulties: An Alternative Way Forward? Paper presented at the National Association of Professionals Concerned with Language Impairment in Children Conference, Oxford, March 2002.

Nash P (2003) Psychosocial implications of experiencing failure at school. Paper presented at the Division of Educational and Child Psychology Conference of the British Psychological Society, 8–10 January, Harrogate.

Nash P, Latham E (in preparation) The Construction and Development of the Life at School Profile (LASP): Assessment for Measuring Children's Perceptions about School.

Nash P, Stengelhofen J, Brown J, Toombs L (2002) Improving Children's Communication, Managing Persistent Difficulties. London: Whurr.

Nash W (1998) At Ease with Stress: The Approach of Wholeness. London: Darton, Longman & Todd.

Nathan L (2002) Functional communication skills of children with speech difficulties: performance on Bishop's Children's Communication Checklist. Child Language Teaching and Therapy 18: 289–313.

Nathan L, Simpson S (2001) Designing a literacy programme for a child with a history of speech difficulties. In: Stackhouse J, Wells B (eds) Children's Speech and Literacy Difficulties, 2 : Identification and Intervention. London: Whurr, pp. 249–98.

Nathan L, Stackhouse J, Goulandris N, Snowling M (2004a) The development of early literacy among children with speech difficulties: a test of the 'critical age hypothesis'. Journal of Speech, Language and Hearing Research 47: 377–91.

Nathan L, Stackhouse J, Goulandris N, Snowling M (2004b) Educational consequences of developmental speech disorder: Key Stage 1 National Curriculum assessment results in English and mathematics. British Journal of Educational Psychology 74: 173–86.

Nation K (1999) Reading skills in hyperlexia: a developmental perspective. Psychological Bulletin 125: 338–55.

Nation K (2005) Children's reading comprehension difficulties. In: Snowling MJ, Hulme C (eds) The Science of Reading. Oxford: Blackwell Publishing, pp. 248–65.

Nation K, Snowling MJ (1997) Assessing reading difficulties: the validity and utility of current measures of reading skill. British Journal of Educational Psychology 67: 359–70.

Nation K, Snowling MJ (1998a) Individual differences in contextual facilitation: evidence from dyslexia and poor reading comprehension. Child Development 69: 996–1011.

Nation K, Snowling MJ (1998b) Semantic processing and the development of word recognition skills: evidence from children with reading comprehension difficulties. Journal of Memory and Language 39: 85–101.

Nation K, Clarke P, Snowling MJ (2002) General cognitive ability in children with poor reading comprehension. British Journal of Educational Psychology 72: 549–60.

Nation K, Clarke P, Marshall C, Durand M (2004) Hidden language impairments in children: parallels between poor reading comprehension and specific language impairment? Journal of Speech, Hearing and Language Research 47: 199–211.

National Back Pain Association (1995) Are You Sure Your Child has a Healthy Back? A Guide for Parents. Twickenham: NBPA.

National Reading Panel (2000) Report of the National Reading Panel: Reports of the Subgroups. Washington, DC: National Institute of Child Health and Human Development Clearing House.

Neale MD (1967) Neale Analysis of Reading Ability Second Edition (NARA-II). Windsor: NFER-Nelson.

Neale MD (1989) Neale Analysis of Reading Ability: Revised British Edition. Windsor: NFER-Nelson.

Neale MD, Whetton C, Caspall L (1999) Neale Analysis of Reading Ability, 2nd revised British edition (NARAII). Windsor: NFER-Nelson.

Nelson D, Stojanovik V (2002) Prelinguistic Primitives and the Evolution of Argument Structure: Evidence from Specific Language Impairment. Paper presented at Evolution of Language, 4th International Conference on Language Evolution at Harvard University, 27–30 March.

Nelson NW (1989) Curriculum-based language assessment and intervention. Language, Speech and Hearing Services in Schools 20: 170–84.

New Zealand Department of Education (1987) Classified Guide of Complementary Reading Materials – Books for Junior Classes: A Classified Guide for Teachers. Wellington: Department of Education.

Nicolson RI, Fawcett AJ (1990) Automaticity: a new framework for dyslexia research? Cognition 35: 159–82.

Nicolson RI, Fawcett AJ (1996) The Dyslexia Early Screening Test. London: Psychological Corporation.

Nippold M (2001) Phonological disorders and stuttering in children: what is the frequency of co-occurrence? Clinical Linguistics and Phonetics 15: 219–28.

Norwich B (1996) Special needs education or education for all: connective specialisation and ideological impurity. British Journal of Special Education 23: 123–456.

Nunes A (2003) The Price of a Perfect System: The Clever Thing about Learning to Talk. PhD thesis, University of Durham, UK.

Oakhill JV (1982) Constructive processes in skilled and less-skilled comprehenders' memory for sentences. British Journal of Psychology 73: 13–20.

Oakhill JV (1984) Inferential and memory skills in children's comprehension of stories. British Journal of Educational Psychology 54: 31–9.

Oakhill JV (1994) Individual differences in children's text comprehension. In: Gernsbacher MA (ed.) Handbook of Psycholinguistics. San Diego, CA: Academic Press, pp. 821–48.

Oakhill J, Kyle F (1999) The relation between phonological awareness and working memory. Journal of Experimental Child Psychology 75: 152–64.

Oakhill JV, Yuill N (1996) Higher order factors in comprehension disability: processes and remediation. In: Cornoldi C, Oakhill JV (eds) Reading Comprehension Difficulties. Mahwah, NJ: Lawrence Erlbaum Associates, pp. 69–92.

Office for Standards in Education (1999) Pupils with Specific Learning Difficulties in Mainstream Schools. London: OFSTED

Olson RK, Forsberg H, Wise B (1994) Genes, environment, and the development of orthographic skills. In: Berninger VW (ed.) The Varieties of Orthographic Knowledge, I: Theoretical and Development Issues. Dordrecht: Kluwer Academic, pp. 27–71.

Olson R, Wise B, Johnson M, Ring J (1997) The etiology and remediation of phonologically based word recognition and spelling disabilities: are phonological deficits the 'Hole' story? In: Blanchman B (ed.) Foundations of Reading Acquisition. Mahwah, NJ: Lawrence Erlbaum, pp. 305–26.

Ostler C (1996) Study Skills – a Pupil's Survival Guide. Surrey: Ammonite Books.

Ostler C, Ward F (2002) Advanced Study Skills. Wakefield: SEN Marketing.

Palincsar AS, Brown AL (1984) Reciprocal teaching of comprehension-fostering and comprehension-monitoring activities. Cognition and Instruction 1: 117–75.

Palmer S (2000a) Working memory: a developmental study of phonological recoding. Memory 8: 179–94.

Palmer S (2000b) Phonological recoding deficit in working memory of dyslexic teenagers. Journal of Research in Reading 23: 28–40.

Palmer S (2000c) Development of phonological recoding and literacy acquisition: a four-year cross-sequential study. British Journal of Developmental Psychology 18: 533–55.

Paris SG, Upton LR (1976) Children's memory for inferential relationships in prose. Child Development 47: 660–8.

Pascoe M, Stackhouse J, Wells B (2005) Phonological therapy within a psycholinguistic framework: promoting change in a child with persisting speech difficulties. International Journal of Language and Communication Disorders 40: 189–220.

Passenger T, Stuart M, Terrell C (2000) Phonological processing and early literacy. Journal of Research in Reading 23: 55–66.

Passy J (1993a) Cued Articulation. Ponteland, Northumberland: STASS Publications.

Passy J (1993b) Cued Vowels. Ponteland, Northumberland: STASS Publications.

Paulesu E, Frith U, Snowling M, Gallagher A, Morton J, Frackowiak FSJ, Frith CD (1996) Is developmental dyslexia a disconnection syndrome? Evidence from PET scanning. Brain 119: 143–57.

Paulesu E, McCrory E, Fazio F, Menoncello L, Brunswick N, Cappa SF, Cotelli M, Cossu G, Corte F, Lorusso M, Pesent S, Gallagher A, Perani D, Price C, Frith CD, Frith U (2000) A cultural effect on brain function. Nature Neuroscience 3: 91–6.

Paulesu E, Démonet J-F, Fazlo F, McCrory E, Chanoine V, Brunswick N, Cappa SF, Habib M, Frith CD, Frith U (2001) Dyslexia: cultural diversity and biological unity. Science 291: 2165–7.

Peer L, Reid G (eds) (2001) Dyslexia – Successful Inclusion in the Secondary School. London: David Fulton.

Pelletier PM, Ahmad SA, Rourke BP (2001) Classification rules for basic phonological processing disabilities and nonverbal learning difficulties: formulation and external validity. Child Neuropsychology 7: 84–98.

Pennington BF, Lefly DL (2001) Early reading development in children at family risk for dyslexia. Child Development 72: 816–33.

Pennington BF, Van-Orden GC, Smith SD, Green PA (1990) Phonological processing skills and deficits in adult dyslexics. Child Development 61: 1753–78.

Perfetti CA (1985) Reading Ability. New York: Oxford University Press.

Perfetti C, Beck I, Bell L, Hughes C (1987) Phonemic knowledge and learning to read are reciprocal: a longitudinal study of first grade children. Merrill-Palmer Quarterly 33: 283–319.

Perin D (1983) Phonemic segmentation and spelling. British Journal of Psychology 74: 129–44.

Pert S, Letts C (2003) Developing an expressive language assessment for children in Rochdale with a Pakistani heritage background. Child Language Teaching and Therapy 1: 291–31.

Phillips BM, Lonigan CJ (2005) Social correlates of emergent literacy. In: Snowling MJ, Hulme C (eds) The Science of Reading: A Handbook. Oxford: Blackwell, pp. 173–87.

Pickering SJ (2001) The development of visuo-spatial working memory. Memory 9: 423–32.

Pickering S, Gathercole S (2001) Working Memory Test Battery for Children. London: Psychological Corporation.

Place M, Reynolds J, Cousins A, O'Neill S (2002) Developing a resilience package for vulnerable children. Child and Adolescent Mental Health 7: 162–7.

Plaut DC, McClelland JL, Seidenberg MS, Patterson K (1996) Understanding normal and impaired word reading: computational principles in quasi-regular domains. Psychological Review 103: 56–115.

Popple J, Wellington W (1996) Collaborative working within a psycholinguistic framework. Child Language Teaching and Therapy 12: 60–70.

Popple J, Wellington W (2001) Working together: the psycholinguistic approach within a school setting. In: Stackhouse J, Wells B (eds) Children's Speech and Literacy Difficulties, 2: Identification and Intervention. London: Whurr, pp. 299–329.

Pressley M, McCormick CB (1995) Advanced Educational Psychology for Educators, Researchers and Policymakers. New York: Harpercollins.

Qualifications and Curriculum Authority (1999) Teaching Speaking and Listening in Key Stage 1 and 2. London: DfES Publications Centre.

Qualifications and Curriculum Authority (2003) Speaking, Listening, Learning: Working with Children in Key Stage 1 and 2. London: DfES Publications Centre.

Quinton D, Pickles A, Maughan B, Rutter M (1993) Partners, peers and pathways: assortative pairing and continuities in conduct disorder. Development and Psychopathology 5: 763–83.

Rack JP (1985) Orthographic and phonetic coding in developmental dyslexia. British Journal of Psychology 76: 325–40.

Rack J, Hatcher J (2002) Spellit Summary Report. The Dyslexia Institute. www.dyslexia-inst.org.uk/spellitsum.htm

Rack J, Hatcher J (2003) Defining and assessing dyslexia: evidence from SPELLIT. Dyslexia Review 14: 9–12.

Rack J, Hulme C, Snowling MJ (1993) Learning to read: a theoretical synthesis. In: Reese H (ed.) Advances in Child Development and Behavior, Vol. 24. New York: Academic Press, pp. 99–132.

Rack J, Snowling M, Olson R (1992) The nonword reading deficit in developmental dyslexia: a review. Reading Research Quarterly 27: 29–53.

Raitano NA, Pennington BF, Tunick RA, Boada R, Shriber L (2004) Pre-literacy skills of subgroups of children with phonological disorder. Journal of Child Psychology and Psychiatry 45: 821–35.

Ramus F, Rosen S, Dakin SC, Day BL, Castellote JM, White S, Frith U (2003). Theories of developmental dyslexia: insights from a multiple case study of dyslexic adults. Brain 126: 841–65.

Rasbash J, Browne W, Goldstein H, Yang M, Plewis I, Healy M, Woodhouse G, Draper D, Langford I, Lewis T (2000) A User's Guide to MLwiN. London: Institute of Education.

Raven JC (1984) Coloured Progressive Matrices. London: HK Lewis.

Read C (1986) Children's Creative Spelling. London: Routledge & Kegan Paul.

Rees R (2002) Language Programmes. In: Kersner M, Wright JA (eds) How to Manage Communication Problems in Young Children, 3rd edn. London: David Fulton, pp. 81–94.

Reid J, Millar S, Tait L, Donaldson M, Dean E, Thomson G, Grieve R (1996) The Role of Speech and Language Therapists in the Education of Pupils with Special Educational Needs. Edinburgh: Centre for Research in Child Development.

Renfrew C (1995) Renfrew Bus Story, UK 3rd Edition. Bicester: Winslow Press.

Rice M (1993) 'Don't talk to him; he's weird.' A social consequences account of language and social interactions. In: Kaiser AP, Gray DB (eds) Enhancing Children's Communication: Research Foundations for Intervention. Baltimore: Paul H Brookes.

Rice ML, Wexler K (2001) Rice–Wexler Test of Early Grammatical Impairment. London: Psychological Corporation.

Richman LC, Wood KM (2002) Learning disability subtypes: classification of high functioning hyperlexia. Brain and Language 82: 10–21.

Riddick B (2002) Researching the social and emotional consequences of dyslexia. In: Wearmouth J, Soler J, Reid G (eds) Addressing Difficulties in Literacy Development. London: Routledge-Falmer, pp. 282–302.

Rinaldi W (1992) Working with Language Impaired Teenagers with Moderate Learning Difficulties. London: ICAN.

Rohl M, Pratt C (1995) Phonological awareness, verbal working memory and acquisition of literacy. Reading and Writing 7: 327–60.

Roodenrys S, Hulme C, Alban J, Ellis A, Brown GDA (1994) Effects of word frequency and age of acquisition on short-term memory span. Memory and Cognition 22: 695–701.

Rourke BP (1989) Nonverbal Learning Difficulties: The Syndrome and the Model. New York: Guildford Press.

Rust J, Golombok S, Trickey G (1993) Wechsler Objective Reading Dimensions (WORD). London: Psychological Corporation.

Rustin L, Kuhr A (1999) Social Skills and the Speech Impaired, 2nd edn. London: Whurr.

Rutter M (1985) Resilience in the face of adversity: protective factors and resistance to psychiatric disorder. British Journal of Psychiatry 147: 598–611.

Rutter M, Rutter M (1993) Developing Minds: Challenge and Continuity Across the Life Span. London: Penguin.

Rutter M, Yule W (1975). The concept of specific reading retardation. Journal of Child Psychology and Psychiatry 16: 181–97.

Santrock JW (1994) Child Development, 6th edn. Wisconsin: Brown & Benchmark.

Sawyer D (1987) Test of Awareness of Language Segments (TALS). Austin, TX: Pro-Ed.

Scarborough H (1990) Very early language deficits in dyslexic children. Child Development 61: 1728–43.

Scarborough H (1991) Antecedents to reading disability: pre-school language development and literacy experiences of children from dyslexic families. Reading and Writing 3: 219–33.

Scarborough H (1998) Early identification of children at risk for reading disabilities. In: Shapiro BK, Accardo PJ, Capute AJ (eds) Specific Reading Disability: A View of the Spectrum. Timonium, MD: York Press, pp. 75–119.

Schaffer HR (1996) Social Development. Oxford: Blackwell.

Schneider W, Naslund JC (1993) The impact of metalinguistic competencies and memory capacity on reading and spelling in elementary schools: results of the Munich longitudinal study on the genesis of individual competencies (LOGIC). European Journal of Psychology of Education 8: 273–87.

Schneider W, Sodian B (1997) Memory strategy development: lessons from longitudinal research. Developmental Review 17: 442–61.

Schonell F (1971) Graded Word Reading Test. Edinburgh: Oliver & Boyd.

Schonell FJ, Schonell FE (1956) Diagnostic and Attainment Testing: Including a Manual of Tests, their Nature, Use, Recording and Interpretation. London: Oliver & Boyd.

Scottish Council for Research in Education (1974) Burt Rearranged Word Reading Test. London: Hodder & Stoughton.

Searleman A, Herrman D (1994) Memory From a Broader Perspective. Singapore: McGraw-Hill.

Seidenberg MS, McClelland JL (1989) A distributed, developmental model of word recognition and naming. Psychological Review 96: 523–68.

Semel E, Wiig EH, Secord WA (1995) Clinical Evaluation of Language Fundamentals, 3rd edn. London: Psychological Corporation.

Semel E, Wiig EH, Secord WA (2000) Clinical Evaluation of Language Fundamentals (CELF-III). London: Psychological Corporation.

Share DL, Jorm AF, Maclean R, Matthews R (1984) Sources of individual differences in reading acquisition. Journal of Educational Psychology 76: 1309–24.

Shaw R (2000) Test of Word and Grammatical Awareness (TOWGA). Windsor: NFER-Nelson.

Shaywitz BA, Fletcher JM, Holahan JM, Shaywitz SE (1992) Discrepancy compared to low achievement definitions of reading disability: results from the Connecticut longitudinal study. Journal of Learning Disabilities 25: 639–48.

Shaywitz SE, Shaywitz BA, Pugh KR, Fulbright RK, Constable RT, Mencl WE, Shankweiler DP, Liberman AM, Skudlarski P, Fletcher JM, Katz L, Marchione KE, Lacadie C, Gatenby C, Gore JC (1998) Functional disruption in the organisation of the brain for reading in dyslexia. Proceedings of the National Academy of Sciences of the USA 95: 2636–41.

Shaywitz SE, Shaywitz BA, Fulbright RK, Skudlarski P, Mencl WE, Constable RT, Pugh KR, Holahan JM, Marchione KE, Fletcher JM, Lyon GR, Gore JC (2003) Neural systems for compensation and persistence: young adult outcome of childhood reading disability. Biological Psychiatry 54: 25–33.

Sheridan MD (1975) From Birth to Five Years: Children's Developmental Progress. Windsor: NFER-Nelson.

Shriberg L, Tomblin JB, McSweeny JL (1999) Prevalence of speech delay in 6-year old children and co-morbidity with language impairment. Journal of Speech, Language and Hearing Research 42: 1461–81.

Shriberg LD, Flipsen P, Thielke H, Kwiatowski J, Kertoy M, Nellis R, Block M (2000a) Risk for speech disorder associated with recurrent otitis media effusion: two retrospective studies. Journal Speech and Hearing Research 43: 79–99.

Shriberg LD, Friel-Patti S, Flipsen P, Brown RL (2000b) Otitis media, fluctuant hearing loss and speech–language delay: a preliminary structural equation model. Journal of Speech, Language and Hearing Research 43: 100–20.

Simos PG, Breier JI, Fletcher JM, Bergman E, Papanicolaou AC (2000) Cerebral mechanisms involved in word reading in dyslexic children: a magnetic source imaging approach. Cerebral Cortex 10: 809–16.

Simos PG, Fletcher JM, Bergman E et al. (2002) Dyslexia-specific brain activation profile becomes normal following successful remedial training. Neurology 58: 1203–13.

Simpson J, Everatt J (2005) Reception class predictors of literacy skills. British Journal of Educational Psychology 75: 171–88.

Simpson S (2000) Dyslexia: a developmental language disorder. Child: Health, Care and Development 26: 355–80.

Singleton C, Thomas K, Horne J (2000) Computer-based cognitive assessment and the development of reading. Journal of Research in Reading 23: 158–80.

Singleton CH, Thomas KV, Leedale RC (1996) Cognitive Profile System. Beverley, East Yorks: Lucid Research.

Skuse DH (1991) Deprivation, physical growth and language development. In: Fletcher P, Hall D (eds) Specific Speech and Language Disorders in Children. London: Whurr, pp. 29–50.

Smith F (1971) Understanding Reading: A Psycholinguistic Analysis of Reading and Learning to Read. New York: Holt Rinehart & Winston.

Snow CE, Juel C (2005) Teaching children to read: what do we know about how to do it? In: Snowling MJ, Hulme C (eds) The Science of Reading: A Handbook. Oxford: Blackwell, pp. 501–20.

Snowling MJ (1985) Children's Written Language Difficulties. Windsor: NFER-Nelson.

Snowling MJ (1987) Dyslexia. A Cognitive Developmental Perspective. Oxford: Basil Blackwell.

Snowling MJ (2000) Dyslexia, 2nd edn. Oxford: Blackwell.

Snowling MJ, Frith U (1986) Comprehension in 'hyperlexic' readers. Journal of Experimental Child Psychology 42: 392–415.

Snowling M, Hulme C (1994) The development of phonological skills. Philosophical Transactions of the Royal Society of London Series B: Biological Sciences 346: 21–7.

Snowling M, Stackhouse J (1983) Spelling performance of children with developmental verbal dyspraxia. Developmental Medicine and Child Neurology 25: 430–7.

Snowling MJ, Bishop DVM, Stothard SE (2000) Is pre-school language impairment a risk factor for dyslexia in adolescence? Journal of Child Psychology and Psychiatry 41: 587–600.

Snowling MJ, Chiat S, Hulme C (1991) Words, nonwords and phonological processes: some comments on Gathercole, Ellis, Emslie and Baddeley. Applied Psycholinguistics 12: 369–73.

Snowling MJ, Gallagher A, Frith U (2003) Family risk of dyslexia is continuous: individual differences in the precursors of reading skill. Child Development 74: 358–73.

Snowling MJ, Goulandris N, Defty N (1996) A longitudinal study of reading development in dyslexic children. Journal of Educational Psychology 88: 653–69.

Snowling MJ, Stackhouse J, Rack J (1986). Phonological dyslexia and dysgraphia: a developmental analysis. Cognitive Neuropsychology 3: 309–39.

Snowling M, Stothard S, McLean J (1996) The Graded Nonword Reading Test. Bury St Edmunds: Thames Valley Test Company.

Snowling MJ, Hulme C, Smith A, Thomas J (1994) The effects of phonetic similarity and list length on children's sound categorization performance. Journal of Experimental Child Psychology 58: 160–80.

Stackhouse J (1992) Developmental verbal dyspraxia: a longitudinal case study. In: Campbell R (ed.) Mental Lives: Cases Studies in Cognition. Oxford: Blackwell, pp. 84–98.

Stackhouse J (2000) Barriers to literacy development in children with speech and language difficulties. In: Bishop DVM, Leonard L (eds) Speech and Language Impairments in Children: Causes, Characteristics, Intervention and Outcome. Hove: Psychology Press, pp. 73–97.

Stackhouse J, Wells B (1993) Psycholinguistic investigation of developmental speech disorders. European Journal of Disorders of Communication 28: 331–48.

Stackhouse J, Wells B (1997) Children's Speech and Literacy Difficulties, 1: A Psycholinguistic Framework. London: Whurr.

Stackhouse J, Wells B (eds) (2001) Children's Speech and Literacy Difficulties, 2: Identification and Intervention. London: Whurr.

Stackhouse J, Wells B, Pascoe M, Rees R (2002) From phonological therapy to phonological awareness. Seminars in Speech and Language 23: 27–42.

Stainthorp R, Hughes D (1995) The cognitive characteristics of young early readers. In: Rabin-Bisby B, Brokes G, Wolfensdale S (eds) Developing Language and Literacy. Stoke on Trent: Tretham Books, pp. 99–113.

Stanovich KE, Siegel LS (1994) The phenotypic performance profile of reading-disabled children: a regression-based test of the phonological-core variable-difference model. Journal of Educational Psychology 86: 24–53.

Stein J, Talcott J (1999) Impaired neuronal timing in developmental dyslexia – the magnocellular hypothesis. Dyslexia 5: 59–77.

Stein J, Walsh V (1997) To see but not to read: the magnocellular theory of dyslexia. Trends in the Neurosciences 20: 147–52.

Stothard SE, Hulme C (1991) A note of caution concerning the Neale Analysis of Reading Ability (Revised). British Journal of Education Psychology 61: 226–9.

Stothard SE, Hulme C (1992) Reading comprehension difficulties in children: the role of language comprehension and working memory skills. Reading and Writing 4: 245–56.

Stothard SE, Hulme C (1995) A comparison of phonological skills in children with reading comprehension difficulties and children with decoding difficulties. Journal of Child Psychology and Psychiatry 36: 399–408.

Stothard SE, Snowling MJ, Bishop DVM, Chipchase B, Kaplan C (1998) Language impaired pre-schoolers: a follow-up in adolescence. Journal of Speech, Language and Hearing Research 41: 407–18.

Stuart M, Coltheart M (1988) Does reading develop in a sequence of stages? Cognition 30: 139–81.

Stuart M, Dockrell J, King D (in press) Language intervention in preschool. Talking time – evidence for the development of oral language skills in classrooms. In: Maridaki K (ed.) Children's Understanding of Mind: Empirical and Theoretical Approaches.

Sturner R, Kunze L, Funk S, Green J (1993) Elicited imitation its effectiveness for speech and language screening. Developmental Medicine and Child Neurology 35: 715–26.

Swanson HL (1993) Working memory and learning disabilities. Journal of Experimental Child Psychology 65: 87–114.

Tabachnick B, Fidell L (1989) Using Multivariate Statistics. New York: Harper Collins.

Tallal P, Miller S, Fitch RH (1993) Neurobiological basis of speech: a case for the pre-eminence of temporal processing. Annals of the New York Academy of Sciences 682: 27–47.

Temple E, Poldrack RA, Salidis J et al. (2001) Disrupted neural responses to phonological and orthographic processing in dyslexic children: an fMRI study. Neuroreport 12: 299–307.

Temple E, Deutsch GK, Poldrack RA et al. (2003) Neural deficits in children with dyslexia ameliorated by behavioral remediation: evidence from functional MRI. Proceedings of the National Academy of Sciences of the USA 100: 2860–5.

Thompson T (1999) Underachieving to Protect Self Worth: Theory, Research and Interventions. Aldershot: Ashgate

Thomson M (1991) The teaching of spelling using techniques of simultaneous oral spelling and visual inspection. In: Snowling M, Thomson M (eds) Dyslexia: Integrating Theory and Practice. London: Whurr, pp. 244–50.

Tod J (2002) Individual education plans and dyslexia: some principles. In: Reid G Wearmouth J (eds) Dyslexia and Literacy: Theory and Practice. Chichester: Wiley, pp. 251–70.

Tomblin JB, Buckwater PR (1994) Studies of genetics in specific language impairment. In: Watkins RV, Rice ML (eds) Specific Language Impairments in Children. Baltimore, MD: Paul Brookes, pp. 17–34.

Torgesen J, Bryant B (1994) Test of Phonological Awareness (TOPA). Austin, TX: Pro-Ed.

Torgesen J, Wagner RK, Rashotte CA (1999) Test of Word Reading Efficiency (TOWRE). London: Psychological Corporation.

Torgesen JK, Alexander AW, Wagner RK, Rashotte CA, Voeller KKS, Conway T (2001) Intensive remedial instruction for children with severe reading disabilities: immediate and long-term outcomes from two instructional approaches. Journal of Learning Disabilities 34: 33–58, 78.

Townend J, Turner M (eds) (2000) Dyslexia in Practice: A Guide for Teachers. New York: Plenum.

Treiman R (1985) Onsets and rimes as units of spoken syllables: evidence from children. Journal of Experimental Child Psychology 39: 161–81.

Treiman R (1993) Beginning to Spell. A Study of First Grade Children. New York: Oxford University Press.

Treiman R, Weatherston S, Berch D (1994) The role of letter names in children's learning of phoneme–grapheme relations. Applied Psycholinguistics 15: 97–122.

Troia GA (1999) Phonological awareness intervention research: a critical review of the experimental methodology. Reading Research Quarterly 34: 28–52.

Tuley AC (1998) Never Too Late to Read. Language Skills for the Adolescent with Dyslexia. Maryland: York Press.

Tunmer WE (1989) The role of language-related factors in reading disability. In: Shankweiler D, Liberman IY (eds) Phonology and Reading Disability: Solving the Reading Puzzle. Ann Arbor: University of Michigan Press, pp. 91–131.

Tunmer WE (1994) Phonological processing skills and reading remediation. In: Hulme C, Snowling M (eds) Reading Development and Dyslexia. London: Whurr, pp. 147–62.

Tunmer WE, Chapman JW (1998) Language prediction skill, phonological recoding, and beginning reading. In: Hulme C, Joshi R (eds) Reading and Spelling: Development and Disorders. Mahwah, NJ: Lawrence Erlbaum Associates, pp. 33–67.

Tunmer WE, Herriman ML, Nesdale AR (1988) Metalinguistic abilities and beginning reading. Reading Research Quarterly 23: 134–58.

Turley-Ames K, Whitfield MM (2003) Strategy training and working memory performance. Journal of Memory and Language 49: 446–68.

Van der Lely H, Herzog C, Froud K, Gardner H (in press) Grammar and Phonology Screen (GAPS). London: University College London.

Van der Lely HKJ, Ullman MT (2001) Past tense morphology in specifically language impaired and normally developing children. Language and Cognitive Processes 16: 177–217.

Van der Lely HKJ, Rosen S, McClelland A (1998) Evidence for a grammar specific deficit in children. Current Biology 8: 1253–8 .

Van Ijzendoorn MH, Bus AG (1994) Meta-analytic confirmation of the nonword reading deficit in developmental dyslexia. Reading Research Quarterly 29: 267–75.

Vance M (2001) Speech Processing and Short-term Memory in Children with Normal and Atypical Speech and Language Development. PhD thesis, University of London.

Varnhagen CK, McCallum M, Burstow M (1997) Is Children's Spelling Naturally Stage-like? Reading and Writing 9: 451–81.

Vellutino FR (1979) Dyslexia: Research and Theory: Cambridge, MA: MIT Press.

Vellutino F, Scanlon D (1991) The pre-eminence of phonologically based skills in learning to read. In: Brady S, Shankweiler D (eds) Phonological Processes in Literacy: A Tribute to Isabelle Y. Liberman. Hillsdale, NJ: Lawrence Erlbaum Associates, pp. 237–52.

Vellutino FR, Fletcher JM, Snowling MJ, Scanlon DM (2004) Specific reading disability (dyslexia): what have we learned in the past four decades? Journal of Child Psychology and Psychiatry 45: 2–40.

Vernon PE (1977) Graded Word Spelling Test. London: Hodder & Stoughton.

Vernon PE (1998) Graded Word Spelling Test, 2nd edn. London: Hodder & Stoughton.

Vincent D, Clayton D (1982) Diagnostic Spelling Tests. Basingstoke: Macmillan.

Vincent D, De la Mare M (1989) New Macmillan Reading Analysis. Basingstoke: Macmillan Education.

Vitale BM, Bullock WB (1996) Ann Arbor Learning Inventory. Northumberland: Ann Arbor Publishers.

Wade B, Moore M (1998) An early start with books: literacy and mathematical evidence from a longitudinal study. Educational Review 50: 135–45.

Wagner RK, Torgesen JK (1987) The nature of phonological processing and its causal role in the acquisition of reading skills. Psychological Bulletin 101: 192–212.

Wagner RK, Torgesen JK, Rashotte CA (1994) The development of reading-related phonological processing abilities: new evidence of bi-directional causality from a latent variable longitudinal study. Developmental Psychology 30: 73–87.

Wagner RK, Torgesen JK, Rashotte CA (1999) CTOPP: Comprehensive Test of Phonological Processing. Austin, TX: Pro-Ed.

Wagner RK, Torgesen JK, Rashotte CA, Hecht SA, Barker TA, Burgess SR, Donahue J, Garon T (1997) Changing relations between phonological processing abilities and word-level reading as children develop from beginning to skilled readers: a 5-year longitudinal study. Developmental Psychology 33: 468–79.

Walker J, Brooks L et al (1993) Dyslexia Institute Literacy Programme. Staines: Dyslexia Institute.

Watson BU, Miller TK (1993) Auditory perception, phonological processing and reading ability/disability. Journal of Speech and Hearing Research 36: 850–63.

Webster PE, Plante AS (1992) Effects of phonological impairment on word, syllable, and phoneme segmentation and reading. Language, Speech and Hearing Services in Schools 23: 176–82.

Wechsler D (1992) Wechsler Intelligence Scale for Children (WISC-III UK). New York: Harcourt Brace Jovanovich.

Weiss C, Gordon ME, Lillywhite HS (1987) Clinical Management of Articulation Disorders. St Louis, MO: Mosby.

Wellington W, Wellington J (2002) Children with communication difficulties in mainstream science classrooms. School Science Review 83: 81–92.

Wells B (1994) Junction in developmental speech disorder: a case study. Clinical Linguistics and Phonetics 8: 1–25.

Wernham S, Lloyd S (1993) Jolly Phonics. Chigwell: Jolly Learning.

Westwood P (1997) Commonsense Methods for Children with Special Needs. London: Routledge.

Whitehurst GJ, Zevenbergen AA, Crone DA, Schultz MD, Velting ON, Fischel JE (1999) Outcomes of an emergent literacy intervention from Head Start through second grade. Journal of Educational Psychology 91: 261–72.

Whitmarsh E (1988) First Year Secondary School Children's Attitudes to Handwriting. London: Whurr.

Wiig EH, Secord WA (1992) Test of Word Knowledge (TOWK). London: Psychological Corporation.

Wilkinson G (1993) Wide Range Achievement Test 3 (WRAT 3). Wilmington, DE: Wide Range.

Williams D (1995) Early Listening Skills. Bicester: Speechmark.

Williams P (2004) Nuffield Dyspraxia Programme. Windsor: Miracle Factory.

Williams P, Stackhouse J (2000) Rate, accuracy and consistency: diadochokinetic performance of young, normally developing children. Clinical Linguistics and Phonetics 14: 267–93.

Wilson BA, Moffat N (1984) Clinical Management of Memory Problems. London: Croom Helm.

Wilson J (1993) Phonological Awareness Training Programme. London: Educational Psychology Publishing.

Witruk E, Ho CSH, Schuster U (2002) Working memory in dyslexic children: how general is the deficit? In: Witruk E, Friederici A, Lachmann T (eds) Basic Functions of Language, Reading and Reading Disability. Neuropsychology and Cognition, Vol. 20. Dordrecht: Kluwer Academic, pp. 281–97.

Wolf MA (1982) The word retrieval process and reading in children and aphasics. In: Nelson K (ed.) Children's Language. Hillsdale, NJ: Lawrence Erlbaum Associates, pp. 437–92.

Wolf M (1997) A provisional, integrative account of phonological and naming-speed deficits in dyslexia: implications for diagnosis and intervention. In: Blachman B (ed.) Foundations of Reading Acquisition in Dyslexia. Hillsdale, NJ: Lawrence Erlbaum Associates, pp. 67–92.

Wolf M, Bowers P (1999) The double deficit hypothesis for the developmental dyslexias. Journal of Educational Psychology 9: 1–24.

Wolf M, O'Brien B (2001) On issues of time, fluency and intervention. In Fawcett A (ed.) Dyslexia: Theory and Good Practice. London: Whurr, pp. 124–40.

Wood J, Wright JA, Stackhouse J (2000) Language and Literacy: Joining Together Reading: British Dyslexia Association.

Worling DE, Humphries T, Tannock R (2001) Spatial and emotional aspects of language inferencing in nonverbal learning difficulties. Brain and Language 70: 220–39.

Wright JA (1996) Teachers and therapists: the evolution of a partnership. Child Language Teaching and Therapy 12: 3–16.

Wright JA, Kersner M (2004) Short term projects: the Standards Fund and collaboration between speech and language therapists and teachers. Support for Learning 19: 19–23.

Wright JA, Wood J, Stackhouse J (2004) Early years language and literacy. In: Dyslexia: Perspectives for Classroom Practitioners. Reading: British Dyslexia Association.

Yopp HK (1988) The validity and reliability of phonemic awareness tests. Reading Research Quarterly 23: 159–77.

Young D (1978) SPAR Spelling and Reading Tests. London: Hodder & Stoughton.

Young D (1983) The Parallel Spelling Tests A and B. London: Hodder & Stoughton.

Yuill N, Oakhill JV (1991) Children's Problems in Text Comprehension. Cambridge: Cambridge University Press.

Ziegler JC, Goswami U (2005) Reading acquisition, developmental dyslexia and skilled reading across languages: a psycholinguistic grain size theory. Psychological Bulletin 131: 3–29.

Zivianni J (1998) Some elaborations on handwriting speed in 7–14 year old school students using modern cursive script. Australian Occupational Therapy 45: 59–64.

Author index

Subject index